AF598056

Perioperative Kidney Injury

Charuhas V. Thakar • Chirag R. Parikh
Editors

Perioperative Kidney Injury

Principles of Risk Assessment, Diagnosis and Treatment

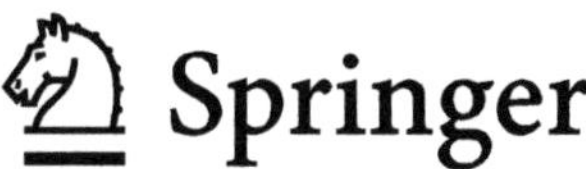

Editors
Charuhas V. Thakar, MD, FASN
Division of Nephrology and Hypertension
University of Cincinnati
Cincinnati, OH, USA

Chirag R. Parikh, MD, PhD, FASN
Program of Applied Translational Research
Department of Medicine
Yale University School of Medicine
New Haven, CT, USA

ISBN 978-1-4939-1272-8 ISBN 978-1-4939-1273-5 (eBook)
DOI 10.1007/978-1-4939-1273-5
Springer New York Heidelberg Dordrecht London

Library of Congress Control Number: 2014944534

Printed on acid-free paper

Springer is part of Springer Science+Business Media (www.springer.com)

Foreword

Perioperative changes in renal function cause anxiety in both the care provider and the patient as it imparts significant risk for adverse outcomes. Over the last decade, the Risk, Injury, Failure, Loss, and End-Stage Kidney Disease (RIFLE), Acute Kidney Injury Network (AKIN), and Kidney Disease: Improving Global Outcomes (KDIGO) criteria have standardized the diagnosis and staging of acute kidney injury and facilitated the recognition and management of acute kidney injury (AKI). As surgical techniques have evolved, it has become evident that the kidney can be affected through more than one mechanism and at different time points in relation to surgery. Several studies, largely focused on cardiovascular surgery, have provided insights into potential patient and process of care factors influencing renal function in the perioperative period. There is now increased recognition of the need for multidisciplinary approaches for managing patients at high risk for kidney injury. However, there has been a relative paucity of information on risk assessment, recognition, targeted interventions, renal support, and rehabilitation of patients with kidney injury across the spectrum of surgical procedures. Drs. Thakar and Parikh have filled this gap in knowledge with the compilation of chapters in this book.

Drs. Thakar and Parikh are both internationally recognized clinician investigators who have contributed widely to the field of AKI. Charuhas has published extensively on the epidemiology of postoperative AKI and developed risk scores for need for dialysis post-cardiac surgery. Chirag leads the National Institutes of Health (NIH) funded Translational Research Investigating Biomarker End-Points (TRIBE) consortium evaluating biomarkers post-cardiac surgery and the ASsessment, Serial Evaluation, and Subsequent Sequelae in Acute Kidney Injury (ASSESS-AKI) study evaluating the natural history of AKI in hospitalized patients. Both share a passion for evidence-based practice for clinical excellence and bring their expertise and experience to bear in editing this book. They have assembled an international group of contributors with the intellectual strength, clinical expertise, and research experience to address the wide range of subjects across different surgical procedures. The excellent reviews and timely discussions of topics are very relevant and address emerging tools that will influence patient management. The editors have wisely incorporated scientific evidence with pragmatic practical advice to improve patient management.

Given the fundamental importance of this area, I believe that Drs. Thakar and Parikh have provided a unique comprehensive resource that will prove invaluable to anyone involved in the care of surgical patients. Emerging technology, minimally invasive surgery, and use of implantable devices will continue to shape the perioperative landscape and will undoubtedly provide new challenges for the management of kidney injury in this setting. In the meantime, I am confident that this book will allay some of the trepidation clinicians face in facing an elevated creatinine or reduced urine output in a surgical patient. I congratulate the editors and the authors on an excellent resource that will certainly be referred to often in my library.

San Diego, CA, USA Ravindra L. Mehta, MD

Foreword

This new book edited by Thakar and Parikh fills an important niche in providing bedside clinical resources for the care of patients at risk for and who develop acute kidney injury (AKI) after surgery. Advances in surgical techniques and perioperative care since World War II have revolutionized medical care, providing life-enhancing and sustaining therapies to millions of patients. It is estimated that more than 50 million operations are performed annually in the United States, and the average American can expect to undergo at least 7 operations over the course of a lifetime. Yet despite these many successes, postoperative sepsis and organ system failure, including the development of AKI, continue to be feared complications that contribute to substantial patient morbidity and mortality.

AKI is defined as a rapid and often reversible decline in kidney function. In the twenty-first century, there have been major advances in understanding the epidemiology, diagnosis, prevention, and treatment of acute kidney injury, perhaps catalyzed most prominently by achieving a broad consensus on definitions and terminology for AKI. Current definitions also redefine the full spectrum of AKI, encompassing early and mild AKI all the way to severe disease requiring urgent use of renal replacement therapy. These consensus definitions were prompted by recognition that even relatively modest acute changes in kidney function (most commonly measured by changes in serum creatinine) are highly associated with adverse outcomes in hospitalized patients, including increased mortality, health-care utilization, and length of hospital stay. We know that the incidence of AKI is increasing rapidly (rates between 10 and 11 % per year in national surveys) in hospitalized patients in the United States. A major recent development is that the long-standing classical understanding that AKI is a reversible condition without long-term effects on kidney function has been challenged by data demonstrating the frequent persistence of chronic kidney disease (CKD) months to years after AKI. However, the mechanisms by which AKI may cause acceleration of chronic kidney disease are not well understood and are currently being intensively studied. This dynamic field of knowledge about AKI is undergoing rapid change, and Thakar and Parikh have captured the knowledge base required for clinicians.

By focusing on the diverse and unique surgical settings associated with AKI, *Perioperative Kidney Injury: Principles of Risk Assessment, Diagnosis and Treatment* will help those involved in patient care – including surgeons, hospitalists, anesthesiologists, and nephrologists – and provide the most comprehensive and up-to-date best practices for their patients.

Seattle, WA, USA Jonathan Himmelfarb, MD

Preface

The kidneys participate in all vital processes of the body to maintain overall homeostasis and health. These organs receive 20 % of cardiac output and, in return, maintain fluid and electrolyte balance, control blood pressure, and assist with detoxification and excretion of metabolites and drugs. The kidneys also orchestrate communication with other organs, such as the heart and liver, and compensate the internal environment when these organs go into states of dysfunction. Thus, it is no surprise that during surgical interventions, when kidneys are injured, metabolic and hemodynamic control is disrupted. Advances in surgical techniques, medical devices, and anesthetic procedures have allowed clinicians to perform organ transplants, insert artificial devices, and conduct complex surgeries that not too long ago would have been considered high risk to perform, particularly in older patients with multiple comorbidities. Now, over 200 million surgical procedures are performed worldwide. However, as a consequence, the number of hospitalizations that include acute kidney injury have risen to epidemic proportions, with an over eight-fold increase in last decade. With the central role of kidneys in precisely maintaining the internal milieu, it follows that surgeries complicated by kidney injury and dysfunction are associated with greater perioperative mortality, length of hospital stay, and cost.

The involvement of multidisciplinary physicians (internist, anesthesiologist, surgeon, hospitalist, critical care specialist, etc.), anticipating and collaborating to address the problems and challenges in complex cases, fosters successful outcomes after surgery. As a result, the knowledge, evolving practices, and advancements in medical care within each specialty must be disseminated to the multidisciplinary team. This handbook is a humble attempt to outline the concepts and principles of care to prevent kidney complications during surgical procedures and arm healthcare providers with strategies to manage acute kidney injury and associated complications when they occur. In this book, we have attempted to blend the established standards of care with cutting-edge advances in the field and also provide the reader with a peek into innovations on the horizon.

Across the 18 chapters, we cover diverse surgical settings, ranging from the more common, such as abdominal, cardiac, and vascular surgeries, to the intricately complex, including the use of the left ventricular assist device and organ transplants. Each chapter highlights the key principles, with frequent use of algorithms, which we hope will assist clinicians at the bedside with a sound evidence-based approach to anticipate and manage kidney injury and the associated complications. Despite the common approach to acute kidney injury in the hospitalized patient, each surgical setting offers a unique opportunity to "fine-tune" surgical management, such as the use of hypertonic saline in neurosurgical cases to improve cerebral perfusion. In addition, in the early portion of the book, we devote chapters to summarize the current definitions of kidney injury, discuss traditional and novel diagnostic tools, and enumerate principles of volume and electrolyte management as they relate to different surgical settings. Concepts surrounding the initiation of dialysis, appropriate modality, and associated challenges of anticoagulation after surgery are also discussed by experts in the field. We also reviewed important topics that often do not receive optimal consideration, such as kidney injury after surgeries in children, nutrition during the period of kidney failure, assessment of intra-abdominal hypertension and the effects on the kidney, and intraoperative anesthesia considerations as they relate to kidney function.

We are grateful to all of the contributing authors, who are leaders in their respective areas, for their time and effort. We acknowledge and are thankful for their thoughtful and excellent contributions to this book. We also thank the team from Springer who supported our mission and assisted in the development of this book.

Cincinnati, OH, USA Charuhas V. Thakar, MD, FASN
New Haven, CT, USA Chirag R. Parikh, MD, PhD, FASN

Acknowledgments

To our teachers, peers, trainees, and patients, from whom we have gained knowledge.

To our educational institutions, upon which we have depended during this journey.

To our family members who inspire and allow us to dedicate time towards such important contributions.

Contents

Contributors

Shamsuddin Akhtar, MD Department of Anesthesiology, Yale University School of Medicine, New Haven, CT, USA

Krishna P. Athota, MD Department of Surgery, University of Cincinnati, Cincinnati, OH, USA

Sherif Awad, FRCS, PhD Division of Gastrointestinal Surgery, Nottingham Digestive Diseases Centre NIHR Biomedical Research Unit, Queen's Medical Centre, Nottingham, UK

Justin M. Belcher, MD Program of Applied Translational Research, Yale-New Haven Medical Center, New Haven, CT, USA

Meredith A. Brisco, MD, MSCE Division of Cardiology, Section of Advanced Heart Failure and Cardiac Transplantation, Medical University of South Carolina, Charleston, SC, USA

Jeremiah R. Brown, PhD, MS The Dartmouth Institute for Health Policy and Clinical Practice, and the Departments of Medicine and Community and Family Medicine, Audrey and Theodore Geisel School of Medicine at Dartmouth, Lebanon, NH, USA

Lakhmir S. Chawla, MD Department of Anesthesiology and Critical Care Medicine, George Washington University, Washington, DC, USA

Michael J. Connor Jr., MD Division of Pulmonary, Allergy, and Critical Care Medicine, Department of Medicine, Emory University, Atlanta, GA, USA

Steven Deitelzweig, MD, MMM, FACP, SFHM Department of Hospital Medicine, Ochsner Clinic Foundation, New Orleans, LA, USA

Stuart M. Flechner, MD, FACS Department of Urology, Glickman Urologic and Kidney Institute, Cleveland Clinic Lerner College of Medicine, Cleveland, OH, USA

Krishnanath Gaitonde, MD Division of Urology, University of Cincinnati, Cincinnati, OH, USA

Section of Urology, Cincinnati VA Medical Center, Cincinnati, OH, USA

Susan Garwood, MBChB Department of Anesthesiology, Yale New Haven Hospital, Yale University School of Medicine, New Haven, CT, USA

T. Alp Ikizler, MD Division of Nephrology, Department of Medicine, Vanderbilt University Medical Center, Nashville, TN, USA

Catherine D. Krawczeski, MD Department of Cardiology, Lucile Packard Children's Hospital, Palo Alto, CA, USA

David M. Kwiatkowski, MD The Heart Institute, Cincinnati Children's Hospital Medical Center, Cincinnati, OH, USA

Christophe Legendre, MD Department of Nephrology and Transplantation, Necker Hospital, Paris, France

Kelly Liang, MD Renal-Electrolyte Division, Department of Medicine, University of Pittsburgh, Pittsburgh, PA, USA

Dileep N. Lobo, MS, DM, FRCS, FACS, FRCPE Division of Gastrointestinal Surgery, Nottingham Digestive Diseases Centre NIHR Biomedical Research Unit, Nottingham University Hospitals, Queen's Medical Centre, Nottingham, UK

Anju Oommen, MD Division of Nephrology, Department of Medicine, Emory University, Atlanta, GA, USA

Paul M. Palevsky, MD Renal Section, VA Pittsburgh Healthcare System, Pittsburgh, PA, USA

Department of Medicine, University of Pittsburgh School of Medicine, Pittsburgh, PA, USA

Chirag R. Parikh, MD, PhD, FASN Program of Applied Translational Research, Department of Medicine, Yale University School of Medicine, New Haven, CT, USA

Lakshmi Narasimha Prasad Ravipati, MD, MBBS, MRCP, FACP Department of Hospital Medicine, Ochsner Clinic Foundation, New Orleans, LA, USA

Anna Parker Sattah, MD Department of Anesthesiology and Critical Care Medicine, George Washington University Medical Center, Washington, DC, USA

Bernd Schröppel, MD Division of Nephrology, University of Ulm, Ulm, Germany

Lori Shutter, MD, FCCM, FNCS Department of Critical Care Medicine, University of Pittsburgh Medical Center, Pittsburgh, PA, USA

Edward D. Siew, MD, MSCI Division of Nephrology and Hypertension, Department of Medicine, Vanderbilt University Medical Center, Nashville, TN, USA

Titte R. Srinivas, MD Section of Transplant Nephrology, Division of Nephrology, Medical University of South Carolina, Charleston, SC, USA

Jeffrey M. Testani, MD, MTR Program of Applied Translational Research, Yale University, New Haven, CT, USA

Charuhas V. Thakar, MD, FASN Division of Nephrology and Hypertension, University of Cincinnati, Cincinnati, OH, USA

Section of Nephrology, Cincinnati VA Medical Center, Cincinnati, OH, USA

Ashita J. Tolwani, MD, MSE Department of Medicine, University of Alabama at Birmingham, Birmingham, AL, USA

Betty J. Tsuei, MD Department of Surgery, University of Cincinnati, Cincinnati, OH, USA

William R. Zhang, BS Yale Program of Applied Translational Research, Section of Nephrology, Yale University School of Medicine, New Haven, CT, USA

Part I
Perioperative Acute Kidney Injury: Overview and Approach

Chapter 1
Incidence, Trends, and Diagnosis of Perioperative Acute Kidney Injury

Justin M. Belcher and Chirag R. Parikh

Objectives

- To understand the modern definitions of acute kidney injury (AKI).
- To understand the impact of AKI definition on published incidence rates for postoperative AKI.
- To appreciate the rising incidence of postoperative AKI.

Introduction

Acute kidney injury (AKI) refers to a sudden loss of kidney function and is associated with significant morbidity, mortality, and health care costs. In addition to contributing to elevated in-hospital mortality, AKI is associated with increased incident and progressive chronic kidney disease (CKD) as well as deceased long-term survival. Those patients suffering the most severe form of AKI, that which requires dialysis, have particularly high rates of adverse outcomes during their hospitalization and following discharge. Though outcomes in patients with AKI have improved modestly [1], efforts toward significant reductions in morbidity and mortality have been stymied by a lack of effective therapies for the most common cause

J.M. Belcher, MD (✉)
Program of Applied Translational Research, Yale-New Haven Medical Center, 60 Temple Street Suite 6C, New Haven, CT 06510, USA
e-mail: justin.belcher@yale.edu

C.R. Parikh, MD, PhD, FASN
Program of Applied Translational Research, Department of Medicine, Yale University School of Medicine, New Haven, CT, USA
e-mail: chirag.parikh@yale.edu

C.V. Thakar, C.R. Parikh (eds.), *Perioperative Kidney Injury: Principles of Risk Assessment, Diagnosis and Treatment*, DOI 10.1007/978-1-4939-1273-5_1

of hospital-based AKI, acute tubular necrosis (ATN). One of the primary reasons for this failure is that treatment is often delayed as the exact timing of the insult that precipitates AKI is typically unknown. AKI has long been recognized as a common and severe complication of surgery [2] with approximately 35 % of hospitalized AKI occurring in the postoperative setting [3]. Though the majority of literature on postoperative AKI has focused on cardiac surgery, AKI is strongly associated with poor outcomes and increased costs in multiple surgical areas [4]. Interest in research around postoperative AKI is rapidly expanding with the recognition that the setting presents tremendous opportunity for advances in both therapeutic options and epidemiologic understanding of AKI. Multiple potentially modifiable preoperative and perioperative risk factors for AKI have been identified (see Chap. 2) and present attractive targets for interventions designed to ameliorate the risk of AKI. In addition, surgery represents a known, timed insult and when concern exists for incipient AKI, either due to technical aspects of an operation or measurement of novel, rapidly expressed kidney biomarkers (see Chap. 3), treatments may be given immediately following surgery or even intraoperatively. Such rapid application of therapeutics may in fact temporize the pathophysiologic injury associated with AKI and prevent or at least moderate its clinical manifestation. With the opportunity for both interventions geared toward minimizing the risk of AKI and immediate treatment should injury occur, postoperative AKI may not only be an ideal setting to evaluate new therapeutics but may also allow for more precise elucidation of the causal association between AKI and subsequent CKD and end-stage kidney disease (ESRD). Figure 1.1 depicts a framework where, with known risk factors and a timed insult, the study of AKI following cardiovascular surgery may facilitate advances in the prevention, treatment, and outcomes of AKI. This chapter will present how AKI is defined and diagnosed in the modern age, examine the incidence of postoperative AKI in both the cardiovascular and non-cardiovascular surgical settings, and discuss the available data on temporal trends in the incidence of postoperative AKI.

Definition

Research in AKI was long hampered by a lack of a standardized definition of what, in fact, constituted acute kidney injury. Reviews of the literature revealed at least 30 definitions meaning that epidemiologic assessment of AKI incidence and trends was virtually impossible [5]. In 2004, the Acute Dialysis Quality Initiative workgroup proposed a set of criteria to standardize the definition of AKI. The Risk, Injury, Failure, Loss, and End-stage kidney disease (RIFLE) criteria defined AKI both by changes in serum creatinine and urine output [6] (Table 1.1). The RIFLE criteria stratify AKI by degrees of severity (Risk, Injury, Failure) and outcomes (Loss, End-Stage Kidney Disease). Patients can be diagnosed with AKI through fulfilling either the serum creatinine or urine output criteria or both. The mildest

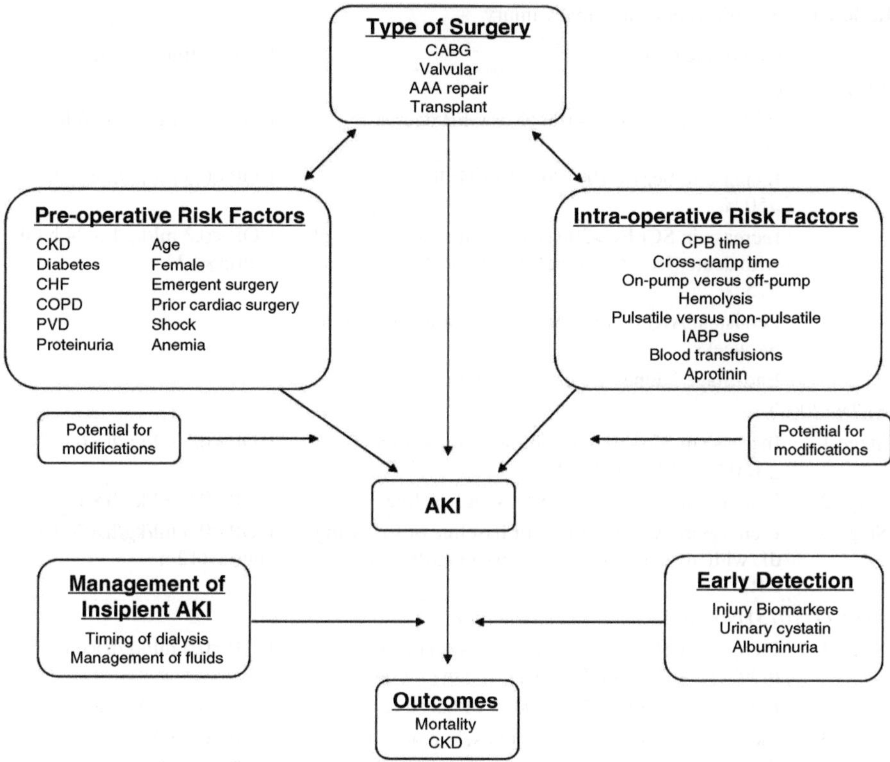

Fig. 1.1 Opportunities and strategies for prevention and treatment of AKI following cardiovascular surgery. Patients undergoing cardiovascular surgery are at risk for acute kidney injury (*AKI*) based on the specific type of surgery and multiple preoperative and perioperative risk factors. Understanding and intervening on modifiable risk factors may reduce the incidence of AKI. In addition, with a timed insult, novel, rapidly expressed biomarkers may allow for the rapid detection of kidney injury and early therapeutic intervention. In addition to ameliorating AKI severity, trials using such interventions may help elucidate the strength of the causal association between transient AKI and long-term chronic kidney disease and end-stage kidney disease

category of AKI, Risk, is defined by an increase in creatinine of 50–100 % from baseline and a fall in glomerular filtration rate (GFR) of 25–50 % from baseline or urine output <0.5 ml/kg/h for at least 6 consecutive hours. RIFLE stipulates that the changes in creatinine have to occur over fewer than 7 days and be sustained for greater than 24 h. Patients who fulfill both categories of criteria are assigned the most severe classification. Following RIFLE, multiple studies demonstrated that even very small acute changes in serum creatinine, potentially as small as 0.1 mg/dL, were associated with adverse outcomes [7]. In light of this data on the significance of small changes, an updated set of diagnostic criteria were proposed by the Acute Kidney Injury Network (AKIN) [8]. AKIN maintained the framework where

Table 1.1 Definitions of acute kidney injury

	Creatinine criteria	Urine output criteria
RIFLE (2004)		
R	Increase in Scr by 50–100 % or GFR decrease >25 %	UOP <0.5 ml/kg/h × 6 h
I	Increase in Scr by 100–200 % or GFR decrease >50 %	UOP <0.5 ml/kg/h × 12 h
F	Increase in SCr by >200 % or creatinine ≥ 4 mg/dL with acute rise ≥0.5 mg/dL OR GFR decrease >75 %	UOP <0.3 ml/kg/h × 24 h OR anuria × 12 h
L	Persistent AKI = complete loss of kidney function >4 weeks	
E	End-Stage Kidney Disease >3 months	
AKIN (2007)		
Stage 1	Increase in SCr ≥0.3 mg/dL or increase in SCr to ≥150 %–200 % of baseline	UOP <0.5 ml/kg/h × 6 h
Stage 2	Increase in SCr to >200–300 % of baseline	UOP <0.5 ml/kg/h × 12 h
Stage 3	Increase in SCr to >300 % of baseline or to ≥4 mg/dL with an acute increase of ≥0.5 mg/dL or on RRT	UOP <0.3 ml/kg/h × 24 h OR anuria × 12 h
KDIGO (2013) current recommended definition		
Stage 1	Increase in SCr ≥0.3 mg/dL with 48 h or increase in SCr to ≥150–200 % of baseline over 7 days	UOP <0.5 ml/kg/h × 6 h
Stage 2	Increase in SCr to ≥200–300 % of baseline	UOP <0.5 ml/kg/h × 12 h
Stage 3	Increase in SCr to ≥300 % of baseline or to ≥4 mg/dL or on RRT	UOP <0.3 ml/kg/h × 24 h OR anuria × 12 h

Abbreviations: *RIFLE* Risk, Injury, Failure, Loss, and End-Stage kidney disease, *GFR* glomerular filtration rate, *UOP* urine output, *Scr* serum creatinine, *AKI* acute kidney injury, *AKIN* Acute Kidney Injury Network, *RRT* renal replacement therapy, *KDIGO* Kidney Disease: Improving Global Outcomes

AKI is stratified by severity and diagnosed either by a rise in serum creatinine or fall urine output, with AKIN stages 1, 2, and 3 roughly equating to RIFLE, R, I, and F. However, stage 1, while still containing the criteria of a rise in serum creatinine by 50–100 %, can also be fulfilled by an increase in creatinine of ≥0.3 mg/dL from baseline. The criteria relating to changes in GFR were not included in AKIN. In addition, the AKIN criteria require that changes in creatinine must occur over a 48-h period and the "Loss" and "End-Stage" categories were eliminated. In 2012, the Kidney Disease: Improving Global Outcomes (KDIGO) clinical practice guidelines were published which attempt to meld the strengths of RIFLE and AKIN [9]. As with AKIN, the KDIGO guidelines stratify AKI into three stages of severity and maintain the minimum creatinine threshold for the diagnosis of AKI as a rise of 0.3 mg/dL or 50 % from baseline. However, while an absolute rise is required to occur in <48 h, the 50 % rise from baseline may occur over 7 days, as with RIFLE.

Future Definitions

The introduction of the RIFLE, AKIN, and KDOQI guidelines has codified standardized definitions for AKI and is invaluable for research into its epidemiology and treatment. However, by focusing their classifications of AKI simply on its peak severity, these definitions as currently constituted may miss an opportunity to refine their prognostic utility. Several studies have found that the duration of AKI, independent of its severity, strongly associates with outcomes [10]. It may be that future definitions incorporating both severity and duration will demonstrate enhanced prognostic performance. Even more fundamentally, all three definitions are dependent of changes in serum creatinine and urine output, which are imperfect markers of kidney injury and renal dysfunction. Fluid shifts and the provision of intravenous fluids and volume expanding agents intraoperatively may impact urine output outside of any changes in glomerular filtration rate, and dilution of serum creatinine levels due to expansion of intravascular volume may mask the presence of a true acute decline in filtration. An explosion of research interest has focused on novel urinary biomarkers of kidney (primarily tubular) injury which directly reflect structural damage and are not beholden to the vagaries of fluid balance. Such biomarkers, which will be addressed in depth in Chap. 3, include interleukin-18 (IL-18) [11], neutrophil gelatin-associated lipocalin (NGAL) [11], kidney injury molecule-1 (KIM-1) [12], and liver-type fatty acid-binding protein (L-FABP) [12]. A recent consensus conference recommended that such biomarkers of structural injury be combined with creatinine-based criteria to enhance the early detection and differential diagnosis of AKI [13]. In addition to urinary biomarkers, serum markers potentially more sensitive to alteration in glomerular filtration than creatinine have been evaluated for the detection of postoperative AKI. Cystatin C is a low-molecular-weight cysteine proteinase inhibitor synthesized at a constant rate by all nucleated cells. Cystatin C is freely filtered by the glomerulus, nearly completely reabsorbed and catabolized by the proximal tubule, does not undergo secretion, and is less influenced by nonrenal factors than creatinine. Several studies suggest that AKI defined as requiring increases in both serum creatinine and cystatin C may associate more strongly with adverse outcomes than when defined by either marker alone [14]. Future incorporation of novel urinary and serum biomarkers in the definition and diagnosis of AKI may facilitate both increased sensitivity for kidney injury as well as earlier diagnosis.

Incidence of AKI

Cardiovascular

The reported incidence of AKI following cardiovascular surgery varies markedly based upon the AKI definition and the type of surgery under study. Prior to the introduction of the recent standardized guidelines, AKI was often defined as creatinine rising above a (frequently quite high) set cutoff. Other studies, often to facilitate retrospective chart review, have defined AKI by the need for acute dialysis. While such definitions are quite specific, they are significantly lacking in sensitivity. Predictably, when defined by the requirement for dialysis, the incidence of AKI following cardiovascular surgery is quite low, ranging from 0.6 % to 1.5 % [11, 15–17]. The incidence of AKI would be expected to change with evolutions in patients selected for surgery and surgical techniques (see section "Trends in incidence and outcomes of AKI" below), and past estimates of the incidence of acute dialysis following cardiovascular surgery may no longer be valid. Unsurprisingly, when diagnostic thresholds for AKI are more lenient, the incidence has been found to be significantly higher, with an incidence of 4.9 % [11], 16.4 % [18], and 24 % [19] when AKI is defined by a rise in creatinine of 100 %, 50 %, or 25 %, respectively.

Within the setting of cardiovascular surgery, the incidence of AKI varies with the type of surgery, i.e., coronary artery bypass graft (CABG), valvular repair, aortic aneurysm repair, or cardiac transplantation. The incidence of AKI following aortic aneurysm repair is dependent both upon the surgical technique and the anatomical location of the aneurysm. In a study of 6,516 patients from the National Inpatient Sample undergoing abdominal aortic aneurysm repair (AAA), the overall incidence of AKI (diagnosed via hospital discharge codes) was 6.7 %, but the adjusted odds ratio (95 % confidence interval) for AKI was 0.42 (0.33–0.53) for patients undergoing endovascular as opposed to open repair [20]. This distinction remained significant after adjustment for propensity scores. In contrast, the overall incidence of AKI following thoracic aortic aneurysm surgery, defined as either a postoperative serum creatinine concentration greater than 1.7 mg/dL in patients with normal preoperative renal function or an increase in postoperative serum creatinine concentration greater than 30 % in patients with preoperative chronic kidney disease, is as high as 25 % [21]. In a cohort of 2,843 patients who underwent CABG, AKI, defined as a rise in serum creatinine of >1 mg/dl above baseline, occurred in 7.9 % patients [15]. When defined as a rise on creatinine of >50 % from baseline, the incidence of AKI following CABG has been noted to be as high as 42 % [22]. However, in a large study by Chertow et al. of 42,773 patients undergoing CABG, the incidence of dialysis was only 1.1 % [23]. The incidence of AKI rises with increasing surgical complexity. While patients undergoing CABG and valvular surgery alone had AKI incidences of 1.9 % and 4.4 %, respectively, those receiving a combined CABG and valvular surgery had an elevated incidence of 7.5 % [24]. AKI is especially prevalent following cardiac transplantation where the incidence of severe AKI requiring dialysis can be as high as 5.8 % [25].

Non-cardiovascular

The incidence of AKI following non-cardiovascular surgery is less well establish than that for cardiovascular surgery. Within this broad range of surgical settings, the incidence again varies by AKI definition and type of surgery. Kheterpal et al. evaluated 15,000 patients undergoing a non-cardiovascular "major" surgery, defined as a surgery with a duration of stay of 2 or more days, with an estimated preoperative creatinine clearance of greater than 80 ml/min [26]. With AKI defined as a calculated creatinine clearance of ≤50 ml/min within 7 days postoperatively, the incidence of postoperative AKI was only 0.8 %. Among intensive care unit (ICU) patients undergoing non-cardiovascular surgery, the incidence of AKI is significantly higher (Fig. 1.2). Orthopedic and abdominal surgeries in particular are frequently complicated by AKI, with an incidence in the ICU of 20–25 % [27]. Gastric bypass surgery, increasingly common as a treatment for obesity, is associated with an 8.5 % incidence of postoperative AKI, defined as either a 50 % increase in serum creatinine or dialysis requirement [4]. As AKI incidence is highest in cardiovascular surgery among patients receiving a cardiac transplant, AKI is also extremely common following other solid organ transplants. In the first month following liver transplantation, the overall incidence of AKI can be as high as 48 %, with up to 17 % of patients requiring dialysis [28]. In this setting, AKI may develop in the immediate postoperative time period, where it is often secondary to prerenal azotemia and acute tubular necrosis, as well as several weeks after surgery, where sepsis associated with immunosuppression and calcineurin inhibitor toxicity may predominate as etiologies [28].

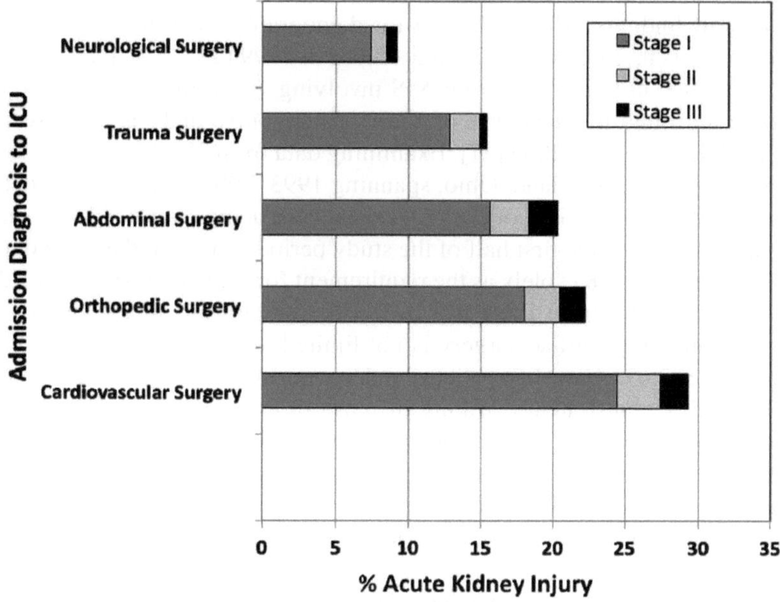

Fig. 1.2 Incidence of AKI in major surgical settings in the intensive care unit (*ICU*). Incidence of acute kidney injury (*AKI*), as staged by the Acute Kidney Injury Network (*AKIN*) criteria, in ICU patients undergoing various types of surgery (Reprinted from Thakar [27], copyright 2013, with permission from Elsevier)

Trends in Incidence and Outcomes of AKI

The incidence of AKI in general, as well as AKI requiring dialysis, is increasing, but the primary factors behind this trend remain unclear. In a general population study, old age, male sex, and black race were associated with higher incidence of dialysis-requiring AKI [29]. However, temporal changes in these as well as other risk factors including sepsis, acute heart failure, cardiac catheterization, and mechanical ventilation accounted for only 30 % of the observed rise in dialysis-requiring AKI from 2000 to 2009. Additionally, similar increases in dialysis incidence were noted across all age, sex, and racial subgroups. It is possible that alterations in physicians' prescription patterns rather than patient characteristics have driven the increased incidence of dialysis-requiring AKI. Evaluation of trends over time in the overall incidence of postoperative AKI is difficult due to changing definitions. In a study of approximately 600,000 patients undergoing CABG or valvular surgery utilizing the National Inpatient Sample (NIS), Lenihan et al. found postoperative AKI, as defined by discharge codes, increased from 4.5 % in 1999 to 12.8 % in 2008 [30]. Analysis of trends utilizing discharge codes however runs the risk of bias via "code creep" where increased recognition of the clinical importance of a condition leads to a rise in the frequency of its documentation. Alternatively, focusing on AKI requiring dialysis allows for the assessment of an objectively documented hard outcome. In the same cohort, incidence of dialysis also increased, from 0.45 % to 1.28 % over the same time period, lending credence to the overall findings. When adjusted for demographic and clinical factors, the odds for dialysis in 2008 were 2.23 times those in 1999 (95 % CI: 1.78–2.80). In a larger study also utilizing data from NIS involving 7.3 million cardiac surgeries, Nicoara et al. found the incidence of acute postoperative dialysis increased from 0.2 % in 1988 to 0.6 % in 2003 [31]. Examining data from 33,217 cardiac surgeries at a single center in Cleveland, Ohio, spanning 1993–2002, Thakar et al., defining AKI as a >50 % fall in GFR or the requirement for acute dialysis, documented a rise in incidence from the first half of the study period, 5.1 %, to the second, 6.6 % [32]. When defining AKI solely as the requirement for acute dialysis, the incidence was also noted to rise from 1.5 % to 2.0 %. The trend toward an apparent increase in dialysis following cardiac surgery is not limited to the United States. Siddiqui et al. studied 552,672 Canadian patients undergoing elective surgery between 1995 and 2009 and demonstrated a striking increase in the incidence of postoperative AKI requiring dialysis [17]. The increase was present across all age strata and remained significant after adjustment for patient and surgical characteristics. During the study period, the incidence of acute dialysis following cardiac surgery increased from 1 in 390 to 1 in 80 and following vascular surgery from 1 in 230 to 1 in 85.

Many of the risk factors for postoperative AKI (and indeed for AKI in most settings) including advanced age, diabetes, and chronic kidney disease have increased in the population. It is likely that some component of the rise in dialysis requiring postoperative AKI is relating to this increasingly aged and comorbid population. However, the trend noted by Siddiqui et al. is independent of changes in these and other risk factors. The introduction of numerous percutaneous and endovascular procedures has meant that increasingly only more complex and severe disease ends up being triaged to surgery, potentially increasing the likelihood of complications such as AKI through selection bias. However, surgical techniques have also continued to improve, and this may be expected to drive complications down. In addition, specifically as regards to AKI requiring dialysis, it is possible that alterations in physicians' prescription patterns rather than patient or surgical characteristics have driven the increased incidence of dialysis-requiring postoperative AKI. Such a change could take the form either of physicians initiating dialysis earlier in the course of AKI, in which case mortality rates for dialyzed patients would be expected to have decreased as more patients with less severe disease were dialyzed, or through the more liberal offering of dialysis to critically ill or elderly patients who previously would have been deemed futile, in which case mortality would be expected to have increased. Studies evaluating trends in mortality for patients with postoperative AKI have produced disparate findings. While some have found falling mortality associated with both all postoperative AKI and that which requires dialysis despite rising incidence [30–32], others have noted no change in mortality rates for patients requiring dialysis even as the incidence has risen [17]. Trends in the incidence and associated mortality of postoperative AKI in the United States and Canada are shown in Fig. 1.3. Further elucidation of the reasons behind the increasing incidence of AKI and of the impact greater dialysis usage has on mortality will be critical as physicians come under increasing pressure to minimize resource utilization while optimizing outcomes.

Key Messages

- Modern definitions for AKI, including RIFLE, AKIN, and KDIGO, have increased sensitivity and have standardized understanding of AKI, allowing improved epidemiologic study.
- The reported incidence of AKI following cardiac surgery historically has varied by AKI definition from <1.5 % for cases requiring dialysis to 25 % when AKI is defined as a rise in creatinine of 25 %.
- AKI rates in noncardiac surgery are significantly lower with the exception of patients in the intensive care unit and those receiving solid organ transplants.
- The incidence of all postoperative AKI, as well as the subset requiring dialysis, is increasing.
- Despite rising AKI incidence, multiple studies have found mortality rates in postoperative patients with AKI to either be stable or falling.

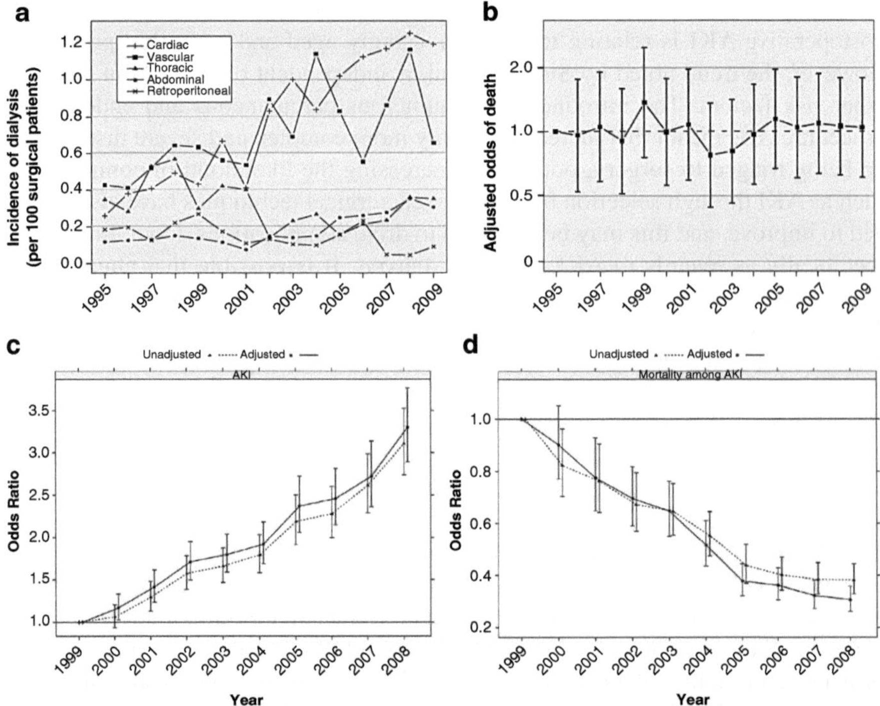

Fig. 1.3 Trends in the incidence of postoperative AKI and associated mortality in Canada and the United States. Figure depicts trends in the incidence of (**a**) AKI requiring dialysis following major surgery in Ontario, Canada, (**b**) adjusted odds of death for patients requiring acute dialysis, (**c**) adjusted and unadjusted odds ratio for all AKI following cardiovascular surgery diagnosed by discharge code relative to 1999 from the Unites States Nationwide Inpatient Sample, and (**d**) adjusted and unadjusted odds ratio for death with postoperative AKI relative to 1999. (**b**) Is adjusted for year, age, Charlson Comorbidity Index, comorbid medical conditions (diabetes mellitus, peripheral vascular disease, chronic obstructive pulmonary disease, hypertension, coronary artery disease, chronic kidney disease, liver dysfunction, cancer, congestive heart failure) and type of surgery. (**c**) and (**d**) are adjusted for age, sex, surgery type, heart failure, diabetes mellitus, hypertension, pulmonary disease, peripheral vascular disease, cerebrovascular disease, obesity, sepsis, and use of intra-aortic balloon pump and mechanical ventilation (*$\mathbf{a}$ and **b** reprinted with permission from Siddiqui et al. [17]. **$\mathbf{c}$ and **d** reprinted from Lenihan et al. [30], copyright 2013, with permission from Elsevier)

References

1. Waikar SS, Curhan GC, Wald R, McCarthy EP, Chertow GM. Declining mortality in patients with acute renal failure, 1988 to 2002. J Am Soc Nephrol. 2006;17(4):1143–50.
2. Taylor WH, Reid JV. Acute renal failure after surgical operation and head injury. Br J Surg. 1958;46(196):136–40.
3. Uchino S, Kellum JA, Bellomo R, Doig GS, Morimatsu H, Morgera S, et al. Acute renal failure in critically ill patients: a multinational, multicenter study. JAMA. 2005;294:813–8.
4. Thakar CV, Kharat V, Blanck S, Leonard AC. Acute kidney injury after gastric bypass surgery. Clin J Am Soc Nephrol. 2007;2:426–30.

5. Mehta RL, Chertow GM. Acute renal failure definitions and classification: time for change? J Am Soc Nephrol. 2003;14(8):2178–87.
6. Bellomo R, Ronco C, Kellum JA, Mehta RL, Palevsky P. Acute renal failure – definition, outcome measures, animal models, fluid therapy and information technology needs: the Second International Consensus Conference of the Acute Dialysis Quality Initiative (ADQI) Group. Crit Care. 2004;8:R204–12.
7. Newsome BB, Warnock DG, McClellan WM, Herzog CA, Kiefe CI, Eggers PW, et al. Long-term risk of mortality and end-stage renal disease among the elderly after small increases in serum creatinine level during hospitalization for acute myocardial infarction. Arch Intern Med. 2008;168:609–16.
8. Mehta RL, Kellum JA, Shah SV, Molitoris BA, Ronco C, Warnock DG, et al. Acute Kidney Injury Network: report of an initiative to improve outcomes in acute kidney injury. Crit Care. 2007;11:R31.
9. Kellum JA, Lameire N, KDIGO AKI Guideline Work Group. Diagnosis, evaluation, and management of acute kidney injury: a KDIGO summary (Part 1). Crit Care. 2013;17(1):204.
10. Brown JR, Kramer RS, Coca SG, Parikh CR. Duration of acute kidney injury impacts long-term survival after cardiac surgery. Ann Thorac Surg. 2010;90(4):1142–8.
11. Parikh CR, Coca SG, Thiessen-Philbrook H, Shlipak MG, Koyner JL, Wang Z, et al. Postoperative biomarkers predict acute kidney injury and poor outcomes after adult cardiac surgery. J Am Soc Nephrol. 2011;22:1748–57.
12. Parikh CR, Thiessen-Philbrook H, Garg AX, Kadiyala D, Shlipak MG, Koyner JL, et al. Performance of kidney injury molecule-1 and liver fatty acid-binding protein and combined biomarkers of AKI after cardiac surgery. Clin J Am Soc Nephrol. 2013;8(7):1079–788.
13. McCullough PA, Bouchard J, Waikar SS, Siew ED, Endre ZH, Goldstein SL, et al. Implementation of novel biomarkers in the diagnosis, prognosis, and management of acute kidney injury: executive summary from the tenth consensus conference of the Acute Dialysis Quality Initiative (ADQI). Contrib Nephrol. 2013;182:5–12.
14. Spahillari A, Parikh CR, Sint K, Koyner JL, Patel UD, Edelstein CL, et al. Serum cystatin C-versus creatinine-based definitions of acute kidney injury following cardiac surgery: a prospective cohort study. Am J Kidney Dis. 2012;60(6):922–9.
15. Conlon PJ, Stafford-Smith M, White WD, Newman MF, King S, Winn MP, et al. Acute renal failure following cardiac surgery. Nephrol Dial Transplant. 1999;14:1158–62.
16. Mangano CM, Diamondstone LS, Ramsay JG, Aggarwal A, Herskowitz A, Mangano DT. Renal dysfunction after myocardial revascularization: risk factors, adverse outcomes, and hospital resource utilization. Ann Intern Med. 1998;128:194–203.
17. Siddiqui NF, Coca SG, Devereaux PJ, Jain AK, Li L, Luo J, et al. Secular trends in acute dialysis after elective major surgery–1995 to 2009. CMAJ. 2012;184(11):1237–45.
18. Andersson LG, Ekroth R, Bratteby LE, Hallhagen S, Wesslen O. Acute renal failure after coronary surgery: a study of incidence and risk factors in 2009 consecutive patients. J Thorac Cardiovasc Surg. 1993;41:237–41.
19. Karkouti K, Wijeysundera DN, Yau TM, Callum JL, Cheng DC, Crowther M, et al. Acute kidney injury after cardiac surgery: focus on modifiable risk factors. Circulation. 2009;119:495–502.
20. Wald R, Waikar SS, Liangos O, Pereira BJ, Chertow GM, Jaber BL. Acute renal failure after endovascular vs open repair of abdominal aortic aneurysm. J Vasc Surg. 2006;43:460–6.
21. Godet G, Fleron MH, Vicaut E, Zubicki A, Bertrand M, Riou B, et al. Risk factors for acute postoperative renal failure in thoracic or thoracoabdominal aortic surgery: a prospective study. Anesth Analg. 1997;85:1227–32.
22. Li S, Krawczeski CD, Zappitelli M, Devarajan P, Thiessen-Philbrook H, Coca SG, et al. Incidence, risk factors, and outcomes of acute kidney injury after pediatric cardiac surgery: a prospective multicenter study. Crit Care Med. 2011;39(6):1493–9.
23. Chertow GM, Levy EM, Hammermeister KE, Grover F, Daley J. Independent association between acute renal failure and mortality following cardiac surgery. Am J Med. 1998;104(4): 343–8.
24. Grayson AD, Khater M, Jackson M, Fox MA. Valvular heart operation is an independent risk factor for acute renal failure. Ann Thorac Surg. 2003;75:1829–35.

25. Boyle JM, Moualla S, Arrigain S, Worley S, Bakri MH, Starling RC, et al. Risks and outcomes of acute kidney injury requiring dialysis after cardiac transplantation. Am J Kidney Dis. 2006;48:787–96.
26. Kheterpal S, Tremper KK, Englesbe MJ, O'Reilly M, Shanks AM, Fetterman DM, et al. Predictors of postoperative acute renal failure after noncardiac surgery in patients with previously normal renal function. Anesthesiology. 2007;107:892–902.
27. Thakar CV. Perioperative acute kidney injury. Adv Chronic Kidney Dis. 2013;20(1):67–75.
28. Cabezuelo JB, Ramírez P, Ríos A, Acosta F, Torres D, Sansano T, et al. Risk factors of acute renal failure after liver transplantation. Kidney Int. 2006;69:1073–80.
29. Hsu RK, McCulloch CE, Dudley RA, Lo LJ, Hsu CY. Temporal changes in incidence of dialysis-requiring AKI. J Am Soc Nephrol. 2012;24:37–42.
30. Lenihan CR, Montez-Rath ME, Mangano CTM, Chertow GM, Winkelmayer WC. Trends in acute kidney injury, associated use of dialysis, and mortality after cardiac surgery, 1999 to 2008. Ann Thorac Surg. 2013;95(1):20–8.
31. Nicoara A, Patel UD, Phillips-Bute BG, Shaw AD, Stafford-Smith M, Milano CA, et al. Mortality trends associated with acute renal failure requiring dialysis after CABG surgery in the United States. Blood Purif. 2009;28(4):359–63.
32. Thakar CV, Worley S, Arrigain S, Yared JP, Paganini EP. Improved survival in acute kidney injury after cardiac surgery. Am J Kidney Dis. 2007;50(5):703–11.

Chapter 2
Serious Perioperative Complications: Hospital Medicine Perspectives

Steven Deitelzweig and Lakshmi Narasimha Prasad Ravipati

Objectives

- To recognize potential perioperative medical complications
- To identify patients at risk of perioperative complications
- To understand preventive perioperative care

Introduction

In the present health-care delivery system, patients who are admitted to hospitals with surgical problems are comanaged by hospitalists [1] and their surgical colleagues, along with the assistance of subspecialists. The clinical settings are diverse, ranging from emergent surgery for a hip fracture to admission for an elective surgery, such as oncosurgery or cardiovascular surgery. Hospitalists are also involved in evaluation and optimization of medical conditions in the preoperative clinic setting for elective procedures and in the hospital setting for emergent procedures. An increasing proportion of patients seeking acute care, including surgical care, are older adults [2]. These patients are likely to have multiple comorbid conditions, and a comprehensive evaluation of these conditions and their implications on surgical outcomes warrants serious consideration.

Perioperative surgical complications are often related to the surgical procedure, the anesthesia, and/or the techniques used to administer anesthesia. In addition, a multitude of medical complications may occur in patients, particularly in

S. Deitelzweig, MD, MMM, FACP, SFHM (✉) • L.N.P. Ravipati, MD, MBBS, MRCP, FACP
Department of Hospital Medicine, Ochsner Clinic Foundation,
1514 Jefferson Highway, New Orleans, LA 70121, USA
e-mail: sdeitelzweig@ochsner.org; lravipati@ochsner.org; prasadrln@yahoo.com

C.V. Thakar, C.R. Parikh (eds.), *Perioperative Kidney Injury: Principles of Risk Assessment, Diagnosis and Treatment*, DOI 10.1007/978-1-4939-1273-5_2

those of advanced age with multiple comorbid conditions. Perioperative medical complications can involve almost every organ system. The degree of severity of organ dysfunction in the immediate perioperative period has short- and long-term consequences to both the patients' health and the health-care system. A significant number of these complications are preventable by a careful preoperative risk evaluation and optimization of certain comorbid conditions prior to surgery.

The following is a brief overview of the various postoperative medical complications the hospitalist is likely to encounter. Our goal is to highlight the most common and important complications.

Classification of Surgical Complications

As indicated in Table 2.1, a contemporary classification system has been developed for gradation of severity of postoperative complications to compare quality of care across different hospitals [3]. This nomenclature allows some degree of standardization when describing surgical and postoperative care across the world. According to this nomenclature, the complexity of surgery is classified as: (1) type A, surgical procedures without opening of the abdominal cavity (e.g., soft tissue surgery, thyroid surgery, excision of nodes); (2) type B, abdominal procedures except liver surgery and major surgery in the retroperitoneum (e.g., small bowel and colon surgery, cholecystectomy); and (3) type C, liver surgery and operations on the esophagus, pancreas, rectum, and retroperitoneum.

It is important to recognize the complex interplay between organ systems. In particular, renal function or dysfunction in the postoperative period is intricately

Table 2.1 Grading of postoperative complications

	Description	Excludes	Examples
Grade I	Deviation from expected/routine postoperative care: antiemetics, antipyretics, analgesics, electrolytes, rehabilitation, and physical/occupational therapy	Pharmacologic, surgical, or radiological intervention	Transient confusion, prolonged noninfectious diarrhea, transient atrial fibrillation, wound drainage at bedside
Grade II	Pharmacologic treatment beyond what is acceptable in Grade I	Surgical or radiologic intervention	UTI, infectious diarrhea, TIA requiring anticoagulation
Grade III	Surgical or radiologic intervention	Organ failure, ICU care	Reoperation for bleeding, wound debridement, radiologic embolization
Grade IV	Life-threatening organ failure	Death	Kidney failure requiring dialysis, cardiac intervention for acute infarction, respiratory failure requiring re-intubation, ICU care
Grade V	Death		

Abbreviations: *ICU* intensive care unit, *TIA* transient ischemic attack, *UTI* urinary tract infection linked to other organ system functions (e.g., the heart, liver, and lung). Thus, reducing the risk of postoperative organ failure, including kidney failure, requires a "holistic" approach, which includes optimal preoperative assessment, anticipation of morbidity, and timely intervention. A multidisciplinary collaborative approach involving the surgeon, anesthesiologist, primary care provider, hospitalist, and subspecialist will help ensure proper risk assessment and optimization.

Cardiac Complications

Postoperative cardiac complications are significant causes of morbidity after noncardiac surgery. They include nonfatal myocardial infarction, heart failure, serious arrhythmia-like ventricular tachycardia, and cardiac death. Patients with preexisting cardiovascular disease are at a higher risk of cardiac complications during the perioperative period. A number of tools for preoperative cardiac evaluation exist [4, 5]. Independent risk predictors of cardiac complications that are included in the Revised Cardiac Risk index (Table 2.2) include high-risk type surgery, history of ischemic heart disease, history of congestive heart failure, history of cerebrovascular disease, preoperative treatment with insulin, and preoperative serum creatinine >2.0 mg/dl [4].

Table 2.2 Independent risk factors of major cardiac event

Independent risk factors	Clinical events
1. High-risk surgical procedures	Intraperitoneal
	Intrathoracic
	Suprainguinal vascular
2. History of ischemic heart disease	Myocardial infarction
	Positive stress test
	Current angina
	Use of nitrate
	ECG with abnormal Q waves
3. History of congestive heart failure	Pulmonary edema
	Paroxysmal nocturnal dyspnea
	Bilateral rales/S3 gallop
	Chest radiograph with pulmonary congestion
4. History of cerebrovascular disease	TIA or stroke
5. Preoperative use of insulin	
6. Preoperative serum creatinine > 2.0 mg/dl	
Risk of major cardiac event	
Point (class)[a]	**Risk**
0 (I)	0.4 %
1 (II)	0.9 %
2 (III)	6.6 %
3 or more (IV)	11 %

Abbreviation: *ECG* electrocardiogram
[a]Each risk factor equals 1 point

Notably, coronary artery disease may be asymptomatic in patients who have functional limitations from their comorbid conditions, such as degenerative arthritis, obesity, and advanced age. In such patients, if indicated, anatomical or functional evaluation for coronary artery disease should be considered preoperatively. Particular attention also needs to be paid to previous history of cardiac stenting and type (drug eluting, bare metal stent) and date of the stent. Prior revascularization will have implications for perioperative management, such as need for antiplatelet agent therapy. Inappropriate interruption of antiplatelet therapy within the recommended duration of treatment after the stenting procedure may lead to stent thrombosis, a very serious complication.

Heart failure is a common postoperative cardiac complication. Patients with preexisting heart disease are predisposed to heart failure during the postoperative period and should be considered for therapeutic optimization by balancing the specific surgical setting. Patients with heart failure and those receiving vasoactive drugs are at an increased risk for hemodynamic fluctuations, leading to impairment in tissue perfusion during the postoperative period.

Pulmonary Complications

Postoperative pulmonary complications are common, associated with high morbidity and mortality, and lead to expensive care in ICU [6–8]. Postoperative pulmonary complications include atelectasis, aspiration, pneumonia, and respiratory failure [6]. Patient-related risk factors include obesity, preoperative functional limitation, advanced age, chronic obstructive pulmonary disease, sleep apnea, tobacco use, and pulmonary hypertension [7]. Procedure-related risk factors include surgeries close to the diaphragm, open versus laparoscopic procedures, and duration of surgery [7]. Tobacco cessation, breathing exercises, and incentive spirometry reduce the risk of postoperative pulmonary complications.

Sleep apnea has particular implications in the perioperative period with its potential to cause hypoxia that can contribute to cardiac complications. Sleep apnea is often an underdiagnosed and undertreated problem, and vigilance during the preoperative evaluation is suggested to identify patients who are at risk for sleep apnea [9]. Typically, it is reasonable to allow patients who wear noninvasive ventilation devices to use their machinery during their hospital stay. End-tidal CO_2 monitoring is useful in the perioperative period for detecting respiratory complications early as abnormalities of end-tidal CO_2 occur before oxygen desaturation and hypoventilation [10]. End-tidal CO_2 may possibly be used in monitoring patients with sleep apnea [11].

Endocrine Complications

Uncontrolled diabetes mellitus can contribute to multiple postoperative complications [12]. The presence of insulin requiring diabetes is a risk factor for postoperative morbidity and mortality [13]. Diabetic patients are also at a risk for longer hospital

Table 2.3 Common scenarios of impairments in glucose control

	Hypoglycemia	Hyperglycemia
Patient factors	Fasting, loss of appetite	Illness, adherence
Surgery/procedure related	Adrenal insufficiency, inadequate caloric intake	Surgical stress and stress hormones, pain, inappropriate nutrition
Drug related	Oral hypoglycemic agents; chronic steroid therapy	Changes in home regimens, steroid therapy

length of stay. Surgery often disrupts the patient's usual home diabetic regimen [14]. Oral hypoglycemic, non-insulin injectable agents are typically held and replaced with a physiological insulin regimen which consists of basal and prandial insulin during the immediate perioperative period. A basal prandial insulin regimen is more effective than supplemental (sliding scale) insulin.

Several factors influence glucose control in the perioperative period (Table 2.3). Factors that contribute to hyperglycemia during this time include the insulin counter regulatory hormones: growth hormone, cortisol, epinephrine, and glucagon. On the other hand, fasting status and decreased appetite contribute to hypoglycemia. The use of perioperative steroids in surgeries that involve immune suppression (such as organ transplants) and steroid use for neurosurgical conditions can also lead to uncontrolled glucose. Maintaining euglycemia during the perioperative period is an attempt to balance the above factors. Insulin is likely to be used for better flexibility of glucose control perioperatively, even in type 2 diabetics who are on oral agents.

Another area of concern is perioperative adrenal insufficiency. Chronic administration of glucocorticoid therapy can suppress the hypothalamic pituitary adrenal axis that can lead to adrenal gland hypofunction during the stressful perioperative period. A focused preoperative endocrine evaluation should involve inquiry about the use of steroids for conditions that the surgery might be addressing such as intra-articular steroid injections for osteoarthritis of the knees and hips, epidural steroid injections for spinal conditions, and other common conditions such as obstructive airway disease and immunological conditions. In selected patients, a stress dose of steroids is indicated in the perioperative period.

In addition to glycemic control, thyroid hormone homeostasis is also important in the perioperative period. Particular preparation is required for surgeries involving the thyroid gland for hyperthyroidism to avoid thyroid storm. Similarly, surgeries involving the adrenal gland for pheochromocytoma require specific pretreatment to avoid hypertensive crisis.

Hematopoietic and Vascular Complications

Acute expected blood loss and related anemia is not uncommon with most inpatient surgeries. The decision to transfuse packed red blood cells should be based on the symptoms of anemia and both the anticipated extent and rate of drop in the hemoglobin and hematocrit. Underlying cardiopulmonary conditions such as coronary artery disease and systolic and diastolic heart failure should also be taken into account. The threshold for blood transfusion has risen (restrictive versus liberal strategy) compared to the past [15].

Other important hematologic complications that can occur are associated with the use of heparin for thromboembolic prophylaxis during the perioperative period. These include heparin-induced thrombocytopenia (HIT type 2) and heparin-induced thrombocytopenia and thrombosis (HITT) in which the thrombocytopenia is associated with arterial and venous thrombosis [16]. HIT type 2 is an immune-mediated disorder in which antibodies form against the heparin-platelet factor 4 complex. The incidence is higher in patients treated with unfractionated heparin rather than low molecular weight heparin and is also more common in females compared to males and in surgical patients compared to medical patients.

Venous thromboembolism is another well-recognized complication of the perioperative state. Without prophylaxis, the risk of deep vein thrombosis (DVT) is very high [17] among patients undergoing surgery. Patients undergoing surgery should thus be evaluated for their risk of DVT, and prophylaxis should be administered based on the patients' risk. Patients at high risk for venous thromboembolism include those who have undergone major orthopedic procedures such as total hip and total knee replacements, hip fracture surgery, and abdominal or pelvic cancer surgery. They benefit from extended venous thromboembolism prophylaxis and with a longer duration of pharmacotherapy; for example, up to 4 weeks of treatment is advantageous for patients undergoing hip replacement.

Management of patients receiving anticoagulation is critically important during the perioperative period. The factors that need to be considered to manage perioperative anticoagulation include the indication for anticoagulation (commonly atrial fibrillation, venous thromboembolism, and mechanical heart valves), the type of surgery/procedure, and the comorbid conditions. Some procedures, such as gastrointestinal luminal endoscopic studies without biopsies, minor skin procedures, and joint aspirations, do not require interruption of anticoagulation. When anticoagulation needs to be interrupted, the safety of this interruption needs to be evaluated. Bridging anticoagulation should be considered for patients with conditions that are at high risk for thromboembolism, such as atrial fibrillation, recent thromboembolism, and thrombophilic conditions with recurrent thrombotic events, and in patients with certain types of mechanical heart valves.

It is becoming increasingly common to manage patients on newer or novel oral anticoagulants in the preoperative as well as the postoperative period. The available agents include direct factor Xa inhibitors, rivaroxaban and apixaban, and direct thrombin inhibitor dabigatran [18]. It is important that the hospitalists are aware of the pharmacokinetics of these agents, especially in instances of renal or liver dysfunction, to determine the appropriate dosage and duration of treatment. Currently, there are no specific antidotes available for the reversal of anticoagulation effect of many of these agents, making it challenging to use these agents in the immediate postoperative period. Of particular importance is balancing the risk and benefit of their use in neurosurgical procedures.

Neuropsychiatric Complications

A common neurological complication during the perioperative period is delirium [19]. It is associated with delay in overall postoperative recovery and length of hospitalization. Delirium can be hypoactive or hyperactive. Postoperative pain and analgesics can be associated with postoperative delirium.

Patient-related predisposing risk factors for delirium include older age [20] (>75 years), cognitive impairment, anxiety, depression, sedation, alcohol excess, reduced functional status, and abnormal glucose control. Precipitating factors for delirium include uncontrolled pain and medications such as Demerol (opioids), anticholinergics, antihistamines, and benzodiazepines. Procedure-related risk factors include hip fracture surgery and emergent surgeries versus elective surgeries.

There are various tools available for detection of delirium. The Confusion Assessment Method (CAM) is a bedside method that helps clinicians rapidly diagnose delirium [21]. Early detection of delirium is needed to enable prompt initiation of treatment. It is suggested that clinicians caring for patients who are at risk of delirium look for signs and symptoms of delirium by incorporating bedside delirium evaluation tools in their daily assessments as delirium is often underdiagnosed.

Surgery can create anxiety among patients that can affect blood pressure and heart rate in the perioperative period, particularly on the day of surgery. Preexisting psychiatric illnesses including anxiety and depression are likely to identify patients at risk of poor outcomes after surgery [22].

Gastrointestinal/Hepatic Complications

Because of reduced postoperative mobility and the administration of opioid analgesics, constipation and ileus are commonly encountered during the perioperative period. Preemptive use of a bowel regimen that might include a combination of laxatives may be required. Postoperative nausea and vomiting is another common complication that can be a side effect of medications as well as part of the medical condition. Vomiting in the postoperative period can be complicated by aspiration and pneumonia. Anticipating these events and using prophylaxis are considered to be the best approach in prevention.

There are certain perioperative complications specific to patients with preexisting liver disease [23]. They include infections, hepatorenal syndrome, and decompensated liver disease. Hepatic decompensation can occur in patients who may not have an established liver disease. A careful preoperative evaluation focusing on the presence of risk factors for chronic liver disease such as chronic viral hepatitis, alcohol excess, and nonalcoholic steatohepatitis should be performed for patients in whom chronic liver disease is suspected. Particular attention needs to be paid to clinical signs and symptoms of chronic liver disease and laboratory studies to help identify patients who may have undiagnosed chronic liver disease. Given the complexity, it is usually recommended to involve a subspecialist when managing perioperative patients at risk of or with liver disease.

Urinary Complications

Urinary retention can occur postoperatively and is a common preventable and treatable problem. Procedure-related risk factors include orthopedic surgeries, hernia repair, and surgeries involving perineum and rectum [24]. Older men are at a higher risk of retention, likely because of the preexisting prostatic hypertrophy. Urinary retention can be associated with constipation and can lead to urinary tract infection. Certain medications such as anticholinergics, antihistamines, and opioids, particularly when administered during the perioperative state, can predispose to urinary retention. Awareness of this problem and identifying the risk factors are the key to addressing urinary retention.

Perioperative Pharmacotherapy

It is of utmost importance that information be obtained about the medications that the surgical patient is taking including prescribed medications, over-the-counter medications, and supplements including herbal remedies. One of the roles of the hospitalist is to make recommendations about the perioperative use of the medication [25] as some of the medications may have to be held (if appropriate). It is advisable to have a consultation with a dedicated pharmacist who has a thorough understanding of the efficacy and adverse reactions in patients being prepared for surgery. Moreover, titration of pharmacotherapy is equally important during the hospital course in patients with liver or renal dysfunction. And lastly, medication reconciliation is essential at the time of discharge, which may reduce the risk of readmissions.

Conclusion

Hospitalists involved in the care of a patient undergoing a surgical procedure should be aware of the potential medical complications that are likely to occur in the perioperative period. A significant number of complications are predictable and preventable with the knowledge of the patient's risk factors for those complications. A comprehensive preoperative evaluation, postoperative care regimen, and a collaborative approach with the surgeon and anesthesiologist will help in reducing the risk of vital organ damage and achieve better patient outcomes.

Key Messages

- Vital organ dysfunction, including renal dysfunction, is not uncommon and leads to increased morbidity and mortality in the postoperative period.
- Cardiac and metabolic derangements are among the most common complications in the postoperative period.
- Careful organ-specific assessment of the patient in the preoperative period is essential.
- A collaborative approach for risk evaluation, optimization, and management by a multidisciplinary team involving the primary care provider, hospitalist, subspecialist, anesthesiologist, and surgeon during the perioperative period is likely to provide better patient outcomes.

References

1. Hinami K, Whelan CT, Konetzka RT, Meltzer DO. Provider expectations and experiences of comanagement. J Hosp Med. 2011;6(7):401–4.
2. Doerflinger DM. Older adult surgical patients: presentation and challenges. AORN J. 2009;90(2):223–40, quiz 241–4.
3. Demartines N, Clavien PA. Classification of surgical complications: a new proposal with evaluation in a cohort of 6336 patients and results of a survey. Ann Surg. 2004;240(2):205–13.
4. Lee TH, Marcantonio ER, Mangione CM, et al. Derivation and prospective validation of a simple index for prediction of cardiac risk of major noncardiac surgery. Circulation. 1999;100(10):1043–9.
5. Fleisher LA, Beckman JA, Brown KA, et al. ACC/AHA 2007 Guidelines on Perioperative Cardiovascular Evaluation and Care for Noncardiac Surgery. Executive Summary: A Report of the American College of Cardiology/American Heart Association Task Force on Practice Guidelines (Writing Committee to Revise the 2002 Guidelines on Perioperative Cardiovascular Evaluation for Noncardiac Surgery) developed in collaboration with the American Society of Echocardiography, American Society of Nuclear Cardiology, Heart Rhythm Society, Society of Cardiovascular Anesthesiologists, Society for Cardiovascular Angiography and Interventions, Society for Vascular Medicine and Biology, and Society for Vascular Surgery. J Am Coll Cardiol. 2007;50(17):1707–32. Erratum in: J Am Coll Cardiol. 2008;52(9);794–7.
6. Sachdev G, Napolitano LM. Postoperative pulmonary complications: pneumonia and acute respiratory failure. Surg Clin North Am. 2012;92(2):321–44, ix.
7. Canet J, Gallart L. Predicting postoperative pulmonary complications in the general population. Curr Opin Anaesthesiol. 2013;26(2):107–15.
8. Shander A, Fleisher LA, Barie PS, Bigatello LM, Sladen RN, Watson CB. Clinical and economic burden of postoperative pulmonary complications: patient safety summit on definition, risk-reducing interventions, and preventive strategies. Crit Care Med. 2011;39(9):2163–72.
9. Kaw R, Michota F, Jaffer A, Ghamande S, Auckley D, Golish J. Unrecognized sleep apnea in the surgical patient: implications for the perioperative setting. Chest. 2006;129(1):198–205.
10. Kierzek G, Jactat T, Dumas F, Pourriat JL. End-tidal carbon dioxide monitoring in the emergency department. Acad Emerg Med. 2006;13(10):1086.
11. Chen WH, Ye JY, Zhang YH, Wang JY. Application of pressure of end-tidal carbon dioxide concentration in polysomnography. [Chinese]. Zhonghua Er Bi Yan Hou Tou Jing Wai Ke Za Zhi. 2013;48(2):158–60.

12. Meneghini LF. Perioperative management of diabetes: translating evidence into practice. Cleve Clin J Med. 2009;76 Suppl 4:S53–9.
13. Rittler P, Broedl UC, Hartl W, Goke B, Jauch K. Diabetes mellitus – perioperative management [in German]. Chirurg. 2009;80(5):410, 412–5.
14. Rizvi AA, Chillag SA, Chillag KJ. Perioperative management of diabetes and hyperglycemia in patients undergoing orthopaedic surgery. J Am Acad Orthop Surg. 2010;18(7):426–35.
15. Carson JL, Terrin JL, Noveck ML, et al FOCUS Investigators. Liberal or restrictive transfusion in high-risk patients after hip surgery. N Engl J Med. 2011;365(26):2453–62.
16. Battistelli S, Genovese A, Gori T. Heparin-induced thrombocytopenia in surgical patients. Am J Surg. 2010;199(1):43–51.
17. Grant PJ, Brotman DJ, Jaffer AK. Perioperative anticoagulant management. Anesthesiol Clin. 2009;27(4):761–77.
18. Levy JH, Key NS, Azran MS. Novel oral anticoagulants: implications in the perioperative setting. Anesthesiology. 2010;113(3):726–45.
19. Allen SR, Frankel HL. Postoperative complications: delirium. Surg Clin North Am. 2012; 92(2):409–31.
20. Brooks PB. Postoperative delirium in elderly patients. Am J Nurs. 2012;112(9):38–49, quiz 51.
21. Sieber FE. Postoperative delirium in the elderly surgical patient. Anesthesiol Clin. 2009;27(3):451–64, table of contents.
22. Trief PM, Grant W, Frederickson B. A prospective study of psychological predictors of lumbar surgery outcome. Spine (Phila Pa 1976). 2000;25(20):2616–21.
23. Pandey CK, Karna ST, Pandey VK, Tandon M, Singhal A, Mangla V. Perioperative risk factors in patients with liver disease undergoing non-hepatic surgery. World J Gastrointest Surg. 2012;4(12):267–74.
24. Darrah DM, Griebling TL, Sliverstein JH. Postoperative urinary retention. Anesthesiol Clin. 2009;27(3):465–84.
25. Mercado DL, Petty BG. Perioperative medication management. Med Clin North Am. 2003; 87(1):41–57.

Chapter 3
Role of Novel Kidney Injury Biomarkers in Perioperative Acute Kidney Injury

Chirag R. Parikh and William R. Zhang

Objectives

- To address the pressing need for a more specific and sensitive paradigm for AKI detection and risk stratification, especially in the perioperative setting.
- To provide the basic science background and foundation of several novel kidney injury biomarkers.
- To highlight the findings of these biomarkers in the large-scale clinical validation studies carried out by the TRIBE-AKI Consortium.

Introduction

Acute kidney injury (AKI) after major surgery is a serious complication that is associated with significant morbidity and mortality and a poor prognosis. Previously known as acute renal failure (ARF), this relatively new term encompasses a constellation of renal pathologies, which often manifests in clinically silent steps and leads to irreversible damage. With AKI after surgery reaching epidemic proportions worldwide, the insidious nature of this condition is especially concerning as it outpaces our current paradigms for treatment [1].

C.R. Parikh, MD, PhD, FASN (✉)
Program of Applied Translational Research, Department of Medicine, Yale University School of Medicine, New Haven, CT, USA
e-mail: chirag.parikh@yale.edu

W.R. Zhang, BS
Yale Program of Applied Translational Research, Section of Nephrology, Yale University School of Medicine, 60 Temple Street, Suite 6C, New Haven, CT 06510, USA
e-mail: williamrzhang@gmail.com

C.V. Thakar, C.R. Parikh (eds.), *Perioperative Kidney Injury: Principles of Risk Assessment, Diagnosis and Treatment*, DOI 10.1007/978-1-4939-1273-5_3

For almost a century, clinicians have used serum creatinine as the gold standard for assessing glomerular filtration and the primary means for evaluating renal function [2]. While this traditional biomarker detects renal filtering capacity, it may not be adequate to detect different forms of AKI that do not involve impaired filtering, such as structural tubular injury [3]. Many other conditions, including volume depletion, alterations in the afferent arterioles leading to the glomerulus, and urinary tract obstructions, may be the underlying cause of a serum creatinine increase, while the intrinsic structure of the kidney remains unaffected. In other words, serum creatinine may, at best, only be a nonspecific marker of kidney injury. Several nonrenal factors also influence serum creatinine concentrations, including body weight, race, age, gender, hydration status, drug usage, muscle mass and metabolism, and diet, thus compromising the sensitivity of this metric [4].

Further, even when this biological signal does detect significant renal disease, it is often too late. Studies have shown that over 50 % of renal function may be lost before serum creatinine rises are detectable above the upper reference limit and may not be elevated until days after injury [5–7]. And in the case of kidney injury, timing is absolutely critical. After an injury is well established, there is little that can be done for patients. Serum creatinine thus may only be providing what clinicians refer to as "the tip of the iceberg" of the AKI landscape, with subclinical diagnoses still to be uncovered underneath the surface. This pressing need to predict AKI before the increase in serum creatinine has been driving the search for novel disease-specific biomarkers of AKI [8].

Specifically, perioperative AKI is a major area of concern as surgery remains a leading cause of AKI, with an incidence of up to 47 % in hospitalized patients [9, 10]. As procedures of deliberate intervention with established monitoring, the setting of surgery provides especially fertile ground for early detection and implementing catered care regimens following operation. Unfortunately, the translation of the advances on the molecular and cellular fronts of this field have proceeded at a relatively sluggish pace, but there are signs of hope: innovative technologies have uncovered several novel genes and gene products that are produced by and involved in the early stress response of the kidney, which have led to the discovery of novel biomarkers—several of which have recently reached the point of clinical validation [11–13].

Right Place, Right Time: Emerging Biomarkers of AKI

The first efforts to move beyond serum creatinine introduced the usage of fractional excretion of sodium (FeNa) and urine microscopy as signals of kidney injury. FeNa is a fluctuating measure that can distinguish prerenal injury from AKI, while urinary microscopy provides an indication of tubular damage [4]. However, these techniques have been insensitive and nonspecific for early AKI detection and have not advanced the treatment of AKI, which has prompted the search for novel markers [14–16]. By looking for cues at the right place and the right time of the pathophysiologic process, novel AKI biomarkers, some of which are presented below, may collectively provide clinicians greater resolution into disease management and revolutionize treatment regimens. Figure 3.1 provides a graphical summary of these

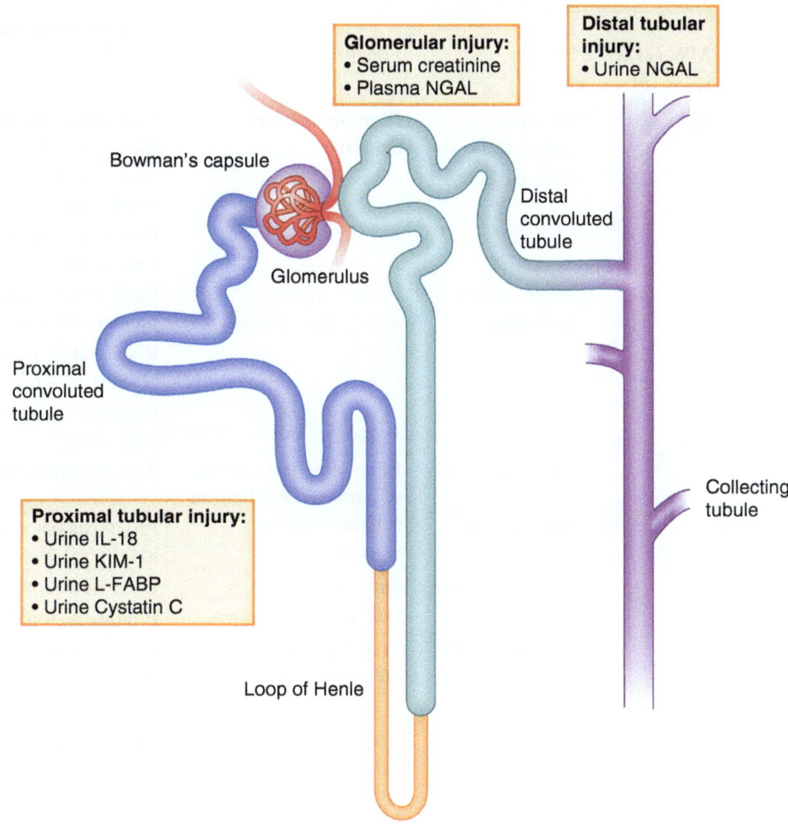

Fig. 3.1 AKI biomarkers along the nephron. Biomarkers of AKI, such as those discussed in the text, can provide information about damage and injury to specific anatomical locations on the nephron

biomarkers in their specific anatomical locations on the nephron, and Table 3.1 lists major characteristics of each of the below biomarkers.

IL-18

Interleukin-18 (IL-18) is a proinflammatory member of the IL-1 cytokine superfamily that is generally produced by macrophages and other immune cells to regulate both the innate and adaptive immune response [17]. Renal proximal tubule cells are thought to be the primary renal source of this cytokine, which is secreted as a precursor, cleaved into the active form, and subsequently released into the urine following the onset of AKI [18–20]. In response to ischemic injury, this molecule is also known to recruit neutrophils, contributing to the development of ischemic acute tubular necrosis (ATN) [21, 22].

Table 3.1 Perioperative kidney injury biomarker characteristics

Name	MW (kDa)	Source	Function	Role in perioperative AKI
Urine biomarkers				
IL-18	18	Proximal tubule cells	Proinflammatory cytokine	Early detection of tubular cell damage
		Immune cells		Risk stratification of severity of AKI
				Prognosis (short and long term)
NGAL	25	Renal tubular epithelium	Bacteriostatic, antioxidant, growth factor	Early detection of tubular cell damage
				Risk stratification of severity of AKI
				Prognosis (short and long term)
KIM-1	90	Proximal tubule epithelium	Regulating remodeling of damaged epithelium/ activate immune response	Risk stratification
		Immune cells		Prognosis (short and long term)
L-FABP	15	Proximal tubule cells	Fatty-acid-binding protein	Early detection
				Prognosis (long term)
Cystatin C	13	All nucleated cells	Transmembrane protein (CAM)	Early detection of tubular dysfunction
Plasma biomarkers				
NGAL	25	Neutrophils	Bacteriostatic, antioxidant, growth factor	Early detection of ischemia reperfusion injury
		Lung		Risk stratification of severity of AKI
		Liver		Prognosis (short term)
Cystatin C	13	All nucleated cells	Cysteine protease inhibitor	Alternate measure of GFR

Accordingly, early evidence for the utility of IL-18 first emerged as a marker for ATN in a study of 72 patients with different forms of kidney injury. Patients with ATN and delayed graft function were found to exhibit significantly greater median urine IL-18 than healthy controls ($p<0.0001$ and $p=0.009$, respectively) [22]. In a subsequent study, the cytokine was also found to be an early predictive biomarker for AKI in a cohort of 55 patients undergoing cardiopulmonary bypass. Detection of IL-18 was feasible 4–6 h following surgery and remained elevated up to 48 h, with peak levels at over 25-fold at 12 h and a corresponding maximum area under the curve (AUC) of 0.75 [23].

NGAL

Neutrophil gelatinase-associated lipocalin (NGAL) is an immunoregulatory peptide associated with gelatinase that is usually expressed at low, undetectable levels by neutrophils but upregulated in models of AKI, especially following ischemia [24–26]. Forms of this protein are also known to be produced by renal tubular epithelial cells. Renal clearance is crucial for maintenance of NGAL levels, and filtered NGAL can be sequestered by the proximal tubules [25, 27].

Readily detected in both the serum and urine, this biomarker has been demonstrated to predict various clinical outcomes, including the need for intensive care unit (ICU) admission and dialysis, as well as mortality for patients in the emergency room (ER) [26, 28]. One early study of NGAL in a cohort of 71 children undergoing cardiopulmonary bypass found this protein to be significantly increased 2 h after surgery in both urine and serum. Following multivariate analysis, urine NGAL emerged as a powerful predictor of AKI that may even serve as a standalone marker with an AUC of 0.998, a sensitivity of 1.00, and a specificity of 0.98 [29].

KIM-1

Kidney injury molecule-1 (KIM-1) is a transmembrane protein that is expressed in immune cells as well as in proximal tubules during times of growth [30]. Following renal injury, especially in the case of ischemia, this protein is overexpressed in the proximal tubule, as the peptide sheds its ectodomain and appears in the urine [31].

While the kinetics of KIM-1 have been reported to be delayed to around 12–24 h, elevated levels have been shown to distinguish ischemic AKI from prerenal azotemia and chronic renal disease, and may also lead to distinguishing AKI subtypes: notably, one early study has shown that elevated urine KIM-1 levels could be specifically predictive of ATN in a cohort of 46 patients [4, 32]. While the pool of KIM-1 research has been relatively limited, another early study corroborated these trends and further concluded that urine KIM-1 predicted AKI with an AUC of 0.83 in a small pediatric cohort undergoing cardiac surgery [33].

L-FABP

Liver-type fatty-acid-binding protein (L-FABP) is a cytoplasmic protein that is involved in fatty-acid metabolism. Not only is this factor expressed in the liver but also in the intestine, pancreases, lung, stomach, and the kidney, where it is produced in the proximal tubules [34, 35]. During times of injury, the protein is known to be transported from the cytoplasm of the proximal tubule cells into the tubular lumen and is thus detected in the urine [35].

Early measurements at 4 and 12 h of urine L-FABP have been shown to predict ischemic AKI with an AUC of 0.81 in a cohort of 40 pediatric patients undergoing cardiopulmonary bypass. In fact, urine L-FABP levels at 4 h following surgery was demonstrated to serve as an independent risk factor for AKI [36].

Cystatin C

Cystatin C (cysC) is an endogenous cysteine protease inhibitor that is secreted by essentially all nucleated cells [37, 38]. While initial studies of plasma cysC demonstrated promise, it has recently been appreciated that plasma cysC may be influenced by inflammatory conditions [39–41]. Normally, plasma cysC is freely filtered by the glomerulus and completely reabsorbed and degraded in the proximal tubules, thus serving as a sensitive marker of glomerular filtration superior to serum creatinine [42]. Despite the fact that this marker is also less influenced by the colluding factors that limit serum creatinine, plasma cysC is not necessarily a holistic marker of kidney injury as it still suffers limitations including the inability to discern different types of AKI. On the other hand, urine cysC, which will appear in the urine due to impaired reabsorption when the proximal tubule is injured, boasts early and sensitive detection of AKI as a sign of tubular dysfunction [43].

In an early study of a cohort of 72 adults undergoing cardiac surgery, urine cysC predicted AKI in all 34 patients that developed the condition 6 h after ICU admission (AUC=0.724, 95 % confidence interval (CI)=0.601–0.846; $p=0.002$) [44]. The study even found that even while the patient is still in the operating room, urine cysC could be predictive of AKI with an over 147-fold increase, compared to an approximately eightfold increase in those that did not develop AKI ($p=0.007$). This marker is emerging as one of the best and most consistently performing biomarkers for identifying established AKI with AUCs of 0.88–0.97 [45–49].

Forging Forward: Clinical Validation in Perioperative Settings

With mounting evidence from these initial studies, larger-scale validation is necessary to confirm the potential of these biomarkers and pave the path for enhanced diagnosis and prognosis of AKI at various points within the span of surgical procedures. The Translational Research Investigating Biomarker Endpoints in Acute Kidney Injury (TRIBE-AKI) consortium has begun to address this very need. The research group has conducted large, prospective, multicenter cohort studies of 1,219 adults and 311 children undergoing cardiac surgery. With patients enrolled from 11 collective medical centers, these studies are manifestations of the first strides to guide translation of these biomarkers for clinical use. Figure 3.2 summarizes the collective data from the TRIBE-AKI studies.

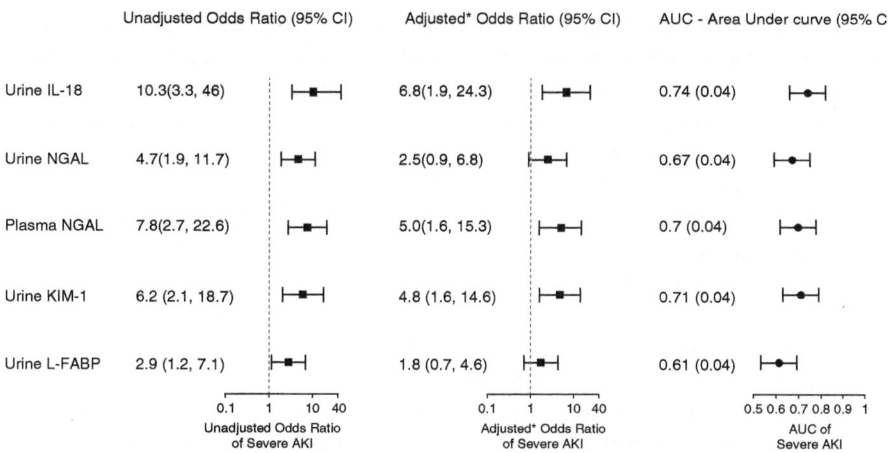

Fig. 3.2 TRIBE-AKI biomarker performance. For each of the discussed biomarkers, both the unadjusted and adjusted odds ratios and area under the curve are included, along with the 95 % confidence interval (95 % *CI*) for each metric in parenthesis

The first TRIBE-AKI study investigated the early predictive potential of urine IL-18 and urine and plasma NGAL in the adult cohort [50]. These biomarkers peaked within 6 h, which was significantly earlier than the rise in serum creatinine occurring at 24–72 h. The highest quintile of IL-18 was associated with an adjusted 6.8-fold higher odds of AKI (95 % CI = 1.9–24.3) compared with the lower quintiles, significantly improved the AKI risk prediction model by the Society of Thoracic Surgeons (STS) from 0.69 to 0.76, and enhanced reclassification (categorical net reclassification index (NRI) = 0.25 (0.1); $p = 0.01$). In the same vein, the highest quintile of serum NGAL was associated with an adjusted 5.0-fold higher odds of AKI (95 % CI = 1.6–15.3) compared to lower quintiles, significantly improved the STS model to an AUC of 0.75, and significantly enhanced reclassification (categorical NRI = 0.18 (0.09); $p = 0.05$). In addition, these biomarkers also forecasted prognostic events: elevated urine IL-18 and urine and plasma NGAL were separately associated with longer length of hospital and ICU duration and higher risk for dialysis and death.

Similar trends were found in the pediatric setting after cardiac surgery [51]. Urine IL-18 and plasma NGAL levels also peaked within 6 h, boasting a significantly earlier rise than serum creatinine. Further, the first measurement of these two biomarkers in the urine was associated with severe AKI. When stratifying the biomarker levels, the highest quintiles of urine IL-18 and urine NGAL were associated with a 6.9- (95 % CI = 1.7–28.8) and 4.1-fold (95 % CI = 1.0–16.3) higher odds of AKI, respectively, compared to the lower quintiles. Both urine IL-18 and urine NGAL exhibited moderate AUCs of 0.72 and 0.71, respectively, and were associated with the prognostic prediction of longer hospital and ICU duration and higher risk for dialysis and death.

Interestingly, for the adult cohort, none of the urine NGAL quintiles were independently associated with the development of AKI, while, for the pediatric cohort, plasma NGAL was not associated with the development of postoperative severe AKI. Such discrepancies point to the need for further studies to validate the current pool of data and call for specific baselines for different clinical settings.

Studies from the TRIBE-AKI consortium have also further examined KIM-1, confirming the markers utility in predicting AKI [52]. KIM-1 was found to peak 2 days after surgery in adults and after 1 day in children. In both cohorts, postoperative KIM-1 levels through 6 h after surgery were significantly higher in patients who developed AKI than those who did not ($p<0.001$ and $p=0.001$, respectively), though these levels were not significantly different from levels prior to surgery. While the biomarker was not able to provide additional resolution in detecting AKI in children, KIM-1 exhibited further prognostic potential in the adult cohort: elevated concentrations of KIM-1 were associated with increased risk of hospital death or dialysis and were able to slightly improve the AUC to 0.73 when added to the clinical model for AKI. In addition, the highest quintile of the KIM-1 was associated with AKI when compared to the lowest quintile up to 6 h following surgery.

L-FABP was examined alongside KIM-1 and shown to peak within 6 h after surgery in both the adult and pediatric cohort, and median levels within this time span were significantly higher in those with AKI than those without AKI ($p<0.001$ for both cohorts) [52]. In other respects, findings of L-FABP appeared to be less robust as the marker did not provide any additional prognostic information in either of the cohorts. However, the addition of L-FABP to the clinical model did slightly increase the AUC to 0.81 in the pediatric cohort. These larger studies begin to shed light on the nuances between adult and children subjects and further emphasize the need for cross-validation of these novel biomarkers.

Delving deeper into their prognostic potential, the most recent TRIBE-AKI study has extended follow-up with the initial cohort and reported that urinary NGAL, IL-18, KIM-1, and L-FABP are associated with long-term outcomes following cardiac surgery [53]. Perhaps most strikingly, this follow-up study, conducted at a median duration of 3 years, showcases the enduring predictive power of these biomarkers not only in patients with AKI but also in those without clinical AKI. Following stratification into tertiles, the highest levels of peak urinary NGAL, IL-18, KIM-1, and L-FABP in AKI patients were independently associated with a 2.0–3.2-fold increased risk for mortality compared to the lowest tertiles. In those that did not develop clinical AKI, comparison of the highest and lowest tertiles of urinary IL-18 and KIM-1 also revealed independent association of these biomarkers with long-term mortality and an improvement in net reclassification for predicting these outcomes. Not only do these findings demonstrate greater predictive utility for these biomarkers but also further reveal the contours of AKI pathology and support the very notion of using biomarkers for disease identification and risk stratification.

Future Directions

The current body of work has laid the foundation for future efforts in establishing these biomarkers as integral components of clinical practice. Yet, while early studies demonstrated great promise, instances of larger studies have yielded only moderate results. So what can we make from these discrepancies?

Relying on serum creatinine as the gold standard for classifying cases of AKI may be at the root of the problem, but perhaps such inconsistencies themselves warrant further research and validation. To this end, there are still hurdles to overcome: crucial to their application is demonstration of the incremental value of these biomarkers over clinical risk prediction models and their ability to guide management with this added information. Newer statistical methods to develop combination of biomarkers to improve their classification potential will also be needed. These biomarkers need to be tested in randomized clinical trials to evaluate the clinical benefits and the cost-effectiveness of these biomarkers compared to the standard of care.

Ultimately, each of these biomarkers, and perhaps others that have yet to be identified, can provide a unique lens to focus the blurred image of perioperative AKI that clinicians are currently trying to grasp. And eventually, this set of novel biomarkers may be used to complement serum creatinine in a biomarker "panel" that can collectively serve as an early predictive model in high-risk surgeries and illuminate various aspects of the heterogeneous disease, from the timing of the initial insult and assessing the duration of disease to distinguishing various AKI phenotypes, which in turn, would lead to the most effective treatment strategies. The trajectory to proceed to this step will require the collaboration between industry and academia to propel the research to large-scale clinical use. There is considerable

Key Messages

- Novel biomarkers that signal renal damage may be able to reform disease detection and management for peri-operative AKI. Notably, these molecules can detect cases of subclinical AKI, which traditional measures may fail to identify.
- Kidney injury biomarkers may also offer a window into earlier diagnosis of AKI, as well as provide clinically valuable prognostic information.
- The Translational Research Investigating Biomarker End-Points in Acute Kidney Injury (TRIBE-AKI) has begun to carry out multi-center validation studies of the following promising AKI biomarker candidates: urine IL-18, NGAL, KIM-1, L-FABP, and urine cystatin C

ground left to cover, but the prospects of uncovering the potential and performance of these novel biomarkers for both diagnosis and prognosis, from quantifying the impact of renal structural injury to predicting long-term mortality, can fuel research endeavors to refine and reform how clinicians approach AKI.

References

1. Nash K, Hafeez A, Hou S. Hospital-acquired renal insufficiency. Am J Kidney Dis. 2002; 39(5):930–6.
2. Colls PC. Notes on creatinine. J Physiol. 1896;20(2–3):107–11.
3. Gwinner W, et al. Acute tubular injury in protocol biopsies of renal grafts: prevalence, associated factors and effect on long-term function. Am J Transplant. 2008;8(8):1684–93.
4. Parikh CR, Devarajan P. New biomarkers of acute kidney injury. Crit Care Med. 2008;36(4):S159–65. doi:10.1097/CCM.0b013e318168c652.
5. Parikh CR, et al. Tubular proteinuria in acute kidney injury: a critical evaluation of current status and future promise. Ann Clin Biochem. 2010;47(4):301–12.
6. Siew ED, Ware LB, Ikizler TA. Biological markers of acute kidney injury. J Am Soc Nephrol. 2011;22(5):810–20.
7. Moran SM, Myers BD. Course of acute renal failure studied by a model of creatinine kinetics. Kidney Int. 1985;27(6):928–37.
8. Wu I, Parikh CR. Screening for kidney diseases: older measures versus novel biomarkers. Clin J Am Soc Nephrol. 2008;3(6):1895–901.
9. Carmichael P, Carmichael AR. Acute renal failure in the surgical setting. ANZ J Surg. 2003;73(3):144–53.
10. Altman RD. Overview of osteoarthritis. Am J Med. 1987;83(4, Supplement 2):65–9.
11. Supavekin S, et al. Differential gene expression following early renal ischemia/reperfusion. Kidney Int. 2003;63(5):1714–24.
12. Devarajan P, et al. Gene expression in early ischemic renal injury: clues towards pathogenesis, biomarker discovery, and novel therapeutics. Mol Genet Metab. 2003;80(4):365–76.
13. Devarajan P. Proteomics for biomarker discovery in acute kidney injury. Semin Nephrol. 2007;27(6):637–51.
14. Diamond JR, Yoburn DC. Nonoliguric acute renal failure associated with a low fractional excretion of sodium. Ann Intern Med. 1982;96(5):597–600.
15. Zarich S, Fang LT, Diamond JR. Fractional excretion of sodium: exceptions to its diagnostic value. Arch Intern Med. 1985;145(1):108–12.
16. Miller TR, et al. Urinary diagnostic indices in acute renal failure: a prospective study. Ann Intern Med. 1978;89(1):47–50.
17. Gracie JA, Robertson SE, McInnes IB. Interleukin-18. J Leukoc Biol. 2003;73(2):213–24.
18. Edelstein CL, et al. Proximal tubules from caspase-1-deficient mice are protected against hypoxia-induced membrane injury. Nephrol Dial Transplant. 2007;22(4):1052–61.
19. Ghayur T, et al. Caspase-1 processes IFN-[gamma]-inducing factor and regulates LPS-induced IFN-[gamma] production. Nature. 1997;386(6625):619–23.
20. Gu Y, et al. Activation of interferon-γ inducing factor mediated by Interleukin-1β converting enzyme. Science. 1997;275(5297):206–9.
21. Melnikov VY, Ecder T, Fantuzzi G, Siegmund B, Lucia MS, Dinarello CA, Schrier RW, Edelstein CL. Impaired IL-18 processing protects caspase-1-deficient mice from ischemic acute renal failure. J Clin Invest. 2001;107:1145–52.
22. Parikh CR, et al. Urinary interleukin-18 is a marker of human acute tubular necrosis. Am J Kidney Dis. 2004;43(3):405–14.

23. Parikh CR, et al. Urinary IL-18 is an early predictive biomarker of acute kidney injury after cardiac surgery. Kidney Int. 2006;70(1):199–203.
24. Kjeldsen L, et al. Isolation and primary structure of NGAL, a novel protein associated with human neutrophil gelatinase. J Biol Chem. 1993;268(14):10425–32.
25. Kuwabara T, et al. Urinary neutrophil gelatinase-associated lipocalin levels reflect damage to glomeruli, proximal tubules, and distal nephrons. Kidney Int. 2008;75(3):285–94.
26. Mishra J, et al. Identification of neutrophil gelatinase-associated lipocalin as a novel early urinary biomarker for ischemic renal injury. J Am Soc Nephrol. 2003;14(10):2534–43.
27. Hvidberg V, et al. The endocytic receptor megalin binds the iron transporting neutrophil-gelatinase-associated lipocalin with high affinity and mediates its cellular uptake. FEBS Lett. 2005;579(3):773–7.
28. Nickolas TL, et al. Sensitivity and specificity of a single emergency department measurement of urinary neutrophil gelatinase–associated lipocalin for diagnosing acute kidney injury. Ann Intern Med. 2008;148(11):810–9.
29. Mishra J, et al. Neutrophil gelatinase-associated lipocalin (NGAL) as a biomarker for acute renal injury after cardiac surgery. Lancet. 2005;365(9466):1231–8.
30. Ichimura T, et al. Kidney injury molecule-1 (KIM-1), a putative epithelial cell adhesion molecule containing a novel immunoglobulin domain, is up-regulated in renal cells after injury. J Biol Chem. 1998;273(7):4135–42.
31. Bailly V, et al. Shedding of kidney injury molecule-1, a putative adhesion protein involved in renal regeneration. J Biol Chem. 2002;277(42):39739–48.
32. Han WK, et al. Kidney injury molecule-1 (KIM-1): a novel biomarker for human renal proximal tubule injury. Kidney Int. 2002;62(1):237–44.
33. Han WK, et al. Urinary biomarkers in the early diagnosis of acute kidney injury. Kidney Int. 2007;73(7):863–9.
34. Corsico B, et al. The helical domain of intestinal fatty acid binding protein is critical for collisional transfer of fatty acids to phospholipid membranes. Proc Natl Acad Sci. 1998;95(21): 12174–8.
35. Yamamoto T, et al. Renal L-type fatty acid–binding protein in acute ischemic injury. J Am Soc Nephrol. 2007;18(11):2894–902.
36. Portilla D, et al. Liver fatty acid-binding protein as a biomarker of acute kidney injury after cardiac surgery. Kidney Int. 2007;73(4):465–72.
37. Grubb A. Cystatin C: properties and use as diagnostic marker. Adv Clin Chem. 2000;35: 63–99.
38. Kaseda R, et al. Megalin-mediated endocytosis of cystatin C in proximal tubule cells. Biochem Biophys Res Commun. 2007;357(4):1130–4.
39. Nejat M, et al. Urinary cystatin C is diagnostic of acute kidney injury and sepsis, and predicts mortality in the intensive care unit. Crit Care. 2010;14(3):1–13.
40. Herget-Rosenthal S, et al. Prognostic value of tubular proteinuria and enzymuria in nonoliguric acute tubular necrosis. Clin Chem. 2004;50(3):552–8.
41. Endre ZH, et al. Improved performance of urinary biomarkers of acute kidney injury in the critically ill by stratification for injury duration and baseline renal function. Kidney Int. 2011;79(10):1119–30.
42. Vanmassenhove J, et al. Urinary and serum biomarkers for the diagnosis of acute kidney injury: an in-depth review of the literature. Nephrol Dial Transplant. 2013;28(2):254–73.
43. Herget-Rosenthal S, et al. Cystatin C: efficacy as screening test for reduced glomerular filtration rate. Am J Nephrol. 2000;20(2):97–102.
44. Koyner JL, et al. Urinary cystatin C as an early biomarker of acute kidney injury following adult cardiothoracic surgery. Kidney Int. 2008;74(8):1059–69.
45. Krawczeski CD, et al. Serum cystatin C is an early predictive biomarker of acute kidney injury after pediatric cardiopulmonary bypass. Clin J Am Soc Nephrol. 2010;5(9):1552–7.
46. Benöhr P, et al. Cystatin C – a marker for assessment of the glomerular filtration rate in patients with cisplatin chemotherapy. Kidney Blood Press Res. 2006;29(1):32–5.

47. Zhu J, et al. Cystatin C as a reliable marker of renal function following heart valve replacement surgery with cardiopulmonary bypass. Clin Chim Acta. 2006;374(1–2):116–21.
48. Biancofiore G, et al. Cystatin C as a marker of renal function immediately after liver transplantation. Liver Transpl. 2006;12(2):285–91.
49. Abu-Omar Y, et al. Evaluation of cystatin C as a marker of renal injury following on-pump and off-pump coronary surgery. Eur J Cardiothorac Surg. 2005;27(5):893–8.
50. Parikh CR, et al. Postoperative biomarkers predict acute kidney injury and poor outcomes after adult cardiac surgery. J Am Soc Nephrol. 2011;22(9):1748–57.
51. Parikh CR, et al. Postoperative biomarkers predict acute kidney injury and poor outcomes after pediatric cardiac surgery. J Am Soc Nephrol. 2011;22(9):1737–47.
52. Parikh CR, et al. Performance of kidney injury molecule-1 and liver fatty acid-binding protein and combined biomarkers of AKI after cardiac surgery. Clin J Am Soc Nephrol. 2013;8(7):1079–88.
53. Coca SG, Garg AX, Thiessen-Philbrook H, Koyner JL, Patel JD, Krumholz HM, Shlipak MG, Parikh CR. Urinary biomarkers of acute kidney injury and mortality 3-years after cardiac surgery. J Am Soc of Nephrol. 2013;25(5):1063–71.

Chapter 4
Clinical Pearls: Renal Replacement Therapy for Acute Kidney Injury in the Postoperative Period

Ashita J. Tolwani and Paul M. Palevsky

Objectives

- To discuss the indications for and appropriate timing of renal replacement therapy (RRT) for acute kidney injury (AKI) in the postoperative period
- To compare and contrast the different types of RRT available for AKI
- To review the critical elements of the RRT prescription for AKI in the postoperative period: modality, dose, and anticoagulation

Introduction

No specific pharmacological therapy is effective in established acute kidney injury (AKI). Renal replacement therapy (RRT) is used as supportive management. At present, there is no consensus regarding when to initiate RRT, resulting in a wide variation in clinical practice. Clear indications include severe hyperkalemia, metabolic acidosis, volume overload, overt uremic manifestations, and intoxications.

A.J. Tolwani, MD, MSE
Department of Medicine, University of Alabama at Birmingham,
1720 2nd Avenue South, ZRB 604, Birmingham, AL 35294, USA
e-mail: atolwani@uab.edu

P.M. Palevsky, MD (✉)
Renal Section, VA Pittsburgh Healthcare System, Room 7E123 (111F-U),
University Drive, Pittsburgh, PA 15240, USA

Department of Medicine, University of Pittsburgh School of Medicine,
Pittsburgh, PA, USA
e-mail: palevsky@pitt.edu

C.V. Thakar, C.R. Parikh (eds.), *Perioperative Kidney Injury: Principles of Risk Assessment, Diagnosis and Treatment*, DOI 10.1007/978-1-4939-1273-5_4

Although observational studies suggest that "early" initiation of RRT in AKI is associated with improved patient survival, these studies have significant limitations and remain to be confirmed by adequately powered randomized trials [1, 2]. Nevertheless, clinicians often start RRT prior to the development of overt complications of AKI, taking into account the overall clinical state of the patient.

All modalities of RRT remove water and solutes by transport across a semipermeable membrane. Ultrafiltration is the removal of water across the membrane. In hemodialysis and hemofiltration, increased hydrostatic pressure on the blood side of the membrane drives plasma water across the membrane; in peritoneal dialysis, high dialysate osmolality provides the driving force. Solute removal during RRT can occur by diffusion and/or convection (Fig. 4.1). In diffusion, solute flux across the membrane is driven by the concentration gradient between blood and dialysate. This concentration gradient can be maximized and maintained throughout the length of the dialysis membrane by running the dialysate countercurrent to the blood flow. Diffusion is dependent on the molecular weight of the solute; membrane characteristics such as pore size, charge and water permeability; and circuit factors such as extracorporeal flow rates. Since diffusivity of a solute is inversely proportional to its molecular weight, dialysis is most efficient for the removal of low-molecular-weight solutes, such as urea, as compared to larger ("middle-molecular-weight") solutes, such as inulin, β2-microglobulin, vitamin B12, tumor necrosis factor, and other cytokines.

Convection is the bulk flow of solute that occurs during ultrafiltration. As plasma water crosses the semipermeable membrane, it "drags" with it both low-molecular-weight (urea, creatinine, potassium) and middle-molecular-weight solutes. Convective flux is not size dependent as long as the molecular diameter of the solute is smaller than the membrane pore diameter. With convection, solute clearance is generally proportional to the ultrafiltration rate. The available RRT modalities use ultrafiltration for fluid removal and either diffusion, convection, or a combination to achieve solute clearance. Options for RRT for AKI include intermittent hemodialysis (IHD), peritoneal dialysis (PD), various forms of continuous renal replacement therapy (CRRT), and "hybrid" therapies known as prolonged intermittent renal replacement therapy (PIRRT). The choice of renal replacement modality depends on patient hemodynamics, goals for solute clearance and volume control, need for anticoagulation, and local expertise (Table 4.1).

Intermittent Hemodialysis (IHD)

Traditionally, nephrologists have managed AKI with IHD, empirically delivered 3–6 times a week, 3–4 h per session, with a blood flow rate of 300–500 mL/min and a dialysate flow rate of 500–800 mL/min. Decisions regarding dialysis duration and frequency are based on the patient's catabolism and metabolic control, volume status, and presence of hemodynamic instability. Advantages of IHD include rapid solute and volume removal. Therefore, IHD may be the preferred treatment in

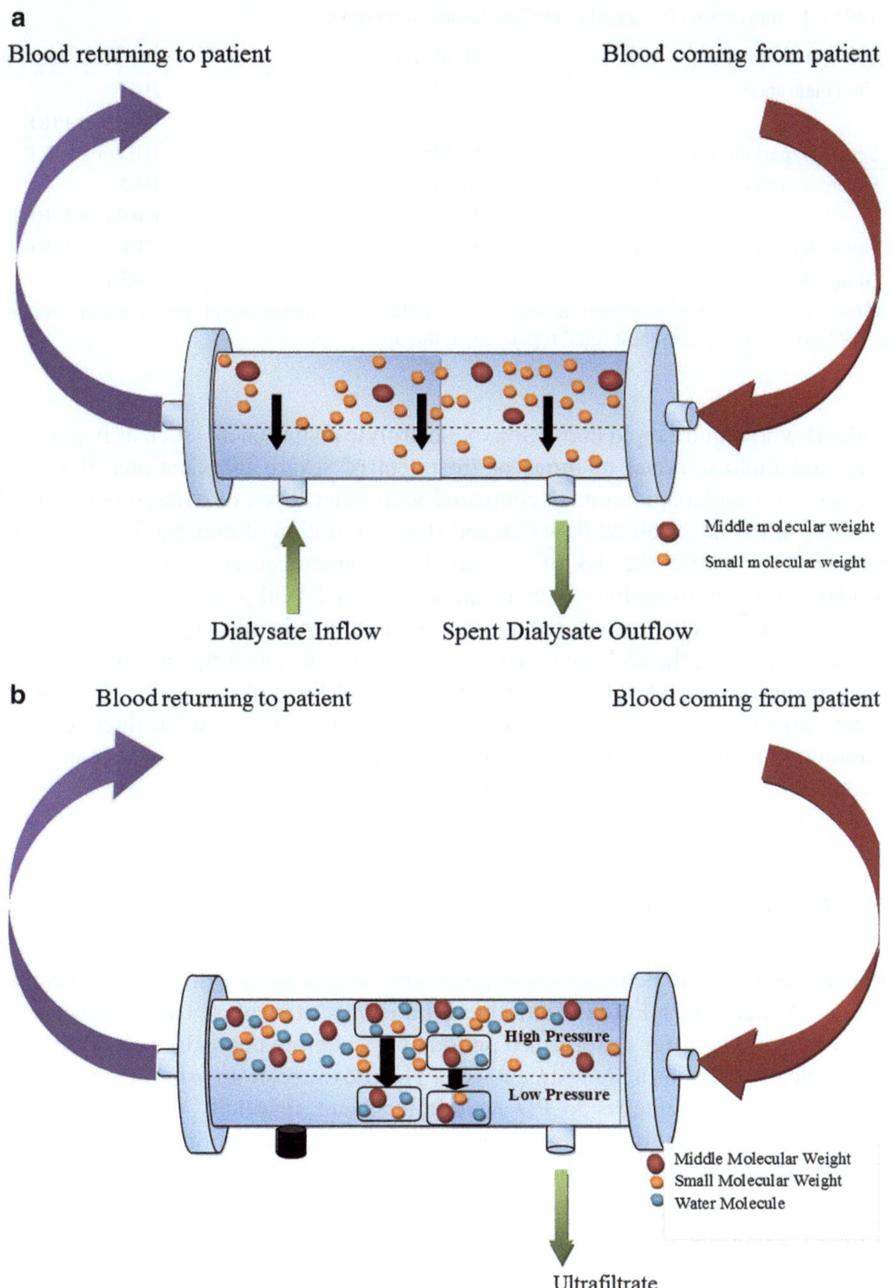

Fig. 4.1 (**a**) Diffusion. (**b**) Convection

Table 4.1 Indications for specific renal replacement therapies

Therapeutic goal	Hemodynamics	Preferred therapy
Urea clearance	Stable	IHD
	Unstable	CRRT or PIRRT
Severe hyperkalemia	Stable or unstable	IHD or PIRRT
Severe metabolic acidosis	Stable	IHD
	Unstable	CRRT or PIRRT
Severe hyperphosphatemia	Stable or unstable	CRRT or PIRRT
Brain edema	Stable or unstable	CRRT

Abbreviations: *IHD* intermittent hemodialysis, *CRRT* continuous renal replacement therapy, *PIRRT* prolonged intermittent renal replacement therapy

patients who require rapid correction of electrolyte disturbances, such as hyperkalemia, and rapid removal of drugs or treatment of severe intoxications. IHD also requires less anticoagulation as compared with other types of extracorporeal RRT because of the faster blood flow rate and shorter duration of therapy. The main disadvantage of IHD is the risk of systemic hypotension caused by rapid solute and fluid removal. Hypotension occurs in approximately 20–30 % of hemodialysis treatments [3, 4]. Mechanisms for improving hemodynamic stability include sodium modeling, cooling the dialysate, increasing the dialysate calcium concentration, and decreasing the rate of solute and volume removal by prolonging the duration or increasing the frequency of treatments or performing additional intermittent ultrafiltration treatments [5]. Despite this, approximately 10 % of AKI patients cannot be treated with IHD because of hemodynamic instability [3, 5–8].

Peritoneal Dialysis (PD)

PD utilizes the peritoneum as a semipermeable membrane for diffusive removal of solutes. A dialysate solution is introduced into the peritoneal cavity through a catheter where it dwells for a prescribed period of time before being drained. The dialysate typically contains a high percentage of glucose to create an osmotic gradient for fluid removal. Advantages to PD include technical simplicity, lack of need for systemic anticoagulation or vascular access, hemodynamic stability, and lower cost. Disadvantages include complications of PD catheter insertion, risk of peritonitis, limited solute clearance in hypercatabolic patients, lack of precise control of ultrafiltration, potential pulmonary restriction due to the expansion of the peritoneal cavity, risk of protein loss, and hyperglycemia [9, 10]. PD is contraindicated in postoperative patients with ileus, recent abdominal surgery, or abdominal drains. In addition, because fluid and solute removal during PD is less predictable, it is used less widely than other therapies in the acute setting. Acute PD may be useful in AKI patients with hemodynamic instability or difficult vascular access issues or who are located in regions with limited resources.

Continuous Renal Replacement Therapy (CRRT)

CRRT modalities use diffusion, convection, or a combination of both and are most commonly employed to manage hemodynamically unstable patients with AKI [11–13]. CRRT is performed in the intensive care unit (ICU) 24 h a day using a venovenous or, less commonly, an arteriovenous extracorporeal circuit. In arteriovenous circuits, blood flow is driven by the gradient between mean arterial and central venous pressure, while in continuous venovenous therapies, a blood pump maintains blood flow and generates hydrostatic pressure across the membrane. Despite their greater technical complexity, arteriovenous therapies have largely been supplanted by venovenous therapies because of the high rate of complications, including clotting, bleeding, and infection, associated with prolonged arterial cannulation.

CRRT is thought to allow for better hemodynamic tolerance than IHD by providing slower solute and fluid removal per unit of time. The gradual continuous volume removal facilitates the administration of medications and nutrition and provides easier control of volume status. Continuous slow solute removal allows for less fluctuation of solute concentrations over time and better control of azotemia, electrolytes, and acid-base status. The main disadvantages of CRRT include access and circuit clotting and the consequent need for anticoagulation. Another disadvantage of CRRT is increased cost and demands on ICU nursing time compared with IHD. Performing CRRT requires the appropriate infrastructure and trained personnel in a multidisciplinary team.

The different CRRT modalities for solute removal include continuous venovenous hemofiltration (CVVH), continuous venovenous hemodialysis (CVVHD), and continuous venovenous hemodiafiltration (CVVHDF) (Table 4.2, Fig. 4.2) [11–13]. In CVVH, solute clearance occurs by convection and is augmented by increasing the volume of ultrafiltrate produced. No dialysate is used. A physiologic crystalloid "replacement fluid" is infused in the blood to replace the excess volume and electrolytes removed by ultrafiltration. In CVVHD, solute removal occurs primarily by diffusion. Unlike IHD, the dialysate flow rate is slower than the blood flow rate, allowing small solutes to equilibrate completely between the blood and dialysate.

Table 4.2 CRRT solute clearance modalities

	Solute transport mechanism			Typical rates used in clinical practice		
	Convection	Diffusion	Replacement fluid	Blood flow rate (mL/min)	Ultrafiltration rate (mL/h)	Dialysate rate (mL/h)
CVVH	++++	–	++++	100–300	500–4,000	0
CVVHD	+	++++	–	100–300	0–350	500–4,000
CVVHDF	+++	+++	++	100–300	500–4,000	500–4,000

CRRT continuous renal replacement therapy, *CVVH* continuous venovenous hemofiltration, *CVVHD* continuous venovenous hemodialysis, *CVVHDF* continuous venovenous hemodiafiltration

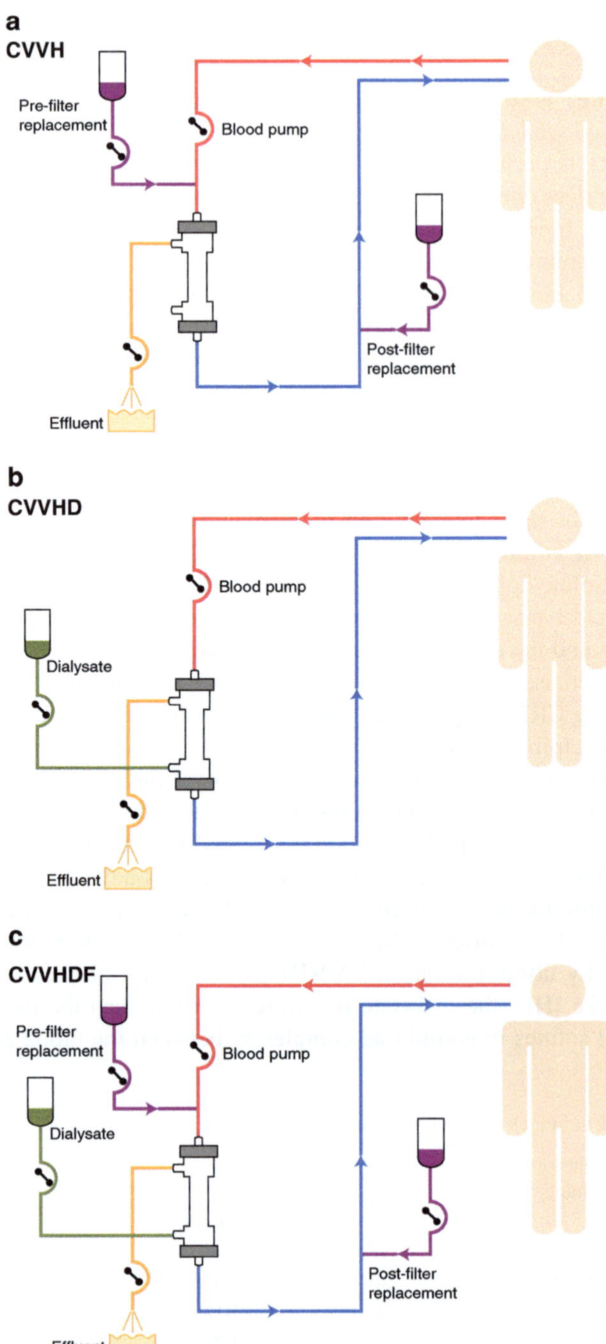

Fig. 4.2 CRRT circuit modality components. (**a**) CVVH uses pre- and/or post-fluid replacement. (**b**) CVVHD uses dialysate. (**c**) CVVHDF uses pre- and/or post-fluid replacement + dialysate

Ultrafiltration is used only for volume control and at rates much lower than required for convective clearance of solutes. CVVHDF combines the convective solute removal of CVVH and the diffusive solute removal of CVVHD. As in CVVH, the high ultrafiltration rates needed for convective clearance require the administration of intravenous replacement fluids.

Many clinicians use a mode of CRRT with at least some hemofiltration (i.e., either CVVH or CVVHDF) in the belief that hemofiltration removes cytokines and thus reduces the effects of the systemic inflammatory response. Although cytokines can be removed by CVVH, most controlled studies have failed to demonstrate a significant and sustained decrease in cytokine plasma concentrations or an improvement in outcome [14–19]. In a recent meta-analysis comparing the outcomes of hemofiltration to hemodialysis in the management of AKI, there was no difference in survival, organ dysfunction, vasopressor use, or renal recovery despite increased clearance of larger molecules with hemofiltration [20]. Presently, there are insufficient data to recommend one type of CRRT modality over another, and the choice of CRRT should be guided by available resources, cost, and expertise of the user.

Prescription orders for initiating CRRT must include mode of therapy, blood flow rate, replacement fluid composition and infusion rate (for CVVH and CVVHDF), dialysate composition and flow rate (for CVVHD and CVVHDF), type and dose of anticoagulation (if used), and net fluid management based on the patient's fluid status. Electrolyte abnormalities can occur due to anticoagulant (i.e., citrate) management or due to excessive losses of electrolytes, such as potassium and phosphorous, from the therapy itself. As a result, specific protocols are needed for frequent monitoring and replacement of electrolytes.

Prolonged Intermittent Renal Replacement Therapy (PIRRT)

PIRRTs, also known as sustained low-efficiency dialysis (SLED) and extended daily dialysis (EDD), are slower dialytic modalities run for prolonged periods using conventional hemodialysis machines with lower blood-pump speeds (e.g., 200 mL/min) and dialysate flow rates (e.g., 100–300 mL/min) for 8–16 h daily. PIRRTs combine the advantages of both CRRT and IHD; they allow for the improved hemodynamic stability that gradual solute and volume removal provide in CRRT while utilizing the less expensive technology for online dialysate generation of conventional IHD. Because they can be performed intermittently based on the needs of the patient, they allow the scheduling of required diagnostic and therapeutic procedures without interruption of therapy. Studies have demonstrated PIRRTs provide hemodynamic control comparable to CRRT [21–24].

Selection of RRT Modality

Evidence for improved outcomes with specific RRT modalities is lacking. Randomized controlled trials (RCTs) have failed to demonstrate any survival advantage for continuous versus intermittent therapies. Several meta-analyses have concluded there were no differences in mortality endpoints in critically ill patients with AKI treated with CRRT and IHD [25–29]. Although observational studies have suggested that surviving patients treated with CRRT are more likely to recover kidney function, a similar benefit has not been observed in randomized trials [30]. CRRT is associated with less need for escalation of vasopressors [25] and with greater net negative fluid balance [31].

Data comparing other modalities of RRT in AKI are sparse. RCTs comparing IHD with PIRRT have not been performed. Clinical experience is more limited with PIRRT as compared to CRRT, and very few RCTs have compared PIRRT to CRRT [23, 32, 33]. Two RCTs have compared PD to other RRT modalities in AKI. In a study from an infectious disease hospital in Vietnam, where the predominant etiology of AKI was malaria, CVVH was associated with better survival than PD, although the applicability of this study in other settings is uncertain [10]. In contrast, there was no difference in survival or renal recovery in an RCT comparing high-volume PD to daily IHD [34]. In the absence of definitive data in support of a particular modality, the modalities of RRT should be viewed as complementary, with the choice of RRT modality in the individual patient influenced by availability, expertise, resources, cost, and physician preference. Transitions between RRT modalities are common and based on the changing clinical status of the patient or technical aspects of the therapy, such as clotting of the circuit.

In patients with acute brain injury or increased intracranial pressure, CRRT is generally preferred over IHD. IHD may worsen neurological status by compromising cerebral perfusion pressure as a result of dialysis-associated hypotension or by increasing cerebral edema and intracranial pressure from rapid intracellular fluid and solute shifts [35–37]. As the rate of volume and solute removal is slower with CRRT, it tends to be better tolerated by patients with brain injury or increased intracranial pressure who are at risk for acute herniation [36, 38].

Anticoagulation

All forms of RRT other than PD may require anticoagulation. Although CRRT without anticoagulation is feasible in patients with coagulopathy, most patients require some form of anticoagulation. Studies have shown that frequent clotting affects treatment efficacy and increases circuit "downtime" which reduces treatment efficacy and increases transfusion requirements and cost [39].

The most commonly used anticoagulant for all modes of extracorporeal RRT, including CRRT, is unfractionated heparin. Unfractionated heparin (UFH) is inexpensive, widely available, easy to administer and monitor, and reversible with protamine. Disadvantages include its unpredictable and complex pharmacokinetics, risk of heparin-induced thrombocytopenia (HIT), heparin resistance due to low patient antithrombin levels, and increased risk of hemorrhage [40]. The incidence of bleeding episodes ranges from 10 % to 50 %, with mortality due to bleeding as high as 15 % [41–43].

In the postoperative setting with a patient at increased risk of bleeding, regional anticoagulation with citrate has been gaining wide acceptance as an anticoagulant for CRRT [44–46]. Citrate is infused into the blood at the beginning of the extracorporeal circuit and chelates ionized calcium necessary for the coagulation cascade [47]. Optimal regional anticoagulation occurs when the ionized calcium concentration in the extracorporeal circuit is <0.35 mmol/L [47, 48]. Part of the calcium-citrate complex is lost across the hemofilter, while the rest of the complex enters the systemic circulation where calcium is released when citrate is metabolized. Calcium is infused back to the patient to replace the calcium lost in the effluent. Citrate is metabolized mainly by the liver to bicarbonate; one citrate molecule can potentially yield three bicarbonate molecules. Advantages of regional citrate anticoagulation (RCA) include the avoidance of systemic anticoagulation and HIT.

A variety of methods of regional citrate anticoagulation are described in the literature [44, 49–59]. However, since citrate is not approved by the FDA as an anticoagulant for CRRT, the commercially available hypertonic citrate solutions must be used with caution as they can result in significant acid-base and electrolyte disturbances, including hypernatremia, hypocalcemia, and metabolic alkalosis. Furthermore, patients with severe liver failure and lactic acidosis may have difficulty metabolizing citrate and can develop citrate accumulation and toxicity, which is characterized by low systemic ionized calcium levels, elevated total serum calcium, metabolic acidosis, and an increased anion gap [60–63]. If properly monitored, complications associated with RCA are uncommon.

Two meta-analyses have concluded that RCA decreased the risk of bleeding as compared to heparin anticoagulation with no significant increase in the incidence of metabolic alkalosis, and one reported improved circuit patency in the citrate groups [64, 65]. Both meta-analyses recommended RCA in patients who require CRRT but are at high risk of bleeding, as long as appropriate protocols and monitoring mechanisms are in place.

Dose of Renal Replacement Therapy

There is no consensus for how dose of RRT should be defined in AKI. Methods used in the chronic dialysis setting such as Kt/V_{urea}—where K is urea clearance, t is treatment time, and V is the volume of distribution of urea—are difficult to apply in the acute setting where V is uncertain and changing. Furthermore, urea clearance may not be the appropriate surrogate for clearance of other molecules that are more important in the toxicity of renal failure. Nevertheless, a suitable alternative for estimating intensity of IHD does not exist. In studies in patients with AKI, the dose (or intensity) of treatment has been assessed by urea clearance in dialysis-based modalities and by effluent volume (a surrogate of urea clearance) in CRRT. The urea clearance achieved during CRRT is approximately equal to the effluent flow rate (the sum of dialysate flow and ultrafiltration rate), expressed as mL/kg/h.

Several small, single center trials suggested that higher doses of IHD and CRRT were associated with improved outcomes [66–68]. However, two large, multicenter RCTs, the Veterans Affairs/National Institutes of Health Acute Renal Failure Trial Network (ATN) Study [69] and the Randomized Evaluation of Normal Versus Augmented Level Renal Replacement Therapy (RENAL) trial [70], did not confirm these findings. In the RENAL trial, patients were randomized to CVVHDF at 25 or 40 mL/kg/h; in the Acute Renal Failure Trial Network Study, patients transitioned between modalities as their hemodynamic status varied, receiving IHD with a target Kt/V_{urea} per treatment of 1.2–1.4 either 3 or 6 times per week when hemodynamically stable and CVVHDF at 20 or 35 mL/kg/h when hemodynamically unstable. In neither study was the more intensive therapy associated with improved survival or recovery of kidney function. However, both trials delivered a higher dose of therapy in the "low-intensity" arms than what is often delivered in clinical practice. For example, 88 % and 95 % of the prescribed dose of CVVHDF was actually delivered in the RENAL trial and Acute Renal Failure Trial Network Study, respectively, and in the Acute Renal Failure Trial Network Study, the mean delivered Kt/V_{urea} was 1.3. Based on these results, the Kidney Disease: Improving Global Outcomes (KDIGO) Clinical Practice Guidelines for Acute Kidney Injury recommend that during CRRT a minimum effluent flow of at least 20–25 mL/kg/h should be provided. Careful attention must be paid to ensuring that the target dose of therapy is actually delivered, addressing technical problems such as poor blood flows, reduced efficiency of the hemofilter over time, or actual filter clotting, which lead to a reduction in delivered dose. Intermittent hemodialysis should be prescribed to deliver a Kt/V_{urea} of at least 1.2–1.4 on a three-time-per-week schedule with more frequent treatments provided if this target dose cannot be achieved. More frequent IHD treatments may also be required to optimize volume management. In both IHD and CRRT, higher doses of therapy may be needed in hypercatabolic patients or for control of severe hyperkalemia or acidemia. Comparable data are not available to guide the dosing of PD or PIRRT.

Key Messages

- *Indications for renal replacement therapy (RRT)*: There is ongoing debate regarding the ideal timing of initiation of RRT in the critically ill patient. RRT should be initiated in life-threatening conditions such as refractory hyperkalemia, acidosis, fluid overload, and uremic symptoms, including refractory uremic bleeding or pericarditis. Initiation should be considered before uremic symptoms develop and take into account the degree of other organ failure and likelihood of rapid renal recovery.
- *Modality choice*: Options for RRT for AKI include intermittent hemodialysis (IHD), peritoneal dialysis (PD), continuous renal replacement therapy (CRRT), and "hybrid" therapies known as prolonged intermittent renal replacement therapy (PIRRT). The choice of modality should be guided by the patient's clinical needs and status, modality availability, and nursing and physician expertise. In general, hemodynamically stable patients are treated with IHD, while hemodynamically unstable patients are treated with CRRT or PIRRT. CRRT should also be considered for patients with brain edema and large fluid removal requirements.
- *Anticoagulation*: In the postoperative setting with a patient at increased risk of bleeding, alternative strategies can be applied, such as regular saline flushes or regional anticoagulation for CRRT.
- *Dose*: The best evidence suggests that patients with dialysis-dependent AKI should receive the equivalent of at least three hemodialysis treatments per week with a delivered Kt/V value of 1.2 or CRRT with an effluent flow of 20–25 mL/kg/h.

References

1. Karvellas CJ, Farhat MR, Sajjad I, et al. A comparison of early versus late initiation of renal replacement therapy in critically ill patients with acute kidney injury: a systematic review and meta-analysis. Crit Care. 2011;15:R72.
2. Seabra VF, Balk EM, Liangos O, Sosa MA, Cendoroglo M, Jaber BL. Timing of renal replacement therapy initiation in acute renal failure: a meta-analysis. Am J Kidney Dis. 2008;52: 272–84.
3. Selby NM, McIntyre CW. A systematic review of the clinical effects of reducing dialysate fluid temperature. Nephrol Dial Transplant. 2006;21:1883–98.
4. Palevsky PM, O'Connor TZ, Chertow GM, Crowley ST, Zhang JH, Kellum JA. Intensity of renal replacement therapy in acute kidney injury: perspective from within the Acute Renal Failure Trial Network Study. Crit Care. 2009;13:310.
5. Emili S, Black NA, Paul RV, Rexing CJ, Ullian ME. A protocol-based treatment for intradialytic hypotension in hospitalized hemodialysis patients. Am J Kidney Dis. 1999;33:1107–14.

6. Conger J. Dialysis and related therapies. Semin Nephrol. 1998;18:533–40.
7. Briglia A, Paganini EP. Acute renal failure in the intensive care unit. Therapy overview, patient risk stratification, complications of renal replacement, and special circumstances. Clin Chest Med. 1999;20:347–66. viii.
8. Paganini EP, Sandy D, Moreno L, Kozlowski L, Sakai K. The effect of sodium and ultrafiltration modelling on plasma volume changes and haemodynamic stability in intensive care patients receiving haemodialysis for acute renal failure: a prospective, stratified, randomized, cross-over study. Nephrol Dial Transplant. 1996;11 Suppl 8:32–7.
9. Steiner RW. Continuous equilibration peritoneal dialysis in acute renal failure. Perit Dial Int. 1989;9:5–7.
10. Phu NH, Hien TT, Mai NT, et al. Hemofiltration and peritoneal dialysis in infection-associated acute renal failure in Vietnam. N Engl J Med. 2002;347:895–902.
11. Cerda J, Ronco C. Modalities of continuous renal replacement therapy: technical and clinical considerations. Semin Dial. 2009;22:114–22.
12. Ronco C, Bellomo R. Basic mechanisms and definitions for continuous renal replacement therapies. Int J Artif Organs. 1996;19:95–9.
13. Ronco C, Ricci Z. Renal replacement therapies: physiological review. Intensive Care Med. 2008;34:2139–46.
14. De Vriese AS, Colardyn FA, Philippe JJ, Vanholder RC, De Sutter JH, Lameire NH. Cytokine removal during continuous hemofiltration in septic patients. J Am Soc Nephrol. 1999;10: 846–53.
15. Farese S, Jakob SM, Kalicki R, Frey FJ, Uehlinger DE. Treatment of acute renal failure in the intensive care unit: lower costs by intermittent dialysis than continuous venovenous hemodiafiltration. Artif Organs. 2009;33:634–40.
16. Heering P, Morgera S, Schmitz FJ, et al. Cytokine removal and cardiovascular hemodynamics in septic patients with continuous venovenous hemofiltration. Intensive Care Med. 1997;23: 288–96.
17. Hoffmann JN, Hartl WH, Deppisch R, Faist E, Jochum M, Inthorn D. Effect of hemofiltration on hemodynamics and systemic concentrations of anaphylatoxins and cytokines in human sepsis. Intensive Care Med. 1996;22:1360–7.
18. Morgera S, Slowinski T, Melzer C, et al. Renal replacement therapy with high-cutoff hemofilters: impact of convection and diffusion on cytokine clearances and protein status. Am J Kidney Dis. 2004;43:444–53.
19. van Deuren M, van der Meer JW. Hemofiltration in septic patients is not able to alter the plasma concentration of cytokines therapeutically. Intensive Care Med. 2000;26:1176–8.
20. Friedrich JO, Wald R, Bagshaw SM, Burns KE, Adhikari NK. Hemofiltration compared to hemodialysis for acute kidney injury: systematic review and meta-analysis. Crit Care. 2012;16:R146.
21. Fieghen HE, Friedrich JO, Burns KE, et al. The hemodynamic tolerability and feasibility of sustained low efficiency dialysis in the management of critically ill patients with acute kidney injury. BMC Nephrol. 2010;11:32.
22. Kumar VA, Yeun JY, Depner TA, Don BR. Extended daily dialysis vs. continuous hemodialysis for ICU patients with acute renal failure: a two-year single center report. Int J Artif Organs. 2004;27:371–9.
23. Kielstein JT, Kretschmer U, Ernst T, et al. Efficacy and cardiovascular tolerability of extended dialysis in critically ill patients: a randomized controlled study. Am J Kidney Dis. 2004;43: 342–9.
24. Wu VC, Wang CH, Wang WJ, et al. Sustained low-efficiency dialysis versus continuous venovenous hemofiltration for postsurgical acute renal failure. Am J Surg. 2010;199:466–76.
25. Rabindranath K, Adams J, Macleod AM, Muirhead N. Intermittent versus continuous renal replacement therapy for acute renal failure in adults. Cochrane Database Syst Rev. 2007;(18): CD003773.

26. Bagshaw SM, Berthiaume LR, Delaney A, Bellomo R. Continuous versus intermittent renal replacement therapy for critically ill patients with acute kidney injury: a meta-analysis. Crit Care Med. 2008;36:610–7.
27. Pannu N, Klarenbach S, Wiebe N, Manns B, Tonelli M. Renal replacement therapy in patients with acute renal failure: a systematic review. JAMA. 2008;299:793–805.
28. Tonelli M, Manns B, Feller-Kopman D. Acute renal failure in the intensive care unit: a systematic review of the impact of dialytic modality on mortality and renal recovery. Am J Kidney Dis. 2002;40:875–85.
29. Kellum JA, Angus DC, Johnson JP, et al. Continuous versus intermittent renal replacement therapy: a meta-analysis. Intensive Care Med. 2002;28:29–37.
30. Schneider AG, Bellomo R, Bagshaw SM, et al. Choice of renal replacement therapy modality and dialysis dependence after acute kidney injury: a systematic review and meta-analysis. Intensive Care Med. 2013;39:987–97.
31. Bouchard J, Soroko SB, Chertow GM, et al. Fluid accumulation, survival and recovery of kidney function in critically ill patients with acute kidney injury. Kidney Int. 2009;76:422–7.
32. Baldwin I, Bellomo R, Naka T, Koch B, Fealy N. A pilot randomized controlled comparison of extended daily dialysis with filtration and continuous veno-venous hemofiltration: fluid removal and hemodynamics. Int J Artif Organs. 2007;30:1083–9.
33. Baldwin I, Naka T, Koch B, Fealy N, Bellomo R. A pilot randomised controlled comparison of continuous veno-venous haemofiltration and extended daily dialysis with filtration: effect on small solutes and acid-base balance. Intensive Care Med. 2007;33:830–5.
34. Gabriel DP, Caramori JT, Martim LC, Barretti P, Balbi AL. High volume peritoneal dialysis vs daily hemodialysis: a randomized, controlled trial in patients with acute kidney injury. Kidney Int Suppl. 2008;73:S87–93.
35. Davenport A. Renal replacement therapy in the patient with acute brain injury. Am J Kidney Dis. 2001;37:457–66.
36. Davenport A. Continuous renal replacement therapies in patients with acute neurological injury. Semin Dial. 2009;22:165–8.
37. Lin CM, Lin JW, Tsai JT, et al. Intracranial pressure fluctuation during hemodialysis in renal failure patients with intracranial hemorrhage. Acta Neurochir Suppl. 2008;101:141–4.
38. Davenport A. Continuous renal replacement therapies in patients with liver disease. Semin Dial. 2009;22:169–72.
39. Venkataraman R, Kellum JA, Palevsky P. Dosing patterns for continuous renal replacement therapy at a large academic medical center in the United States. J Crit Care. 2002;17:246–50.
40. Hirsh J, Warkentin TE, Shaughnessy SG, et al. Heparin and low-molecular-weight heparin: mechanisms of action, pharmacokinetics, dosing, monitoring, efficacy, and safety. Chest. 2001;119:64S–94.
41. Davenport A, Will EJ, Davison AM. Comparison of the use of standard heparin and prostacyclin anticoagulation in spontaneous and pump-driven extracorporeal circuits in patients with combined acute renal and hepatic failure. Nephron. 1994;66:431–7.
42. Martin PY, Chevrolet JC, Suter P, Favre H. Anticoagulation in patients treated by continuous venovenous hemofiltration: a retrospective study. Am J Kidney Dis. 1994;24:806–12.
43. van de Wetering J, Westendorp RG, van der Hoeven JG, Stolk B, Feuth JD, Chang PC. Heparin use in continuous renal replacement procedures: the struggle between filter coagulation and patient hemorrhage. J Am Soc Nephrol. 1996;7:145–50.
44. Tolwani AJ, Prendergast MB, Speer RR, Stofan BS, Wille KM. A practical citrate anticoagulation continuous venovenous hemodiafiltration protocol for metabolic control and high solute clearance. Clin J Am Soc Nephrol. 2006;1:79–87.
45. Morgera S. Regional anticoagulation with citrate: expanding its indications. Crit Care Med. 2011;39:399–400.
46. Oudemans-van Straaten HM, Kellum JA, Bellomo R. Clinical review: anticoagulation for continuous renal replacement therapy–heparin or citrate? Crit Care. 2011;15:202.

47. Calatzis A, Toepfer M, Schramm W, Spannagl M, Schiffl H. Citrate anticoagulation for extracorporeal circuits: effects on whole blood coagulation activation and clot formation. Nephron. 2001;89:233–6.
48. Pinnick RV, Wiegmann TB, Diederich DA. Regional citrate anticoagulation for hemodialysis in the patient at high risk for bleeding. N Engl J Med. 1983;308:258–61.
49. Bagshaw SM, Laupland KB, Boiteau PJ, Godinez-Luna T. Is regional citrate superior to systemic heparin anticoagulation for continuous renal replacement therapy? A prospective observational study in an adult regional critical care system. J Crit Care. 2005;20:155–61.
50. Hofmann RM, Maloney C, Ward DM, Becker BN. A novel method for regional citrate anticoagulation in continuous venovenous hemofiltration (CVVHF). Ren Fail. 2002;24:325–35.
51. Cointault O, Kamar N, Bories P, et al. Regional citrate anticoagulation in continuous venovenous haemodiafiltration using commercial solutions. Nephrol Dial Transplant. 2004;19: 171–8.
52. Bihorac A, Ross EA. Continuous venovenous hemofiltration with citrate-based replacement fluid: efficacy, safety, and impact on nutrition. Am J Kidney Dis. 2005;46:908–18.
53. Kutsogiannis DJ, Mayers I, Chin WD, Gibney RT. Regional citrate anticoagulation in continuous venovenous hemodiafiltration. Am J Kidney Dis. 2000;35:802–11.
54. Mehta RL, McDonald BR, Aguilar MM, Ward DM. Regional citrate anticoagulation for continuous arteriovenous hemodialysis in critically ill patients. Kidney Int. 1990;38:976–81.
55. Monchi M, Berghmans D, Ledoux D, Canivet JL, Dubois B, Damas P. Citrate vs. heparin for anticoagulation in continuous venovenous hemofiltration: a prospective randomized study. Intensive Care Med. 2004;30:260–5.
56. Palsson R, Niles JL. Regional citrate anticoagulation in continuous venovenous hemofiltration in critically ill patients with a high risk of bleeding. Kidney Int. 1999;55:1991–7.
57. Swartz R, Pasko D, O'Toole J, Starmann B. Improving the delivery of continuous renal replacement therapy using regional citrate anticoagulation. Clin Nephrol. 2004;61:134–43.
58. Tobe SW, Aujla P, Walele AA, et al. A novel regional citrate anticoagulation protocol for CRRT using only commercially available solutions. J Crit Care. 2003;18:121–9.
59. Tolwani AJ, Campbell RC, Schenk MB, Allon M, Warnock DG. Simplified citrate anticoagulation for continuous renal replacement therapy. Kidney Int. 2001;60:370–4.
60. Apsner R, Schwarzenhofer M, Derfler K, Zauner C, Ratheiser K, Kranz A. Impairment of citrate metabolism in acute hepatic failure. Wien Klin Wochenschr. 1997;109:123–7.
61. Kramer L, Bauer E, Joukhadar C, et al. Citrate pharmacokinetics and metabolism in cirrhotic and noncirrhotic critically ill patients. Crit Care Med. 2003;31:2450–5.
62. Meier-Kriesche HU, Gitomer J, Finkel K, DuBose T. Increased total to ionized calcium ratio during continuous venovenous hemodialysis with regional citrate anticoagulation. Crit Care Med. 2001;29:748–52.
63. Bakker AJ, Boerma EC, Keidel H, Kingma P, van der Voort PH. Detection of citrate overdose in critically ill patients on citrate-anticoagulated venovenous haemofiltration: use of ionised and total/ionised calcium. Clin Chem Lab Med. 2006;44:962–6.
64. Wu MY, Hsu YH, Bai CH, Lin YF, Wu CH, Tam KW. Regional citrate versus heparin anticoagulation for continuous renal replacement therapy: a meta-analysis of randomized controlled trials. Am J Kidney Dis. 2012;59:810–8.
65. Zhang Z, Hongying N. Efficacy and safety of regional citrate anticoagulation in critically ill patients undergoing continuous renal replacement therapy. Intensive Care Med. 2012;38: 20–8.
66. Ronco C, Bellomo R, Homel P, et al. Effects of different doses in continuous veno-venous haemofiltration on outcomes of acute renal failure: a prospective randomised trial. Lancet. 2000;356:26–30.
67. Schiffl H, Lang SM, Fischer R. Daily hemodialysis and the outcome of acute renal failure. N Engl J Med. 2002;346:305–10.

68. Saudan P, Niederberger M, De Seigneux S, et al. Adding a dialysis dose to continuous hemofiltration increases survival in patients with acute renal failure. Kidney Int. 2006;70:1312–7.
69. Palevsky PM, Zhang JH, O'Connor TZ, et al. Intensity of renal support in critically ill patients with acute kidney injury. N Engl J Med. 2008;359:7–20.
70. Bellomo R, Cass A, Cole L, et al. Intensity of continuous renal-replacement therapy in critically ill patients. N Engl J Med. 2009;361:1627–38.

Chapter 5
Clinical Pearls: Non-dialytic Management of Kidney Complications in the Postoperative Period

Michael J. Connor Jr. and Anju Oommen

Objectives

- To discuss the assessment and maintenance of renal perfusion
- To explain the role of volume expansion in supporting organ and renal function
- To understand the risks of hypervolemia
- To understand the principles of the management of electrolyte and acid/base derangements in patients with AKI

Introduction

Renal complications including derangements in acid/base homeostasis and electrolyte concentrations, volume overload, and acute kidney injury (AKI) are quite common in the postoperative period with AKI incidence of 45–50 % in some populations. These diagnoses are associated with higher morbidity and mortality during the postoperative period and often have a complex and multifactorial etiology. The management of these complications requires a clear understanding of potential contributing factors leading to metabolic derangements, volume overload, and/or AKI. Additionally, it is necessary to have a clear understanding of the limitations of extracorporeal

M.J. Connor Jr., MD (✉)
Division of Pulmonary, Allergy, and Critical Care Medicine, Department of Medicine, Emory University, 550 Peachtree Street, NE, Davis-Fischer Bldg – Room 3243-E, Atlanta, GA 30308, USA
e-mail: michael.connor@emory.edu

A. Oommen, MD
Division of Nephrology, Department of Medicine, Emory University, 1639 Pierce Drive, WMB Suite 3300, Atlanta, GA 30322, USA
e-mail: anju.oommen@emory.edu

C.V. Thakar, C.R. Parikh (eds.), *Perioperative Kidney Injury: Principles of Risk Assessment, Diagnosis and Treatment*, DOI 10.1007/978-1-4939-1273-5_5

(dialysis-based) therapies in the care of the intensive care unit (ICU) patient in the postoperative period.

This chapter will focus on the non-dialytic management of kidney complications with attention to three main areas: (1) determining and maintaining adequate renal perfusion, (2) fluid management with respect to the type of solutions and optimal replacement strategy, and (3) management of acid/base and electrolyte derangements in patients with AKI.

Maintaining Renal Perfusion

Maintaining appropriate renal perfusion is essential to the non-dialytic management of AKI and its associated complications, including efforts to prevent and ameliorate AKI. Depending on the type and complexity of any given surgery, the immediate postoperative course is often notable for a period of hemodynamic instability and impairment in tissue perfusion. Postoperative shock may develop and persist beyond the initial few hours, and maintaining appropriate oxygen delivery and end-organ perfusion is of paramount importance.

Assessment of Renal and Organ Perfusion

Assessment of the adequacy of tissue perfusion and strategies to improve perfusion remains a vexing issue in critical care medicine, especially as it pertains to renal protection and non-dialytic management of AKI. Traditionally, cardiac output via pulmonary artery catheter, central venous pressure (CVP), pulmonary artery occlusion pressure ("wedge pressure"), mean arterial pressure (MAP), physical exam, and acid/base status (base deficit and pH) have been used as surrogate markers of perfusion. However, studies consistently demonstrate that these measurements are of limited utility primarily because they do not address the functional, local effects of perfusion. Absolute lactic acid level and central venous oxygen saturation have been used effectively as functional markers of tissue perfusion during acute resuscitation [1].

More recently, a variety of advanced hemodynamic metrics have been developed, which may be superior functional assessments, thereby improving bedside appraisal of the adequacy of hemodynamic resuscitation. These include: lactate clearance [2], stroke volume variation (SVV) [3], abdominal perfusion pressure (APP) [4], esophageal Doppler or continuous transesophageal echocardiography, and the ratio between the venoarterial carbon dioxide tension gradient and arteriovenous O_2 content gradient [5].

Table 5.1 shows hemodynamic assessment methods and accepted treatment targets. Central venous catheters continue to be nearly ubiquitous in the management of hemodynamically unstable patients. These of pulmonary artery catheters has declined sharply in the last 10 years as it is increasingly recognized that the data they provide are both not essential for management [6] and difficult to interpret in

Table 5.1 Methods of hemodynamic monitoring

Hemodynamic parameter	Accepted Goal Targets
Cardiac output/cardiac index	4–6 l/min OR 2.5–3.0 l/min/m^2
CVP	8–12 cm of H_2O (non-vent) and 10–16 cm of H_2O (ventilated)
SVV	≤15 %
APP	≥60 mmHg
Lactate clearance	>10 % reduction (over 6–12 h)

Abbreviation: *OR* odds ratio

the absence of other variables (ScvO2, serial lactic acid levels, SVV, etc.). Stroke volume variation and noninvasive means of measuring cardiac output yield accurate and dynamic information to guide therapy.

Finally, intra-abdominal hypertension (IAH) and abdominal compartment syndrome (ACS) are increasingly recognized as common complications of modern ICU care. IAH affects 50–60 % and ACS is noted in ~10–20 % of all ICU patients independent of reason for ICU admission [7]. IAH and ACS both compromise abdominal perfusion pressure (APP) especially in the setting of hypotension/shock. A more detailed account of IAH and ACC is discussed in chapter.

Volume Management and Resuscitation

Quantity and Timing of Volume Resuscitation

As discussed above, maintaining appropriate end-organ perfusion in a shock state is essential to optimizing outcomes for the critically ill patient. It is well known that volume expansion plays a key role in the initial resuscitative phase of many patients with shock. Rivers et al. demonstrated that an early goal-directed protocol for the acute resuscitation of patients admitted with community-acquired septic shock improves survival [1]. This trial focused on the early aggressive volume expansion of a patient population known to be volume depleted. The outcome of this study lent credibility to the long-held standard of aggressive volume expansion for the management of shock and/or prevention of AKI. Similarly, goal-directed perioperative fluid resuscitation appears to mitigate AKI risk; however, a recent meta-analysis by Prowle et al. [8] suggested that the quantity of volume given may be less important than simply using a goal-directed approach. Furthermore, this study also suggested that perioperative inotrope use during a goal-directed approach may be the "protective" intervention as the meta-analysis found that only those studies using inotropes showed a benefit of the goal-directed approach [8].

However, subsequently, numerous studies have demonstrated a clear association between volume overload and increased risk of mortality and morbidity among both medical and surgical ICU patients [9, 10]. A liberal approach to fluid management and the presence of hypervolemia (defined as 10 % weight gain from admission) are associated with increased mortality and higher morbidity in sepsis, acute respiratory distress syndrome (ARDS), general surgical patients, trauma, and cardiac surgery [11–16]. The presence of hypervolemia at the time of renal replacement therapy (RRT) initiation in AKI is strongly associated with mortality in both pediatric and adult patient populations [17–22]. Finally, data also suggest a dose and duration response in hypervolemia with a progressive increase in mortality for both a longer duration and escalating degree of hypervolemia [17, 21].

Taken together, the current state of the literature continues to support that a goal-directed approach to volume resuscitation during the acute resuscitative phases of shock or surgical recovery (within the first 6–24 h) is beneficial. However, clinicians are strongly encouraged to convert to a conservative approach to volume management as soon as possible (with a more liberal use of vasopressors) and aggressively avoid volume overload.

Type of Fluid for Volume Resuscitation

Another key question is the choice of fluid to employ for acute volume resuscitation. Isotonic crystalloids are aqueous solutions of mineral salts or other water-soluble molecules. Commonly used solutions in the United States include 0.9 % normal saline, balanced isotonic crystalloids such as lactated Ringer's (LR) or Plasma-Lyte A, dextrose with additives, or rarely other balanced crystalloids (Table 5.2). Colloid solutions consist of homogeneous, noncrystalline molecules suspended in a continuous phase of

Table 5.2 Composition of isotonic crystalloids

Ionic concentration (mmol/l)	0.9 % (normal) saline	Lactated ringer's (LR)	Plasma-Lyte 148 (A)[a]	Hartmann's solution	Isotonic sodium bicarbonate[b]
Sodium	154	130	140	131	150
Potassium		4	5	5	
Chloride	154	109	98	111	
Magnesium			1.5		
Calcium		3		2	
Bicarbonate					150
Lactate		28		29	
Gluconate			23		
Acetate			27		
Osmolarity (mosm/l)	308	273	294	276	300[c]
pH	5.4	6.5	7.4	6.0	8.0[c]

[a]Plasma-Lyte 148 (A) is a commercially available solution (available in most countries) distributed by Baxter in the United States

[b]Prepared by inpatient pharmacy as either 150 meq $NaHCO_3$ (150 cc) added to 1 l D5W or to 850–1,000 ml sterile water for injection (not commercially available in the United States)

[c]Osmolarity and pH will vary slightly depending on method for preparation (D5W or sterile water). These data reflect mixing 150 meq (150 ml) $NaHCO_3$ with 850 ml sterile water for injection

another component and are categorized as blood-derived (i.e., albumin, plasma protein fraction, packed red blood cells, and fresh frozen plasma) or as semisynthetic (hydroxyethylstarch [HES], dextrans, and gelatins). The primary theory in using colloids is that they may remain longer in the intravascular compartment and, by causing a higher intravascular oncotic pressure, promote the movement of interstitial water from the extravascular to intravascular compartment.

Crystalloids vs Colloids

Randomized control trials and meta-analyses no longer support the use of HES for volume expansion in critically ill patients. In the Efficacy of Volume Substitution and Insulin Therapy in Severe Sepsis (VISEP) study, compared to LR, the use of HES was associated with an increased rate of AKI (34.9 vs 22.8 %) and need for RRT (31.0 vs 18.8 %) [23]. The Scandinavian Starch for Severe Sepsis/Septic Shock trial also indicated that HES use is associated with an increased risk of death and need for renal replacement therapy [24]. Finally, the Australian and New Zealand Intensive Care Society (ANZICS) group demonstrated a higher incidence of RRT associated with HES use compared to normal saline but without a difference in mortality [25]. Based on these data, it is recommended that HES-containing fluids should be avoided for volume resuscitation.

With regard to albumin, there are limited data to support the routine use of albumin in critically ill patients. The SAFE (Saline versus Albumin Fluid Evaluation) trial showed no obvious clinical benefit of albumin administration in ICU patients, but albumin use carried increased cost [26]. Subgroup analysis of those with severe sepsis in the SAFE trial as well as a subsequent meta-analysis suggests that albumin use may be associated with a decreased mortality in severe sepsis [27, 28] and there are several ongoing controlled trials investigating this question. Another setting where albumin resuscitation may be beneficial (and is generally recommended) is in patients with advanced liver disease, where albumin-based resuscitation appears to lower the risk of hepatorenal syndrome (HRS) and mortality [29, 30].

Balanced Crystalloids vs 0.9 % (Normal) Sodium Chloride

Debates about the ideal crystalloid for isotonic volume expansion remain at the forefront of critical care medicine. Balanced isotonic crystalloids maintain a near "normal" sodium concentration (130–145), add other cations (potassium, magnesium, calcium), and replace many of the required chloride anions with other anions (bicarbonate, lactate, acetate, or gluconate) (Table 5.2). Historically, hyperchloremic metabolic acidosis has been viewed as a necessary evil of volume resuscitation. However, observational studies increasingly suggest that chloride-rich solutions (0.9 % sodium chloride) have a higher incidence of AKI when compared with balanced salt solutions [31–33]. Given the complex patient population and difficulty in accounting for potential confounders, studies have not been able to demonstrate clear survival benefits of balanced crystalloids. Animal models suggest that hyperchloremia may exacerbate renal ischemia [34]. Small studies of bolus volume expansion in healthy humans demonstrate a less robust increase in urine output (UOP), slower excretion of a volume load, and lower renal perfusion in those receiving chloride-rich compared to balanced crystalloids [35, 36].

Present evidence suggests that balanced crystalloid solutions may be preferable to chloride-rich solutions (0.9 % normal saline), especially for patients requiring large volume expansion and perhaps those predisposed to kidney injury.

Volume Removal

Similar to the challenge of deciding when and how to administer volume expansion, it is just as vexing to determine how and when to remove volume. While there is no benefit for converting oliguric to nonoliguric AKI with the use of diuretics, there is still a role for diuretic or extracorporeal volume removal for symptomatic hypervolemia especially when complicating AKI. As above, hypervolemia should be avoided and volume removal should be considered if patients meet the criteria of either symptomatic hypervolemia or demonstrate that there is a potential for improvement in organ function with volume removal.

Volume Management Summary

Based on the available trials to date, we make the following recommendations:

1. HES should not be used.
2. Isotonic crystalloids are preferred for volume expansion in most (almost all) ICU patients regardless of the ICU setting (medical, surgical, cardiac, neurological).
3. Balanced crystalloids (LR and Plasma-Lyte A) are preferred for large volume resuscitation.
4. Add albumin-based colloid expansion in a balanced approach with isotonic crystalloids in patients with advanced acute or chronic liver disease.
5. Avoid hypervolemia and transition to a conservative approach to fluid management at the earliest possible point in the management of critically ill patients with shock.
6. Consider volume removal via diuresis or RRT if hypervolemia (especially symptomatic volume overload) develops.

Acid/Base Management

A primary function of the kidney is to maintain acid/base homeostasis by excreting organic, nonvolatile, metabolic acids and generate bicarbonate buffer. In AKI, the renal regulatory control of acid/base status decreases, and acid excretion and bicarbonate generation are often disrupted. Furthermore, certain surgeries (especially cardiac, abdominal, and urological surgeries) are associated with worsening metabolic acidosis. Metabolic alkalosis is less common in AKI except in some prerenal causes of AKI.

It should be noted that there are several specific (albeit uncommon) causes of anion gap metabolic acidosis that can be encountered in the ICU, some of which can be fatal. Propofol infusion syndrome is a rare (but possibly underdiagnosed) event which manifests as progressive metabolic acidosis, rhabdomyolysis, lipemia, hyperkalemia, AKI, and arrhythmias leading to cardiovascular collapse. Predisposing factors include young age (especially pediatric patients), severe critical illness of central nervous system or respiratory origin, exogenous catecholamine or glucocorticoid administration, inadequate carbohydrate intake, and subclinical mitochondrial disease [37].

Another rare cause of severe, high anion gap metabolic acidosis in adults is that due to accumulation of 5-oxoproline (pyroglutamic acid). Acetaminophen and several other drugs (vigabatrin and flucloxacillin) have been implicated as causative agents. Patients who have malnutrition, sepsis, chronic alcohol use, underlying liver disease, and/or renal insufficiency and also ingest acetaminophen can develop this due to baseline glutathione deficiency. Treatment consists of discontinuation of the offending agent and supportive care.

Propylene glycol serves as a carrier vehicle for delivery of drugs like lorazepam and phenytoin, which can accumulate resulting in a hyperosmolar anion gap metabolic acidosis. This complication is more common in patients receiving high-dose continuous lorazepam infusions (usually over 10 mg/h) for an extended duration, particularly in the setting of impaired renal function [38].

Finally, a unique form of lactic acidosis known as D-lactic acidosis can occur in patients with jejunoileal bypasses, small bowel resections, or other forms of short-bowel syndrome, which can result in unexplained anion gap metabolic acidosis associated with mental status changes.

When addressing acidemia, urgency of treatment depends on the level of pH. When pH is decreasing, clinicians should consider the following: (1) clearly delineate all acid/base derangements and etiology using the albumin-adjusted anion gap method, strong ion difference, or base excess/deficit model; (2) maximize minute ventilation if coexisting primary respiratory acidosis noted; (3) low threshold for RRT initiation for severe acidemia (pH <7.1–7.15); and (4) limited role for bicarbonate administration as it can worsen volatile acid levels (pCO2) especially when respiratory acidosis is present.

Electrolyte Disturbances

Disturbances in electrolyte concentrations are some of the most frequent disorders in critically ill patients. Electrolyte derangements frequently complicate renal dysfunction and AKI and are independently associated with a worse prognosis. Treatments of electrolyte disturbances are based on few randomized control studies, case reports, expert opinion, and clinical experience. Careful balancing of intravenous solutions and nutrition may prevent the development of electrolyte disturbances. This section will briefly address the implications, causes, and management of the most commonly seen electrolyte disturbances in the ICU. A summary of tests to aid in the evaluation of dysnatremias and dyskalemia is shown in Table 5.3.

Dysnatremias

Disorders of sodium remain the most common electrolyte abnormality in the ICU. Hyponatremia has been reported in about 30–40 % of hospitalized patients [39, 40]. A retrospective analysis by Sakr et al. [41] demonstrated that dysnatremia

Table 5.3 Suggested evaluation for electrolyte imbalances in the ICU

Electrolyte abnormality	Evaluation	Inference
Hyponatremia	1. Serum osmolality	Hypoosmolar or hyperosmolar hyponatremia
	2. Urine osmolality (mosm/kg)	>150 – conditions with impaired water excretion (elevated ADH state)
		<100 – primary polydipsia, volume depletion, reset osmostat
	3. Urine sodium (meq/l)	>40 – conditions with euvolemia (elevated ADH state) or renal salt wasting is present
		<15 – true volume depletion, polydipsia, heart failure, and cirrhosis
		15–40 – saline challenge and retest urine sodium
Hypernatremia	Urine sodium (meq/l)	<10 – extra renal fluid loss
		>20 – renal fluid loss
	Urine osmolality (mosm/kg)	>500–700 – maximally concentrated urine suggesting nonrenal causes
		<300 – inappropriate dilute urine - renal fluid loss
	Electrolyte free water clearance = urine [1 – (UNa + UK)/SNa])	>0 – renal excretion of solute free water
		<0 – renal conservation of water
Dyskalemias	TTKG (urine K * plasma osm)/(plasma K * urine osm)	>7 – renal loss of K (appropriate in hyperkalemia)
		<3 – nonrenal loss of K (appropriate in hypokalemia)

Abbreviations: *ADH* antidiuretic hormone, *SNa* serum concentration of sodium, *TTKG* transtubular potassium gradient, *UK* urinary excretion of potassium, *UNa* urinary excretion of sodium was independently associated with an increased risk of in-hospital death in surgical ICU patients, and dysnatremia at ICU admission was associated with a higher risk of death compared with ICU-acquired dysnatremia.

In general, hyponatremia develops when there is a relative excess of free water in the setting of impaired renal free water excretion. Hypernatremia develops when there is increased free water loss or decreased free water intake, and most commonly it has to be coupled with decreased thirst mechanism or limited access to free water.

The treatment of all dysnatremia should be guided by symptoms and duration. Symptomatic hyponatremia is often a clinical emergency best treated with hypertonic (3 %) saline. The plasma sodium concentration should be corrected by 2–4 meq/l in the first 2–4 h, followed by less than 10 meq/l in any 24 h period and less than 18–20 meq/l in any 48 h period. Overly rapid correction is well known to be harmful by increasing the risk for osmotic demyelination. Slowing the rate of elevation or re-lowering sodium concentration through the addition of free water may be necessary in selected patients who exceed these goals.

Treatment of hypernatremia involves careful assessment of volume status and evaluation of ongoing free water losses (urinary or stool). Free water repletion either via intravenous or enteral route is usually sufficient. The Adrogue-Madias formula can aid the clinician in predicting the expected change in serum sodium with the infusion of any type or volume of intravenous (IV) fluid (assuming a closed system) thereby providing guidance on the initial starting point for the correction of hypo- or hypernatremia [42].

Potassium Disorders

The normal range for potassium is 3.5–5.0 meq/l. Hypokalemia can cause arrhythmias, rhabdomyolysis, gut paralysis, nephrogenic diabetes insipidus, and abnormal neurological functioning. On the other hand, hyperkalemia can cause bradycardia, cardiac arrest, and neurological changes including confusion, flaccid paralysis and also weakness.

In ICU patients, hypokalemia is common due to increased losses in urine and stool, intracellular shifts during alkalosis and drug effects (insulin, catecholamines, and beta-agonists), and inadequate intake. Symptoms and serum levels usually guide dosing for hypokalemia. It has been estimated that for every 0.3 meq/l decrease in serum potassium concentration, the total body potassium deficit in adults is approximately 50–100 meq [43]. It is recommended that repletion of potassium be given via the enteral route whenever possible and that IV potassium with concentrated KCl via central venous line be reserved for severe and symptomatic cases or in those with inadequate enteral function or access.

Hyperkalemia is common in the ICU and is a source of significant anxiety for the clinicians. It is most commonly seen in the setting of renal dysfunction, exuberant supplementation, massive cell necrosis (rhabdomyolysis or tumor lysis syndrome), medications, metabolic acidosis, and hypoaldosteronism. Urgency of treatment should be more based on signs and symptoms (electrocardiogram [EKG] changes such as peaked T waves, lengthening PR interval, loss of P waves, and widening QRS interval.) rather than the absolute level. Bolus IV calcium administration (1–2 g) remains the most important management step for symptomatic hyperkalemia. This should be followed by temporizing measures (insulin, beta-agonists) and augmentation of potassium excretion through diuresis, dialysis, or enteral cation-exchange resins (sodium polystyrene sulfonate). Caution should be advised with cation-exchange resin usage in patients with shock, bowel surgery, trauma, and ileus as this has been associated with bowel necrosis and mesenteric ischemia [44].

Magnesium

Hypomagnesemia is very common in ICU patients and occurs commonly due to inadequate nutrition, enhanced losses due to drugs (diuretics, aminoglycosides, amphotericin B), and cellular uptake as in refeeding syndrome. It commonly occurs in conjunction with hypokalemia and hypocalcemia, and symptoms include tetany, respiratory muscle weakness, fasciculation, arrhythmias, and coronary artery vasospasm. Magnesium excretion is impaired in AKI especially with oliguria, and, thus, hypomagnesemia is less common in AKI. Severe hypermagnesemia can occur in AKI especially with too aggressive supplementation. Symptoms include muscle weakness, hypotension/shock, and depressed neurological function. Symptomatic severe hypermagnesemia in AKI is an indication for acute RRT. In general, it is reasonable to monitor and replace magnesium in AKI, but the dosage and duration of administration should be balanced according to the severity of AKI.

Calcium

Low serum and ionized calcium does occur in ICU patients and can contribute to hemodynamic instability and bleeding. True hypercalcemia is less common in the critically ill and usually results from metastatic disease, medications, and immobilization. Severe hypercalcemia can also cause renal failure by contributing to renal arterial vasoconstriction and polyuria leading to volume depletion. AKI does not usually lead to critically important disorders of calcium levels.

Phosphorus

Hypophosphatemia occurs commonly in the postsurgical patient in the setting of brisk fluid resuscitation and intraoperative bleeding usually as a result of redistribution into intracellular compartment and external losses (urine, blood, cardiopulmonary bypass).

Severe hypophosphatemia is associated with hemodynamic instability, rhabdomyolysis, and respiratory and skeletal muscle weakness from decreased levels of ATP and 2,3 DPG. It is recommended that phosphorus should be checked early in the postoperative course in high-risk patients and levels below 2.0 mg/dl should be repleted.

Hyperphosphatemia is a symptom of AKI as excretion is reduced by impaired renal clearance and glomerular filtration rate (GFR). In general, hyperphosphatemia in AKI does not require specific treatment and is only a rare indication of initiation of RRT. Adjustments to enteral nutrition will limit the rate of accumulation. Various phosphate binders are designed to bind phosphorus in enteral intake (food) and prevent gastrointestinal (GI) absorption. The effectiveness of these agents in ICU patients receiving tube feeds is uncertain; they do not have a role in patients who are not receiving enteral nutrition.

Conclusion

In summary, careful monitoring of filling pressures and maintaining optimal renal perfusion may prevent AKI. Sufficient evidence now exists to guide the choice of fluids to be used during resuscitation, in order to preserve renal function. Additionally, it is important to implement strategies regarding the timing and total volume of resuscitation during critical illness. Patients who develop AKI in ICU are at a high risk of developing electrolyte and metabolic complications. Anticipating these disturbances and careful monitoring may improve patient outcomes.

Key Messages

- Assessment and preservation of renal perfusion is of utmost importance during the postoperative period.
- Volume expansion, when required, should be centered on isotonic crystalloids with preference for balanced crystalloids. HES-based volume expanders lead to increased risk of AKI and should not be used.
- Indiscriminate volume expansion in attempts to reverse AKI should be avoided as hypervolemia is recognized as a serious complication of critical illness and AKI.
- Anticipate key situations in the ICU, which can lead to serious acid/base disturbances.
- Monitoring and aggressive correction of electrolyte abnormalities are essential to prevent morbidity and risk of mortality.

References

1. Rivers E, Nguyen B, Havstad S, et al. Early goal-directed therapy in the treatment of severe sepsis and septic shock. N Engl J Med. 2001;345(19):1368–77.
2. Jones AE. Lactate clearance for assessing response to resuscitation in severe sepsis. Acad Emerg Med. 2013;20(8):844–7. Epub Jul 23 2013.
3. Marik PE, Cavallazzi R, Vasu T, Hirani A. Dynamic changes in arterial waveform derived variables and fluid responsiveness in mechanically ventilated patients: a systematic review of the literature. Crit Care Med. 2009;37(9):2642–7.
4. Cheatham ML, White MW, Sagraves SG, Johnson JL, Block EF. Abdominal perfusion pressure: a superior parameter in the assessment of intra-abdominal hypertension. J Trauma Oct. 2000;49(4):621–6; discussion 626–7.
5. Monnet X, Julien F, Ait-Hamou N, et al. Lactate and venoarterial carbon dioxide difference/arterial-venous oxygen difference ratio, but not central venous oxygen saturation, predict increase in oxygen consumption in fluid responders. Crit Care Med. 2013;41(6):1412–20.
6. Wheeler AP, Bernard GR, Thompson BT, et al. Pulmonary-artery versus central venous catheter to guide treatment of acute lung injury. N Engl J Med. 2006;354(21):2213–24.
7. Mohmand H, Goldfarb S. Renal dysfunction associated with intra-abdominal hypertension and the abdominal compartment syndrome. J Am Soc Nephrol. 2011;22(4):615–21.
8. Prowle JR, Chua HR, Bagshaw SM, Bellomo R. Clinical review: volume of fluid resuscitation and the incidence of acute kidney injury – a systematic review. Crit Care. 2012;16(4):230.
9. Boyd JH, Forbes J, Nakada TA, Walley KR, Russell JA. Fluid resuscitation in septic shock: a positive fluid balance and elevated central venous pressure are associated with increased mortality. Crit Care Med. 2011;39(2):259–65.
10. Wiedemann HP, Wheeler AP, Bernard GR, et al. Comparison of two fluid-management strategies in acute lung injury. N Engl J Med. 2006;354(24):2564–75.
11. Simmons RS, Berdine GG, Seidenfeld JJ, et al. Fluid balance and the adult respiratory distress syndrome. Am Rev Respir Dis. 1987;135(4):924–9.
12. Sakr Y, Vincent JL, Reinhart K, et al. High tidal volume and positive fluid balance are associated with worse outcome in acute lung injury. Chest. 2005;128(5):3098–108.
13. Murphy CV, Schramm GE, Doherty JA, et al. The importance of fluid management in acute lung injury secondary to septic shock. Chest. 2009;136(1):102–9.
14. Toraman F, Evrenkaya S, Yuce M, et al. Highly positive intraoperative fluid balance during cardiac surgery is associated with adverse outcome. Perfusion. 2004;19(2):85–91.
15. Brandstrup B, Tonnesen H, Beier-Holgersen R, et al. Effects of intravenous fluid restriction on postoperative complications: comparison of two perioperative fluid regimens: a randomized assessor-blinded multicenter trial. Ann Surg. 2003;238(5):641–8.
16. Vincent JL, Sakr Y, Sprung CL, et al. Sepsis in European intensive care units: results of the SOAP study. Crit Care Med. 2006;34(2):344–53.
17. Bouchard J, Soroko SB, Chertow GM, et al. Fluid accumulation, survival and recovery of kidney function in critically ill patients with acute kidney injury. Kidney Int. 2009;76(4):422–7.
18. Goldstein SL, Currier H, Graf C, Cosio CC, Brewer ED, Sachdeva R. Outcome in children receiving continuous venovenous hemofiltration. Pediatrics. 2001;107(6):1309–12.
19. Sutherland SM, Zappitelli M, Alexander SR, et al. Fluid overload and mortality in children receiving continuous renal replacement therapy: the prospective pediatric continuous renal replacement therapy registry. Am J Kidney Dis. 2010;55(2):316–25.
20. Bellomo R, Cass A, Cole L, et al. An observational study fluid balance and patient outcomes in the randomized evaluation of normal vs. augmented level of replacement therapy trial. Crit Care Med. 2012;40(6):1753–60.
21. Vaara ST, Korhonen AM, Kaukonen KM, et al. Fluid overload is associated with an increased risk for 90-day mortality in critically ill patients with renal replacement therapy: data from the prospective FINNAKI study. Crit Care. 2012;16(5):R197.

22. Heung M, Wolfgram DF, Kommareddi M, Hu Y, Song PX, Ojo AO. Fluid overload at initiation of renal replacement therapy is associated with lack of renal recovery in patients with acute kidney injury. Nephrol Dial Transplant. 2012;27(3):956–61.
23. Brunkhorst FM, Engel C, Bloos F, et al. Intensive insulin therapy and pentastarch resuscitation in severe sepsis. N Engl J Med. 2008;358(2):125–39.
24. Perner A, Haase N, Guttormsen AB, et al. Hydroxyethyl starch 130/0.42 versus ringer's acetate in severe sepsis. N Engl J Med. 2012;367(2):124–34.
25. Myburgh JA, Finfer S, Bellomo R, et al. Hydroxyethyl starch or saline for fluid resuscitation in intensive care. N Engl J Med. 2012;367(20):1901–11.
26. Finfer S, Bellomo R, Boyce N, French J, Myburgh J, Norton R. A comparison of albumin and saline for fluid resuscitation in the intensive care unit. N Engl J Med. 2004;350(22):2247–56.
27. Finfer S, McEvoy S, Bellomo R, McArthur C, Myburgh J, Norton R. Impact of albumin compared to saline on organ function and mortality of patients with severe sepsis. Intensive Care Med. 2011;37(1):86–96.
28. Delaney AP, Dan A, McCaffrey J, Finfer S. The role of albumin as a resuscitation fluid for patients with sepsis: a systematic review and meta-analysis. Crit Care Med. 2011;39(2):386–91.
29. Sort P, Navasa M, Arroyo V, et al. Effect of intravenous albumin on renal impairment and mortality in patients with cirrhosis and spontaneous bacterial peritonitis. N Engl J Med. 1999;341(6):403–9.
30. Sauneuf B, Champigneulle B, Soummer A, et al. Increased survival of cirrhotic patients with septic shock. Crit Care. 2013;17(2):R78.
31. Yunos NM, Bellomo R, Hegarty C, Story D, Ho L, Bailey M. Association between a chloride-liberal vs chloride-restrictive intravenous fluid administration strategy and kidney injury in critically ill adults. JAMA. 2012;308(15):1566–72.
32. Yunos NM, Bellomo R, Story D, Kellum J. Bench-to-bedside review: chloride in critical illness. Crit Care. 2010;14(4):226.
33. Shaw AD, Bagshaw SM, Goldstein SL, et al. Major complications, mortality, and resource utilization after open abdominal surgery: 0.9% saline compared to plasma-lyte. Ann Surg. 2012;255(5):821–9.
34. Wilcox CS. Regulation of renal blood flow by plasma chloride. J Clin Invest. 1983;71(3): 726–35.
35. Reid F, Lobo DN, Williams RN, Rowlands BJ, Allison SP. (Ab)normal saline and physiological Hartmann's solution: a randomized double-blind crossover study. Clin Sci (Lond). 2003;104(1):17–24.
36. Chowdhury AH, Cox EF, Francis ST, Lobo DN. A randomized, controlled, double-blind crossover study on the effects of 2-L infusions of 0.9% saline and plasma-lyte(R) 148 on renal blood flow velocity and renal cortical tissue perfusion in healthy volunteers. Ann Surg. 2012;256(1): 18–24.
37. Wong JM. Propofol infusion syndrome. Am J Ther. 2010;17(5):487–91.
38. Zar T, Graeber C, Perazella MA. Recognition, treatment, and prevention of propylene glycol toxicity. Semin Dial. 2007;20(3):217–9.
39. Upadhyay A, Jaber BL, Madias NE. Incidence and prevalence of hyponatremia. Am J Med. 2006;119(7 Suppl 1):S30–5.
40. Funk GC, Lindner G, Druml W, et al. Incidence and prognosis of dysnatremias present on ICU admission. Intensive Care Med. 2010;36(2):304–11.
41. Sakr Y, Rother S, Ferreira AM, et al. Fluctuations in serum sodium level are associated with an increased risk of death in surgical ICU patients. Crit Care Med. 2013;41(1):133–42.
42. Adrogue HJ, Madias NE. Hyponatremia. N Engl J Med. 2000;342(21):1581–9.
43. Gennari FJ. Hypokalemia. N Engl J Med. 1998;339(7):451–8.
44. Harel Z, Harel S, Shah PS, Wald R, Perl J, Bell CM. Gastrointestinal adverse events with sodium polystyrene sulfonate (Kayexalate) use: a systematic review. Am J Med. 2013;126(3): 264.e9–24.

Chapter 6
Intraoperative Considerations to Prevent Postoperative Acute Kidney Injury

Susan Garwood

Objectives

- To identify patients at risk for postoperative acute kidney injury (AKI)
- To identify and address modifiable preoperative risk factors for postoperative acute kidney injury
- To plan the intraoperative management of the patient at risk for postoperative acute kidney injury with respect to hemodynamic goals, fluid therapy, and drug administration

Introduction

Intraoperative prevention of postoperative AKI is predicated by an understanding of the unique risk factors presented by the individual patient coming for a particular surgical procedure. Preoperative risk algorithms have been derived from and cross-validated in large databases but differ for patients undergoing subspecialty surgeries, falling broadly into the categories of cardiac surgery [1, 2] and noncardiac major surgery [3, 4]. Similarities exist while others are more specific to the surgery (Table 6.1).

Preoperative risk indices are useful for:

1. Determining the presence of modifiable risk factors which can be optimized prior to surgery
2. Planning the best surgical strategy for the patient
3. Determining the optimal intraoperative management

S. Garwood, MBChB (✉)
Department of Anesthesiology, Yale New Haven Hospital, Yale University School of Medicine, 333 Cedar Street, T#3, New Haven, CT 06510-3206, USA
e-mail: susan.garwood@yale.edu

C.V. Thakar, C.R. Parikh (eds.), *Perioperative Kidney Injury: Principles of Risk Assessment, Diagnosis and Treatment*, DOI 10.1007/978-1-4939-1273-5_6

Table 6.1 Risk factors for acute kidney injury after cardiac and noncardiac surgery

Risk factors common to cardiac and noncardiac surgery	
Older age	
Congestive heart failure	
Decreased left ventricular ejection fraction	
Low cardiac output syndrome	
Renal insufficiency	
Diabetes mellitus	
Peripheral vascular disease	
Chronic obstructive pulmonary disease	
Hypertension	
Anemia	
Increased body mass index	
Preoperative ACE inhibitor/ARB drugs	
Emergency surgery	
Sepsis	
Risk factors unique to cardiac and noncardiac surgery	
Cardiac surgery	**Noncardiac surgery**
Female gender	Male gender
Prolonged CPB/ACC time	Intrathoracic procedures
Need for IABP	Intraperitoneal procedures
Prior cardiac surgery	Suprainguinal vascular procedures
Combined procedures	Ascites
Ventricular assist device procedures	ASA physical status

Adapted from: Karkouti et al. [36], Josephs and Thakar [67], Borthwick and Ferguson [68], Thakar [69], Kheterpal et al. [70]

Abbreviations: *ACE* angiotensin-converting enzyme, *ARB* angiotensin receptor blockade, *ASA* American Society of Anesthesiologists, *IABP* intra-aortic balloon pump, *CPB/ACC* cardiopulmonary bypass/aortic cross-clamp

Preoperative Modifiable Factors

Risk factors for postoperative AKI are predominantly nonmodifiable [1–4], and those that are potentially modifiable may not be practically achievable in the time frame required. However, the following bears consideration:

- *Preoperative hemodynamic optimization*
  A meta-analysis of 20 studies which included both cardiovascular and noncardiovascular surgeries [5] determined that:
  - Preoperative hemodynamic optimization reduced postoperative AKI (odds ratio (OR) 0.70; 95 % confidence interval (CI) 0.53–0.94).
  - Fluid administration alone did not reduce AKI.
  - Fluids plus inotropes significantly decreased the rate of postoperative AKI.

- *Time from contrast dye exposure to surgical procedure*
  Many patients require contrast-enhanced imaging studies prior to surgery and predisposing them to contrast-induced nephropathy (CIN). CIN risk:
  - Profile is very similar to that of perioperative AKI.
  - Is increased in the presence of large doses of contrast.
  - Is increased with hyperosmolar contrast dye.
  - Reduction strategies include hydration, sodium bicarbonate, and pretreatment with N-acetylcysteine (studies of N-acetylcysteine in CIN are inconclusive, but it is commonly used in high-risk patients).
  - The combination of contrast dye exposure and subsequent surgery has been the focus of many studies mainly in cardiac surgery:
  - Most demonstrate an increased risk of postoperative AKI with shorter intervals between exposure and surgery [6, 7].
  - A recent study of >2,000 patients undergoing coronary angiography followed by cardiac surgery found no difference in the incidence of postoperative AKI whether the surgery took place < or >3 days after contrast dye exposure [8].
  - It is advisable to follow CIN risk reduction strategies in high-risk patients and delay surgery (level of evidence B) [9] beyond 3 days if possible.

- *Preoperative medications*
  A number of common medications have been associated with perioperative AKI.

  Drugs associated with increased AKI:

  1. Angiotensin-converting enzyme (ACE) inhibitors and angiotensin II receptor blockers (ARB). The preoperative use of ACE inhibitors/ARB drugs is a risk factor for postoperative AKI in both cardiac surgery [10] and noncardiac surgery [11].
  2. Nonsteroidal anti-inflammatory drugs (NSAID). NSAIDs are associated with renal dysfunction in certain patient populations, and warnings regarding their use in the perioperative period have been issued by UK Regulatory Bodies (www.mhra.gov.uk/Publications/Safetyguidance/DrugSafetyUpdate/CON046451).
  3. Nephrotoxin avoidance and dose reduction/temporary discontinuation of antimicrobial, anticancer or immunosuppressive drugs with known nephrotoxic effects should be considered or substituted with less toxic alternatives if available.

  Drugs associated with decreased AKI:

  1. Aspirin reduces AKI in cardiac surgery [12], and preoperative administration should be considered. Patients who had received aspirin at least once within 5 days prior to cardiac surgery had approximately half the incidence of AKI or new requirement for renal replacement therapy (RRT) than patients who were not taking aspirin (3.7 % vs. 7.1 %; OR 0.38; $p<0.001$).

2. Statins.
   - The evidence from smaller clinical trials supporting the renoprotective effect of statins is contradictory.
   - Large insurance databases show that younger patients (<65 years old) given stains de novo prior to cardiac surgery have less AKI (RR 0.62; 95 % CI, 0.45–0.96) versus those not on statins [13].

- *Sepsis*
  - Is a common risk factor associated with perioperative AKI
  - Is the causative factor of AKI in almost 50 % of critically ill patients [13]

  There are no randomized studies of preoperative treatment of infections to reduce postoperative AKI. An analysis of over 5,000 patients with acute cholecystitis recorded in the American College of Surgeons National Surgical Quality Improvement Program (ACS NSQIP) revealed:

  - There was no association between timing of surgery and renal outcome.
  - Delayed patients were more likely to have an open procedure and require a longer postoperative stay [14].

- *Preoperative hemoglobin levels*
  In a cohort study of 27,381 patients with normal renal function undergoing non-cardiac surgery [15], low preoperative hemoglobin (Hb) levels were associated with postoperative AKI. In comparison to patients with a preoperative Hb >12.0 g/dl:

  - Hb between 10.1 and 12.0 g/dl doubled the risk of AKI.
  - Hb <8.0 g/dl almost quadrupled the risk for AKI.

However, transfusion of blood is also associated with increased postoperative AKI (see below), and other non-transfusion-related therapies to improve preoperative Hb have been advocated.

Surgical Strategy

Since certain surgeries (cardiac, vascular, gastric bypass, intrathoracic, and intraperitoneal) carry a higher risk for postoperative AKI, tailoring the surgical technique to minimize risk should be considered. A fuller discussion of these choices can be found in the pertinent forgoing chapters.

- *Conventional (with cardiopulmonary bypass, CPB) versus off pump (OPCAB) coronary artery bypass graft (CABG) surgery*

  - A meta-analysis of earlier prospective, observational, and randomized trials found a renal advantage with OPCAB surgery [16].
  - Two more recent prospectively randomized trials showed no difference in renal outcomes as defined by the requirement for renal replacement therapy [17] or "renal outcome" [18].

- Results of the CORONARY Study (CABG Off or ON Pump Revascularization Study) of 5,000 prospectively and randomized patients are awaited.
- Evidence exists for better renal outcomes in patients with preoperative chronic kidney disease (CKD) in OPCAB as compared to conventional CABG with CPB [19].
- The American College of Cardiology Foundation/American Heart Association Task Force on Practice Guidelines recommend OPCAB over conventional CABG with CPB for patients with preoperative renal dysfunction but do not favor one approach over the other for those with normal renal function [9].

- *Conventional (with CPB) aortic valve replacement versus transcatheter (endovascular) aortic valve implantation (TAVI)*
  - A review of preliminary trails and national registries of TAVI suggests that a 12–28 % incidence of AKI is seen in these patients which accounts for a 30-day mortality rate of 23–25 % and a 1-year mortality rate of 55–60 % [20].
  - There are no results currently available for prospective randomized trials of TAVI versus conventional aortic valve replacement (AVR).
  - Comparisons with historical case-matched controls [21] or contemporary patient cohorts [22] showed reduced incidence of postoperative AKI in TAVI patients versus surgical AVR with CPB (8.1 % vs. 26.1 %, $p<0.001$ and 9.2 % vs. 25.9 %, $p=0.001$, respectively).
- *Open vascular procedures versus endovascular approach*
  - Early population-based studies of ruptured abdominal aortic aneurysm (AAA) reveal a lower incidence of postoperative AKI in endovascular (23 %) than open surgical repair (30 %, $p<0.01$) [23].
  - Other vascular registries confirm these findings for infrarenal aortic aneurysm repair (0 % vs. 2.6 %, $p<0.05$) [24].
  - A more recent meta-analysis of randomized trials of open versus endovascular repair (endovascular aneurysm repair or EVAR) of AAA showed no advantage of the endovascular approach in low- to medium-risk patients [25] with respect to renal outcome but did confirm an early survival advantage.
  - A meta-analysis and systematic review of nonrandomized studies of descending thoracic aorta EVAR versus open repair conferred an advantage in renal outcome for the EVAR approach (OR 0.40, 95 % CI 0.25–0.63) [26].
- *Laparoscopic versus open gastrointestinal procedures*
  Propensity-matched population database analysis (ACS NSQIP) determined that laparoscopic proctectomy was associated with lower rates of postoperative renal failure (0.8 % vs. 2.0 %, $p=0.007$) [27].
- *Thoracoscopic versus open lung resection surgery* [28]
  - Thoracoscopic lung surgery is independently related to postoperative AKI reduction compared to open thoracotomy (adjusted OR 0.37, 95 % CI 0.15–0.90; $p=0.03$) [26].

- Thoracoscopy has been shown to attenuate the inflammatory response to lung resection when compared to open surgery and may contribute to the reduction in AKI.

Intraoperative Management of Patients at Risk for Postoperative Acute Kidney Injury

The pathophysiology of perioperative AKI is thought to be complex, and the notion of reduced renal blood flow as the predominant factor is now questioned [29]. Nevertheless, the mainstay of intraoperative management in patients at risk for AKI remains the provision of an adequate renal perfusion.

1. Blood pressure
   - In a large database of general surgery patients with normal preoperative renal function [3], the number of intraoperative 5 min epochs with a mean arterial pressure (MAP) <40 mmHg was an independent predictor of postoperative AKI.
   - Interrogation of a database of 33,300 noncardiac surgeries [30] determined:
     - That a MAP <55 mmHg is associated with a higher risk of postoperative AKI
     - The incidence of AKI increases with increasing time spent with MAP <55 mmHg
     - Even short durations of MAP <55 mmHg are associated with AKI
     - A MAP of <55 mmHg for greater than 20 min is significantly associated with a 30-day mortality.
   - A lower limit of mean arterial pressure to prevent AKI may apply in cardiac surgery [31]. By keeping MAP the same and measuring the lower level of *cerebral* autoregulation with near-infrared spectroscopy (NIRS – a noninvasive technique), it was determined that patients with postoperative AKI:
     - Had a higher average baseline pulse pressure
     - Had increased lower limits of cerebral autoregulation
     - Had higher magnitude-duration of MAP below their lower level of cerebral autoregulation
     - Cerebral NIRS may be useful in guiding an appropriate MAP for both cerebral and renal perfusion.
2. Cardiac output and other perfusion parameters
   - Animal data suggests that renal perfusion is dependent upon both MAP and cardiac output (CO) [32].
   - Postoperative general surgery patients managed by monitoring central venous pressure rather than stroke volume had higher rates of AKI despite similar MAP (22 % vs. 8 %; $P=0.03$) [33].

- In two meta-analyses of randomized controlled trials of cardiac and noncardiac surgery [5, 34], goal-directed therapy (monitoring and optimizing hemodynamic parameters using fluids and inotropic drugs to reach normal or supranormal values of cardiac output and oxygen delivery) reduced mortality and AKI (OR 0.64; CI 0.50–0.83; $p=0.0007$) when compared to standard management. Goal-directed therapy was effective:
  - Whether supranormal optimization was used or normal values achieved.
  - Only if vasoactive medications were used with fluid therapy; the use of fluids alone to achieve target values was ineffective.
  - Regardless of the monitoring device or goal parameter utilized (pulmonary artery catheter, esophageal Doppler, FloTrac device (Edwards Lifesciences, Irvine, CA, USA); cardiac output, stroke volume, mixed venous oxygen saturation, lactate or oxygen extraction ratio).
- Current clinical practice guidelines suggest using protocol-based management of hemodynamic and oxygenation parameters to prevent development or worsening of AKI in high-risk patients in the perioperative setting (Level of evidence 2C; Kidney Disease Improving Global Outcomes, www.KIDGO.com accessed 10/5/2013)

3. Intraoperative blood loss and the transfusion of blood
   Anemia contributes to kidney injury by reducing renal oxygen delivery and increasing oxidative stress.
   - In a large database of general surgery patients, postoperative decrease in Hb are associated with increased AKI [15]. A decrease of
     - 1.1–2.0 g/dl was associated with a 50 % increase risk for AKI.
     - >4.0 g/dl was associated with almost five times the risk for AKI.
   - In a retrospective study of 39 Jehovah's Witness patients who died with very low Hb levels (<6 mg/dl) after non cardiac surgery; one third died with a diagnosis of acute renal failure which was the third most common cause of death [35]
   - However, intraoperative transfusion of red blood cells has also been linked to postoperative AKI [36, 37] and:
     - Has been shown to be an independent risk factor for AKI after cardiac surgery [36]
     - Increased the incidence of AKI from 1.8 to 6.6 % in anemic patients compared to those who were not transfused [37]
     - Increased the incidence of AKI from 1.7 to 3.2 % in nonanemic patients compared to those who were not transfused [37]
     - Increased AKI in direct proportion to the number of units transfused
   - Clinical studies indicate that both anemia and blood transfusion are associated with end organ injury across a wide range of disease states and surgical interventions. There is no clear cut algorithm to guide decision making in the intraoperative period [38].

- An alternative strategy in elective surgery is to augment preoperative Hb levels and reduce perioperative losses by
  A. Optimizing hematopoiesis. A single dose of erythropoietin immediately before CABG surgery [39]:
     - Reduced the risk of AKI (8 % vs. 29 %; $p=0.035$)
     - Improved postoperative renal function

     A single dose of erythropoietin plus iron 1 day before valve surgery [40]:
     - Reduced the incidence of AKI from 54 to 24 % ($P=0.017$)
  B. Limiting blood draws and interventional/invasive studies
  C. Using intraoperative antifibrinolytics and blood salvage techniques
  D. Improving tissue oxygenation by other means
  E. Considering the use of investigational therapeutics such as artificial oxygen carrying fluids

4. Crystalloid versus colloid
   Fluid resuscitation is an integral part of goal-directed hemodynamic optimization. There is a long-standing debate over the choice of crystalloid and colloid intraoperatively which has been further confused by the retraction of a number of papers investigating the use of hydroxyethyl starch (HES) in the perioperative period:
   - Clinical trials and meta-analyses of patients with sepsis have shown that the use of synthetic colloids (gelatin, dextran, HES) is associated with increased AKI requiring RRT [41, 42].
   - In a retrospective study of over a thousand patients undergoing lung resection surgery, HES was associated with a higher risk of postoperative AKI (OR 1.5, 95 % CI 1.1–2.1) [28].
   - A recent Cochrane Review determined that all HES products increase the risk in AKI and RRT in all patient populations; a safe volume of any HES solution has yet to be determined, and alternate volume replacement therapies should be used in place of HES products [43, 44].
   - In the absence of hemorrhagic shock, isotonic crystalloids rather than colloids (albumin or starches) are recommended as initial management for expansion of intravascular volume in patients at risk for AKI or with AKI (level of evidence 2B; www.KDIGO.org accessed 10/5/2013).

5. Glucose control
   Following the finding in 2001 that intensive glucose control in patients admitted to the intensive care unit (ICU) reduced overall in-hospital mortality by 34 % and acute renal failure requiring dialysis or hemofiltration by 41 % [45], a large number of studies of intraoperative glucose control have been published:
   - The mean intraoperative glucose level is a significant predictor for renal complications in cardiac surgery patients [46].

- In over 1,000 nondiabetics undergoing cardiac surgery, strict perioperative blood glucose control (<120 mg/dl) was associated with a reduced incidence of renal impairment, failure, and RRT [47].
- The ACCF/AHA 2011 guidelines for CABG surgery recommend the use of insulin to target blood glucose level <180 mg/dl [9] to avoid hypoglycemia and other adverse outcomes [48].
- In considering the large body of literature on glycemic control and AKI, the recommendations are for insulin therapy targeting plasma glucose of 110–149 mg/dl (level of evidence 2C; www.KDIGO.org, accessed 10/5/2013).

6. Intraoperative choice of medications
   There are a few drugs used in the intraoperative period, which are thought to be associated with postoperative AKI:

   - Aprotinin (OR for RRT 2.59; 95 % CI, 1.36–4.95) compared to aminocaproic acid and tranexamic acid [49]
   - Diuretics

     - Intraoperative oliguria is not associated with renal failure in [3].
     - Both mannitol and furosemide increase AKI in general surgery [3].
     - The evidence supporting the benefit of using furosemide in cardiac surgery is weak and in some studies increases AKI [50, 51].

     Current clinical practice guidelines recommend www.KDIGO.org accessed 01/5/13:

     - Not using diuretics to prevent AKI (level of evidence 1B)
     - Not using diuretics to treat AKI, except in the management of volume overload (level of evidence 2C)

   - Dopamine
     While "renal dose" dopamine is not beneficial and may be harmful, the dopamine-1 agonist fenoldopam in smaller cardiac surgery trials:

     - Decreased the risk of AKI and RRT [52]
     - Was protective in a subgroup of patients with low output syndrome (OR 0.14; 95 % CI 0.03–0.7) [53]
     - Was favorable in two meta-analyses [54, 55]

     However, the high potential for causing hypotension particularly in critically ill patients has led to recommendations against the use of fenoldopam to prevent or treat AKI (www.KDIGO.org accessed 10/5/2013).

   - Natriuretic peptides

     1. Atrial natriuretic peptide (NP)

        - Small randomized controlled trials (RCTs) of ANP are inconsistent [56, 57].
        - Recent clinical practice guidelines for AKI (www.KDIGO.org) state "given the potential harm of hypotension and the quality of the positive

studies, the overall recommendation is not to routinely use ANP in the prevention or treatment of AKI (2B/2C recommendation)"

2. Brain natriuretic peptide (BNP, nesiritide)

   - Currently approved for treatment of chronic congestive heart failure and hypertensive crisis
   - Reduced perioperative AKI in clinical trials [58, 59]

   Possible renoprotective agent
   N-acetyl cysteine (NAC) has been most extensively studied in contrast-induced AKI:

   - In major surgery where contrast dye was not used, NAC did not reduce AKI [60].
   - In surgery where contrast dye is required intraoperatively, NAC was no better than hydration alone [61].
   - In liver transplantation where NAC is used to protect against ischemia reperfusion injury, a reduction in the risk for AKI has been reported [62].
   - A Cochrane review of 41 randomized studies of NAC in surgical or critically ill patients did not find any difference in incidence of new organ failure [63]. Because of cardiovascular depression noted in some studies the authors advised against the continued use of NAC in these patient groups

7. Intraoperative monitoring

   - Indices of cardiac performance can be derived from a pulmonary catheter, arterial waveform analysis, echocardiography, and esophageal Doppler. Due to concerns about the complications of invasive monitoring, the National Institute for Health and Clinical Excellence (NICE) in the UK released guidelines advocating the use of esophageal Doppler monitoring, stating that it should be considered for use in patients undergoing major or high-risk surgery or other surgical patients in whom a clinician would consider using invasive cardiovascular monitoring [64].
   - Monitoring of indices renal perfusion has been reported using transesophageal echocardiography [65] and near-infrared spectroscopy [66]. Both of these novel techniques are yet to be studied with respect to postoperative AKI in large patient numbers, and both have significant limitations such as body mass index.

Summary (Table 6.2)

In summary, intraoperative management of the patient at risk for developing perioperative AKI begins with risk stratification in the preoperative period [1–4]. Those at risk for AKI should undergo preoperative optimization which may include

Table 6.2 Summary of pre- and intraoperative strategies to minimize perioperative acute kidney injury

Phase of surgery	Strategy	Comments
Preop	Assess patient for risk of AKI	Apply known risk algorithms
	Stop ACE inhibitor/ARB drugs, nephrotoxins, nonsteroidals; consider giving aspirin, statin	
	Consider delaying surgery after radiocontrast dye exposure	Minimum of 3 days
	Minimize blood draws and invasive procedures	
	Recommend minimally invasive surgery	
	Optimize high-risk patient	Apply goal-directed hemodynamic therapy with appropriate monitoring, fluid, *and* vasoactive drugs
Intraop	Maintain MAP >55 mmHg	May require higher MAPs guided by NIRS
	Consider goal-directed hemodynamic therapy in high-risk patients	Appropriate monitoring, fluid, *and* vasoactive drugs
	Avoid hydroxyethyl starch-based fluids	
	Avoid diuretics to promote urinary flow	Including natriuretic peptides
	Apply blood conservation strategies	Antifibrinolytics
	Avoid blood transfusion whenever feasible	

Abbreviations: *AKI* acute kidney injury, *ACE* angiotensin-converting enzyme, *ARB* angiotensin receptor blocker, *MAP* mean arterial pressure, *NIRS* near-infrared spectroscopy

goal-directed hemodynamic therapy [5], avoidance of anemia [15], consideration of a delay between contrast dye exposure and surgery [6–9], and planning for a minimally invasive procedure [9, 19–24, 26, 27]. Stop drugs associated with postoperative AKI such as ACE inhibitor/ARB drugs [10, 11], nonsteroidals, and nephrotoxic agents and consider giving aspirin [12] and a statin [13].

Goal-directed hemodynamic therapy with fluids *and* vasoactive agents should be continued intraoperatively ([5, 32–34], www.KIDGO.com) in high-risk patients. In all patients, a mean arterial pressure (MAP) of at least 55 mmHg should be maintained [3, 30, 31]. Consideration for higher MAPs in high-risk patients may be appropriate and can be guided by NIRS [32]. Hydroxyethyl starch-based fluids should be avoided [28, 43, 44], and blood preservation strategies are preferable to transfusion of blood products [36–40]. Intraoperative glucose levels have a bearing on renal outcome and should be carefully controlled (<150 mg/dl by KDIGO recommendations; <180 mg/dl by American College of Cardiology Foundation/American Heart Association (ACCF/AHA) recommendations) while avoiding hypoglycemia. Diuretics including natriuretic peptides are not recommended [3, 50, 51]; concerns over the safety of fenoldopam and N-acetyl cysteine have led to recommendation against their use ([63], www.KDIGO.com).

Key Messages

- Patients identified to be at high risk for postoperative AKI should be subjected to careful intraoperative risk reduction strategies, including minimally invasive surgical approaches.
- Key intraoperative renal preservation strategies include: hemodynamic goal-directed therapy by using the right combination of fluids and vasoactive agents, maintaining adequate tissue oxygenation (e.g., optimal hemoglobin levels), and avoidance of known nephrotoxic drugs.
- Both anemia and blood transfusion are associated with increased postoperative AKI. Employ blood preservation strategies such as antifibrinolytics and blood salvage techniques.
- Treatment of oliguria with diuretics should be approached with caution. Routine intraoperative use of dopamine, natriuretic peptides, or N-acetylcysteine is discouraged.

References

1. Wijeysundera DN, Karkouti K, Dupuis JY, Rao V, Chan CT, Granton JT, Beattie WS. Derivation and validation of a simplified predictive index for renal replacement therapy after cardiac surgery. JAMA. 2007;297:1801–9.
2. Thakar CV, Arrigain S, Worley S, Yared J-P, Paganini EP. A clinical score to predict acute renal failure after cardiac surgery. J Am Soc Nephrol. 2005;16:162–8.
3. Kheterpal S, Tremper KK, Englesbe MJ, O'Reilly M, Shanks AM, Fetterman DM, Rosenberg AL, Swartz RD. Predictors of postoperative acute renal failure after noncardiac surgery in patients with previously normal renal function. Anesthesiology. 2007;107:892–902.
4. Kolhe NV, Stevens PE, Crowe AV, Lipkin GW, Harrison DA. Case mix, outcome and activity for patients with severe acute kidney injury during the first 24 hours after admission to an adult, general critical care unit: application of predictive models from a secondary analysis of the ICNARC Case Mix Programme database. Crit Care. 2008;12 suppl 1:S2.
5. Brienza N, Giglio MT, Marucci M, Fiore T. Does perioperative 29 hemodynamic optimization protect renal function in surgical patients? A meta-analytic study. Crit Care Med. 2009;37: 2079–90.
6. Ranucci M, Ballotta A, Kunkl A, De Benedetti D, Kandil H, Conti D, Mollichelli N, Bossone E, Mehta RH. Influence of the timing of cardiac catheterization and the amount of contrast media on acute renal failure after cardiac surgery. Am J Cardiol. 2008;101:1112–8.
7. Medalion B, Cohen H, Assali A, Vaknin Assa H, Farkash A, Snir E, Sharoni E, Biderman P, Milo G, Battler A, Kornowski R, Porat E. The effect of cardiac angiography timing, contrast media dose, and preoperative renal function on acute renal failure after coronary artery bypass grafting. J Thorac Cardiovasc Surg. 2010;139:1539–44.
8. Ko B, Garcia S, Mithani S, Tholakanahalli V, Adabag S. Risk of acute kidney injury in patients who undergo coronary artery angiography and cardiac surgery in close succession. Eur Heart J. 2012;33:2065–70.
9. Hillis LD, Smith PK, Anderson JL, Bittl JA, Bridges CR, Byrne JG, Cigarroa JE, Disesa VJ, Hiratzka LF, Hutter Jr AM, Jessen ME, Keeley EC, Lahey SJ, Lange RA, London MJ, Mack MJ, Patel MR, Puskas JD, Sabik JF, Selnes O, Shahian DM, Trost JC, Winniford MD. 2011

ACCF/AHA guideline for coronary artery bypass graft surgery: a report of the American College of Cardiology Foundation/American Heart Association Task Force on practice guidelines. Circulation. 2011;124(23):e652–735.
10. Coca SG, Garg AX, Swaminatham M, Garwood S, Hong K, Thiessen-Philbrook H, Passik C, Koyner JL, Parikh CR, on behalf of the TRIBE-AKI Consortium. Pre-operative angiotensin converting enzyme inhibitors and angiotensin receptor blocker use and acute kidney injury in patients undergoing cardiac surgery. Nephrol Dial Transplant. 2013;28(11):2787–99.
11. Thakar CV, Kharat V, Blanck S, Leonard AC. Acute kidney injury after gastric bypass surgery. Clin J Am Soc Nephrol. 2007;2:426–30.
12. Cao L, Young N, Liu H, Silvestry S, Sun W, Zhao N, Diehl J, Sun J. Preoperative aspirin use and outcomes in cardiac surgery patients. Ann Surg. 2012;255(2):399–404.
13. Layton JB, Kshirsagar AV, Simpson Jr RJ, Pate V, Jonsson Funk M, Sturmer T, Brookhart MA. Effect of statin use on acute kidney injury following coronary artery bypass grafting. Am J Cardiol. 2013;111(6):823–8.
14. Brooks KR, Scarborough JE, Vaslef N, Shapiro L. No need to wait: an analysis of the timing of cholecystectomy during admission for acute cholecystitis using the American College of Surgeons National Surgical Quality Improvement Program database. J Trauma Acute Care Surg. 2013;74(1):167–73; 173–4.
15. Walsh M, Garg AX, Devereaux PJ, Argalious M, Honar H, Sessler DI. The association between perioperative hemoglobin and acute kidney injury in patients having noncardiac surgery. Anesth Analg. 2013;117(4):924–31.
16. Nigwekar SU, Kandula P, Hix JK, Thakar CV. Off-pump coronary artery bypass surgery and acute kidney injury: a meta-analysis of randomized and observational studies. Am J Kidney Dis. 2009;54(3):413–23.
17. Shroyer AL, Grover FL, Hattler B, Collins JF, McDonald GO, Kozora E, Lucke JC, Baltz JH, Novitzky D, Veterans Affairs Randomized On/Off Bypass (ROOBY) Study Group. On-pump versus off-pump coronary-artery bypass surgery. N Engl J Med. 2009;361:1827–37.
18. Moller CH, Perko MJ, Lund JT, et al. No major differences in 30-day outcomes in high-risk patients randomized to off-pump versus on pump coronary bypass surgery. The best bypass surgery trial. Circulation. 2010;121:498–504.
19. Sajja LR, Mannam G, Chakravarthi RM, Sompalli S, Naidu SK, Somaraju B, Penumatsa RR. Coronary artery bypass grafting with or without cardiopulmonary bypass in patients with preoperative non-dialysis dependent renal insufficiency: a randomized study. J Thorac Cardiovasc Surg. 2007;133(2):378–88.
20. Sinning JM, Werner N, Nickenig G, Grube E. Transcatheter aortic valve implantation: the evidence. Heart. 2012;98 Suppl 4:iv65–72.
21. Latib A, Maisano F, Bertoldi L, Giacomini A, Shannon J, Cioni M, Ielasi A, Figini F, Tagaki K, Franco A, Covello RD, Grimaldi A, Spagnolo P, Buchannan GL, Carlino M, Chieffo A, Montorfano M, Alfieri O, Colombo A. Transcatheter vs surgical aortic valve replacement in intermediate-surgical-risk patients with aortic stenosis: a propensity score-matched case-control study. Am Heart J. 2012;164(6):910–7.
22. Bagur R, Webb JG, Nietlispach F, Dumont E, De Larochelliere R, Doyle D, Masson JB, Gutierrez MJ, Clavel MA, Bertrand OF, Pibarot P, Rodes-Cabau J. Acute kidney injury following transcatheter aortic valve implantation: predictive factors, prognostic value, and comparison with surgical aortic valve replacement. Eur Heart J. 2010;31(7):865–74.
23. Giles KA, Hamdan AD, Pomposelli FB, Wyers MC, Dahlberg SE, Schermerhorn ML. Population-based outcomes following endovascular and open repair of ruptured abdominal aortic aneurysms. J Endovasc Ther. 2009;16(5):554–64.
24. Mehta M, Roddy SP, Darling 3rd RC, Ozsvath KJ, Kreienberg PB, Paty PS, Chang BB, Shah DM. Infrarenal abdominal aortic aneurysm repair via endovascular versus open retroperitoneal approach. Ann Vasc Surg. 2005;19(3):374–8.
25. Dangas G, O'Connor D, Firwana B, Brar S, Ellozy S, Vouyouka A, Arnold M, Kosmas CE, Krishnan P, Wiley J, Suleman J, Olin J, Marin M, Faries P. Open versus endovascular stent

graft repair of abdominal aortic aneurysms: a meta-analysis of randomized trials. JACC Cardiovasc Interv. 2012;5(10):1071–80.
26. Cheng D, Martin J, Shennib H, Dunning J, Muneretto C, Schueler S, Von Segesser L, Sergeant P, Turina M. Endovascular aortic repair versus open surgical repair for descending thoracic aortic disease a systematic review and meta-analysis of comparative studies. J Am Coll Cardiol. 2010;55(10):986–1001.
27. Greenblatt DY, Rajamanickam V, Pugely AJ, Heise CP, Foley EF, Kennedy GD. Short-term outcomes after laparoscopic-assisted proctectomy for rectal cancer: results from the ACS NSQIP. J Am Coll Surg. 2011;212(5):844–54.
28. Ishikawa S, Griesdale DEG, Lohser J. Acute kidney injury after lung resection surgery: incidence and perioperative risk factors. Anesth Analg. 2012;114(6):1256–62.
29. Kellum JA. Invited commentary. Crit Care Med. 2011;39(4):901–3.
30. Walsh M, Devereaux PJ, Garg AX, Kurz A, Turan A, Roseth RN, Cywinski J, Thabane L, Sessler DI. Relationship between intraoperative mean arterial pressure and clinical outcomes after noncardiac surgery. Anesthesiology. 2013;119(3):507–15.
31. Ono M, Arnaoutakis GJ, Fine DM, Brady K, Easly RB, Zheng Y, Brown C, Katz NM, Grams ME, Hogue CW. Blood pressure excursions below the cerebral autoregulation threshold during cardiac surgery are associated with acute kidney injury. Crit Care Med. 2013;41(2):464–71.
32. Rhee CJ, Kibler KK, Easley RB, Andropoulos DB, Czosnyka M, Smielewski P, Brady KM. Renovascular reactivity measured by near-infrared spectroscopy. J Appl Physiol. 2012;113(2):307–14.
33. Jhanji S, Vivian-Smith A, Lucena-Amaro S, Watson D, Hinds CJ, Pearse RM. Haemodynamic optimisation improves tissue microvascular flow and oxygenation after major surgery: a randomised controlled trial. Crit Care (Lond Engl). 2010;14(4):R151.
34. Hamilton MA, Cecconi M, Rhodes A. A systematic review and meta-analysis on the use of preemptive hemodynamic intervention to improve postoperative outcomes in moderate and high-risk surgical patients. Anesth Analg. 2011;112(6):1392–402.
35. Tobian AA, Ness PM, Noveck H, Carson JL. Time course and etiology of death in patients with severe anemia. Transfusion. 2009;49(7):1395–9.
36. Karkouti K, Wijeysundera DN, Yau TM, Callum JL, Cheng DC, Crowther M, Dupuis JY, Fremes SE, Kent B, Laflamme C, Lamy A, Legare JF, Mazer CD, McCluskey SA, Rubens FD, Sawchuk C, Beattie WS. Acute kidney injury after cardiac surgery: focus on modifiable risk factors. Circulation. 2009;119(4):495–502.
37. Karkouti K, Wijeysundera DN, Yau TM, McCluskey SA, Chan CT, Wong PY, Beattie WS. Influence of erythrocyte transfusion on the risk of acute kidney injury after cardiac surgery differs in anemic and nonanemic patients. Anesthesiology. 2011;115(3):523–30.
38. Shander A, Javidroozi M, Ozawa S, Hare GMT. What is really dangerous: anaemia or transfusion? Br J Anaesth. 2011;107(s1):i41–59.
39. Song YR, Lee T, You SJ, Chin HJ, Chae DW, Lim C, Park KH, Han S, Kim JH, Na KY. Prevention of acute kidney injury by erythropoietin in patients undergoing coronary artery bypass grafting: a pilot study. Am J Nephrol. 2009;30(3):253–60.
40. Yoo YC, Shim JK, Kim JC, Jo YY, Lee JH, Kwak YL. Effect of single recombinant human erythropoietin injection on transfusion requirements in preoperatively anemic patients undergoing valvular heart surgery. Anesthesiology. 2011;115(5):929–37.
41. Haase N, Perner A, Hennings LI, Siegemund M, Lauridsen B, Wetterslev M, Wetterslev J. Hydroxyethyl starch 130/0.38–0.45 versus crystalloid or albumin in patients with sepsis: systematic review with meta-analysis and trial sequential analysis. BMJ. 2013;346:f839.
42. Bayer O, Reinhart K, Sakr Y, Kabisch B, Kohl M, Riedemann NC, Bauer M, Settmacher U, Hekmat K, Hartog CS. Renal effects of synthetic colloids and crystalloids in patients with severe sepsis: a prospective sequential comparison. Crit Care Med. 2011;39(6):1335–42.
43. Mutter TC, Ruth CA, Dart AB. Hydroxyethyl starch (HES) versus other fluid therapies: effects on kidney function. Cochrane Database Syst Rev. 2013; (7):CD007594. doi:10.1002/14651858.CD007594.pub3.

44. Thiele RH, Huffmyer JL, Raphael J. Perioperative morbidity: lessons learned from recent clinical trials. Crit Care. 2012;18(4):358–65.
45. van den Berghe G, Wouters P, Weekers F, Verwaest C, Bruyninckx F, Schetz M, Vlasselaers D, Ferdinande P, Lauwers P, Bouillon R. Intensive insulin therapy in critically ill patients. N Engl J Med. 2001;345(19):1359–67.
46. Gandhi GY, Nuttall GA, Abel MD, Mullany CJ, Schaff HV, Williams BA, Schrader LM, Rizza RA, McMahon MM. Intraoperative hyperglycemia and perioperative outcomes in cardiac surgery patients. Mayo Clin Proc. 2005;80(7):862–6.
47. Lecomte P, Van Vlem B, Coddens J, Cammu G, Nollet G, Nobels F, Vanermen H, Foubert L. Tight perioperative glucose control is associated with a reduction in renal impairment and renal failure in non-diabetic cardiac surgical patients. Crit Care (Lond Engl). 2008;12(6):R154.
48. Bhamidipati CM, LaPar DJ, Stukenborg GJ, Morrison CC, Kem JA, Kron IL, Ailawadi G. Superiority of moderate control hyperglycemia to tight control in patients undergoing coronary artery bypass grafting. J Thorac Cardiovasc Surg. 2011;141:543–51.
49. Mangano DT, Tudor IC, Dietzel C. Multicenter study of perioperative ischemia research group. Ischemia research and education foundation. The risk associated with aprotinin in cardiac surgery. N Engl J Med. 2000;354(4):353–65.
50. Lassnigg A, Donner E, Grubhofer G, Presterl E, Druml W, Hiesmayr M. Lack of renoprotective effects of dopamine and furosemide during cardiac surgery. J Am Soc Nephrol. 2000;11(1):97–104.
51. Gandhi A, Husain M, Salhiyyah K, Raja SG. Does perioperative furosemide usage reduce the need for renal replacement therapy in cardiac surgery patients? Interact Cardiovasc Thorac Surg. 2012;15:750–5.
52. Cogliati AA, Vellutini R, Nardini A, Urovi S, Hamdan M, Landoni G, Guelfi P. Fenoldopam infusion for renal protection in high-risk cardiac surgery patients: a randomized clinical study. J Cardiothorac Vasc Anesth. 2007;21(6):847–50.
53. Ranucci M, Soro G, Barzaghi N, Locatelli A, Giordano G, Vavassori A, Manzato A, Melchiorri C, Bove T, Juliano G, Uslenghi MF. Fenoldopam prophylaxis of postoperative acute renal failure in high-risk cardiac surgery patients. Ann Thorac Surg. 2004;78(4):1332–7; discussion 1337–8.
54. Landoni G, Biondi-Zoccai GG, Tumlin JA, Bove T, De Luca M, Calabro MG, Ranucci M, Zangrillo A. Beneficial impact of fenoldopam in critically ill patients with or at risk for acute renal failure: a meta-analysis of randomized clinical trials. Am J Kidney Dis. 2007;49(1): 56–68.
55. Zangrillo A, Biondi-Zoccai GG, Frati E, Covello RD, Cabrini L, Guarracino F, Ruggeri L, Bove T, Bignami E, Landoni G. Fenoldopam and acute renal failure in cardiac surgery: a meta-analysis of randomized placebo-controlled trials. J Cardiothorac Vasc Anesth. 2012;26(3): 407–13.
56. Sward K, Valsson F, Odencrants P, Samuelsson O, Ricksten SE. Recombinant human atrial natriuretic peptide in ischemic acute renal failure: a randomized placebo-controlled trial. Crit Care Med. 2004;32(6):1310–5.
57. Nigwekar SU, Navaneethan SD, Parikh CR, Hix JK. Atrial natriuretic peptide for preventing and treating acute kidney injury. Cochrane Database Syst Rev. 2009;(4):CD006028
58. Mentzer Jr RM, Oz MC, Sladen RN, Graeve AH, Hebeler Jr RF, Luber Jr JM, Smedira NG, NAPA Investigators. Effects of perioperative nesiritide in patients with left ventricular dysfunction undergoing cardiac surgery: the NAPA Trial. J Am Coll Cardiol. 2007;49(6): 716–26.
59. Ejaz AA, Martin TD, Johnson RJ, Winterstein AG, Klodell CT, Hess Jr PJ, Ali AK, Whidden EM, Staples NL, Alexander JA, House-Fancher MA, Beaver TM. Prophylactic nesiritide does not prevent dialysis or all-cause mortality in patients undergoing high-risk cardiac surgery. J Thorac Cardiovasc Surg. 2009;138(4):959–64.
60. Ho KM, Morgan DJ. Meta-analysis of N-acetylcysteine to prevent acute renal failure after major surgery. Am J Kidney Dis. 2009;53(1):33–40.

61. Moore NN, Lapsley M, Norden AG, Firth JD, Gaunt ME, Varty K, Boyle JR. Does N-acetylcysteine prevent contrast-induced nephropathy during endovascular AAA repair? A randomized controlled pilot study. J Endovasc Ther. 2006;13(5):660–6.
62. Hilmi IA, Peng Z, Planinsic RM, Damian D, Dai F, Tyurina YY, Kagan VE, Kellum JA. N-acetylcysteine does not prevent hepatorenal ischaemia-reperfusion injury in patients undergoing orthotopic liver transplantation. Nephrol Dial Transplant. 2010;25(7):2328–33.
63. Szakmany T, Hauser B, Radermacher P. N-acetylcysteine for sepsis and systemic inflammatory response in adults. Cochrane Database Syst Rev. 2012;(9):CD006616. doi:10.1002/14651858.CD006616.pub2.
64. Ghosh S, Arthur B, Klein AA. NICE guidance on CardioQ(TM) oesophageal Doppler monitoring. Anaesthesia. 2011;66:1081–3.
65. Bandyopadhyay S, Kumar Das R, Paul A, Sundar Bhunia K, Roy D. A transesophageal echocardiography technique to locate the kidney and monitor renal perfusion. Anesth Analg. 2013;116(3):549–54.
66. Owens GE, King K, Gurney JG, Charpie JR. Low renal oximetry correlates with acute kidney injury after infant cardiac surgery. Pediatr Cardiol. 2011;32(2):183–8.
67. Josephs SA, Thakar CV. Perioperative risk assessment, prevention, and treatment of acute kidney injury. Int Anesthesiol Clin. 2009;47(4):89–105.
68. Borthwick E, Ferguson A. Perioperative acute kidney injury: risk factors, recognition, management, and outcomes. BMJ. 2010;341:c3365.
69. Thakar CV. Perioperative acute kidney injury. Adv Chronic Kidney Dis. 2013;20(1):67–75.
70. Kheterpal S, et al. Development and validation of an acute kidney injury risk index for patients undergoing general surgery: results from a national data set. Anesthesiology. 2009;110(3):505–15.

Part II
Cardiac and Vascular Surgery

Chapter 7
Acute Kidney Injury After Cardiac Surgery in Adults

Jeremiah R. Brown and Chirag R. Parikh

Objectives

- To describe definition and epidemiology of AKI
- To understand risk factors for AKI and prediction scores
- To discuss prevention and management of AKI

Introduction

Cardiac surgery-associated acute kidney injury (CSA-AKI) has been recognized as a frequent adverse event following cardiac surgery [1–4]. CSA-AKI has nearly doubled over the past decade [5] and strongly associated with increased morbidity, mortality, and length of hospitalization [1–4, 6]. When AKI occurs in the hospital, the approximate additional costs in health-care expenditures amount to $7,500 [7], making AKI a costly complication and an important target for prevention.

J.R. Brown, PhD, MS (✉)
The Dartmouth Institute for Health Policy and Clinical Practice,
and the Departments of Medicine and Community and Family Medicine,
Audrey and Theodore Geisel School of Medicine at Dartmouth, HB 7505 DHMC One Medical Center Drive, Lebanon, NH 03756, USA
e-mail: jbrown@dartmouth.edu

C.R. Parikh, MD, PhD, FASN
Program of Applied Translational Research, Department of Medicine,
Yale University School of Medicine, New Haven, CT, USA
e-mail: chirag.parikh@yale.edu

C.V. Thakar, C.R. Parikh (eds.), *Perioperative Kidney Injury: Principles of Risk Assessment, Diagnosis and Treatment*, DOI 10.1007/978-1-4939-1273-5_7

AKI Epidemiology

AKI is thought to develop as a result of extended cardiopulmonary bypass pump times with paralleled hypoperfusion and reduced oxygen saturation delivery to critical organs including the brain and kidneys.

Common definitions for diagnosing AKI in cardiac surgery have included: the Society for Thoracic Surgeons (STS); the Acute Dialysis Quality Initiative Workgroup for risk, injury, failure, loss, and end-stage kidney disease (RIFLE) criteria [8]; and the Acute Kidney Injury Network (AKIN) [9] definition (Table 7.1). In addition, the duration of AKI using the AKIN definition has also been evaluated as a more sensitive and specific measure of AKI severity after general surgery [10] and cardiac surgery [2].

In cardiac surgery, even small changes in serum creatinine have been associated with poor survivorship [1] and progression of chronic kidney disease and end-stage renal disease [11]. AKI after cardiac surgery has been associated with more rapid progression to incident chronic kidney disease (CKD), progressive CKD, and renal failure (dialysis or kidney transplant) [11]. This evidence suggests that there is a direct correlation between the degree of acute injury to the kidneys during the perioperative period and long-term progression of worsening renal function.

Others have confirmed this phenomenon in other patient populations demonstrating the increase risk of progression to end-stage renal disease (ESRD) and mortality [12–14]. Therefore, patients developing perioperative AKI are at risk for progressing towards worsening renal function and should be monitored following the perioperative period to prevent unnoticed rapid progression to renal failure.

Table 7.1 Incidence of AKI following cardiovascular surgery across AKI definitions

Author	*N*	Year of study	Country	AKI definition	Incidence (%)
Brown [1]	1,391	2001	USA	Scr rise >25 %	27.8
				Scr rise>50 %	11.7
				Scr rise >100 %	4.7
Conlon [65]	2,843	1995–1997	USA	Scr rise >1 mg/dL	7.9
Lassnigg [4]	4,118	2001	Austria	Scr rise >0.5 mg/dL	4.9
Andersson [66]	2,009	1987–1990	Sweden	Scr rise>50 %	16.4
Karkouti [16]	3,500	2004	Canada	Scr rise >25 %	24
				Scr rise >25 %	37.4
Parikh [51]	1,219	2007–2009	USA	Scr rise >100 %	4.9
				Scr rise by 0.3 mg/dL or 50 %	35.2
Brown [2, 35]	4,831	2002–2007	USA	Scr rise by 0.3 or 50 %	39.3
Brown [34]	8,592	2001–2005	USA	eGFR fall by >30 %	2.7
Thakar[a][67]	22,589	1993–2000	USA	GFR fall by >50 %	4.9
Thakar[a][43]	31,677	1993–2002	USA	GFR fall by >30 %	17.4

Abbreviations: *AKI* acute kidney injury, *Scr* serum creatinine, *GFR* glomerular filtration rate, *eGFR* estimate glomerular filtration rate

[a]Patients in cohorts overlap

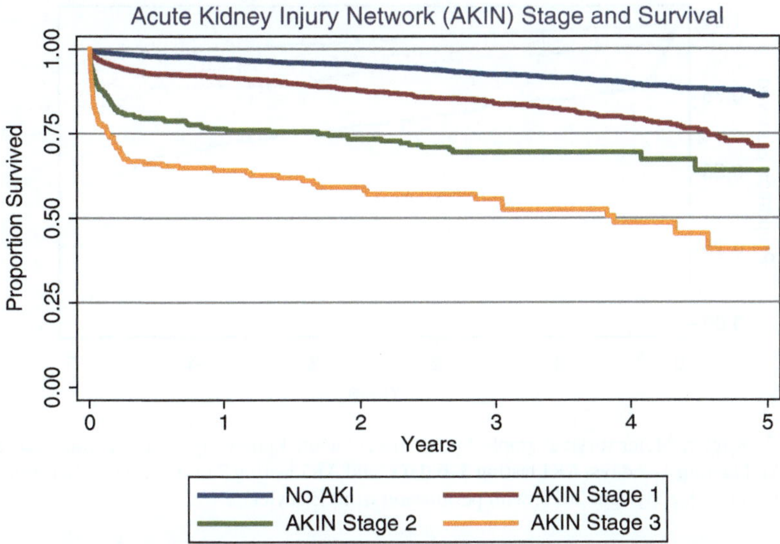

Fig. 7.1 Kaplan-Meier survival graph for cardiac surgery patients by Acute Kidney Injury Network (*AKIN*) stages: no AKI (*blue*), AKIN stage 1 (*red*), AKIN stage 2 (*green*), and AKIN stage 3 or renal failure (*yellow*) (Reprinted by permission of Oxford University Press from Brown and Parikh [68])

The Northern New England Cardiovascular Disease Study Group (NNECDSG, www.nnecdsg.org) has reported on the poor survivorship-associated perioperative changes in serum creatinine [1] and longer durations of AKI [15]. The early findings demonstrated that subtle changes in serum creatinine were directly proportional to increased 90-day mortality [1]. The association between AKIN stages of AKI and survival is consistent with the earlier reports of changes in serum creatinine (Fig. 7.1). More recently, NNECDSG AKI researchers and Translational Research Investigating Biomarker End-Points in Acute Kidney Injury (TRIBE-AKI) investigators jointly evaluated the role of the duration of AKI as a marker for AKI severity and demonstrated the proportionality associated with longer durations of AKI and worse survival (Fig. 7.2). Over 18 % of patients developed AKI for 1–2 days, 11 % for 3–6 days, and 9 % for 7 or more days. AKI duration categories were directly proportional to in-hospital dialysis rates (0.2, 0.5, and 7.2 %) as well as 5-year mortality (13.7, 17.5, and 36.9 %, respectively). These figures demonstrate the severe consequences patients face with the development of AKI and moderate or severe AKI.

Etiology Risk Factors and Prediction of AKI

AKI is postulated to result from various patient and procedural factors. Patient factors include many of the risk factors used the prediction modeling described previously (age, gender, baseline renal function, heart failure, and diabetes).

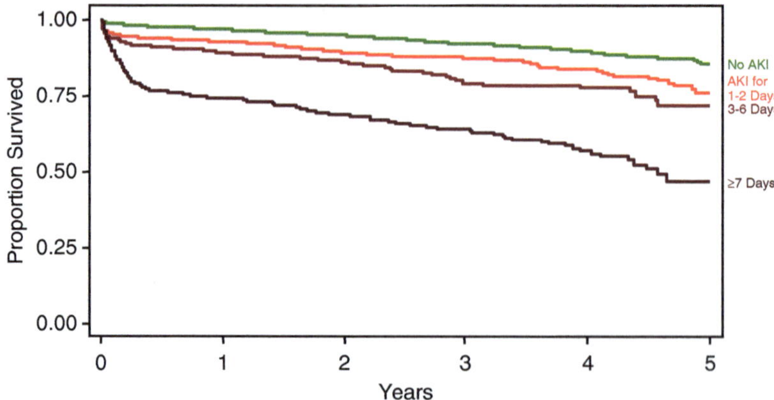

Fig. 7.2 Kaplan-Meier survival graphs by duration of acute kidney injury after cardiac surgery: no AKI, AKI lasting 1–2 days, AKI lasting 3–6 days, and AKI lasting 7 or more days (Reprinted from Brown et al. [2], copyright 2010, with permission from Elsevier)

Preoperative anemia (hemoglobin <14) has also been shown to have an inverse relationship with AKI, whereby each successive drop in hemoglobin under 14 (g/dL) increases the risk of postoperative AKI by 23 % for hemoglobin between 12 and 13.9 (g/dL), by 63 % for hemoglobin 10–11.9 (g/dL), and by 99 % for hemoglobin <10 (g/dL) [16].

Before the patient arrives to the operating room for cardiac surgery, it is most likely the patient has had a recent angiography, or cardiac catheterization. These procedures usually use small amounts of low-osmolar or iso-osmolar contrast; however, sometimes an ad hoc angioplasty (percutaneous coronary intervention, PCI) is performed and stents implanted in the coronary arteries to reestablish or sustain blood flow. During a PCI, larger, and potentially dangerous, volumes of contrast dye are injected to visualize the coronary arteries for the deployment of the devices and stents. It is during this time that patients are likely to develop contrast-induced AKI resulting from acute tubular necrosis and oxidative stress. It has been shown that there is a direct relationship between the dose of contrast and AKI [17, 18]. Others have demonstrated there is direct relationship between the timing of the cardiac catheterization and cardiac surgery, whereby the risk of AKI is higher among patients undergoing cardiac surgery within 24 h of a cardiac catheterization [19–22] with direct ties to the amount of contrast used [19, 20]. In addition, others have reported if the cardiac catheterization was conducted during the same admission as cardiac surgery (including in-patient transfers), the risk of AKI is increased by 54 % [23].

There are several operative factors that should be considered. Cardiopulmonary bypass (pump time) contributes to the development of AKI [1, 16]. Off-pump cardiac surgery has been shown to reduce the incidence of AKI [24, 25]; however, caution should be taken to only incorporate off-pump cardiac surgery as a protective measure against AKI among proficient off-pump surgeons, and the risk-benefit should be weighed against the risk of incomplete revascularization and bleeding [26]. During cardiopulmonary bypass, gaseous or particulate emboli, renal ischemia from hypoperfusion of the kidneys, and myoglobinuria and free hemoglobinuria are proposed causes of AKI [27]. It is thought that the cardiopulmonary bypass pump may result in an imbalance in O_2 supply due to low hematocrit and the need for O_2 by the kidneys. When the O_2 is <260 mL/min/m^2, it can increase lactate levels and increase the risk of AKI. O_2 delivery can be optimized by coupling the pump flow with the hematocrit [28–30]. To counteract these causes, cardiac surgeons and perfusionists have worked together to improve cardiopulmonary bypass management through temperature and blood pressure management and development of mechanisms and filtering devices to reduce gaseous micro-emboli and optimize O_2 delivery through improving the flow rate, hemoglobin levels, and hemodilution [27].

The number of perioperative packed red blood cell (pRBCs) has a direct linear dose-response to the risk of developing AKI. Stored red blood cells have been shown to deteriorate after being frozen and stored for weeks at a lime. It has been demonstrated that these red blood cells develop specula and lose the biconcave disc shape causing inflexibility to travel through the capillaries and result in capillary damage and reduced microcirculation [31]. Others have shown that patients receiving newer blood (pRBC stored for ≤ 14 days) had significantly better survival and a lower incidence of renal failure than patients receiving pRBC transfusions that was stored for more than 14 days [32]. A similar effect was reported in pediatric cardiac surgery for AKI whereby AKI was reduced by 4.4 % [30].

In Table 7.2, we summarize the various etiologies of factors contributing to cardiac surgery-associated AKI in adults including patient factors, medication,

Table 7.2 Factors of cardiac surgery-associated with acute kidney injury

Patient	Medication	Prior procedures	Procedure
Advanced age	NSAIDs	Contrast dye volume	Cardiopulmonary bypass
Female gender	ACE	Contrast agent	Pump times >120 min
Diabetes	ARB	Timing from cardiac catheterization and surgery	Volume of fluids on bypass
Hypertension		Sepsis	Hypotension
Obesity		Endotoxins	Emboli
Albuminuria		Preoperative AKI	IABP
Chronic kidney disease		IABP	Low output failure
Congestive heart failure		Prior cardiac surgery	Reoperation
Peripheral vascular disease		RBC units	Return to bypass during procedure
Anemia			RBC
Inflammation			Nadir hematocrit on bypass
White blood cell count >12,000			Ultrafiltration
Rhabdomyolysis			Use of inotropes
Myoglobin			Warm cardioplegia
			Reperfusion injury
			Change in mean arterial pressure >=26 (mm Hg)
			Oxygen delivery (DO_2) <262 (mL/min/m2)

Reprinted from Huen and Parikh [48], copyright 2012 with permission from Elsevier
NSAIDs nonsteroidal antiinflammatory drugs, *ACE* angiotensin-converting enzyme, *ARB* angiotensin receptor blockers, *DO_2* oxygen delivery = pump flow (hemoglobin $\times 1.3 \times O_2$ saturation $+ 0.003 \times pO_2$) [1, 2, 28, 33–40]

in-hospital and prior procedural risks, as well as cardiac surgery procedural risk factors [1, 2, 28, 33–40].

Identifying risk factors for AKI and establishing prediction models are necessary to risk-stratify patients before, during, and immediately after cardiac surgery. However, most of the prediction modeling efforts have investigated the ability of patient and procedural risk factors to predict the occurrence of renal failure [41–44]. These models have also performed well for predicting severe AKI using the STS definitional of acute renal failure, defined as a 2.0 mg/dL or twofold increase in serum creatinine or new dialysis [42–45]. Yet, other investigators have developed models in predicting immediate postoperative declines in creatinine clearance (CrCl) or estimate glomerular filtration rate (eGFR) [34, 46, 47]. One example is the NNECDSG's approach to predict at least a 30 mL/min/m2 drop in eGFR among patients with normal or near-normal renal function (eGFR ≥60) [34]. Recent investigations have incorporated additional perioperative risk factors from the procedure and complications from the procedure as an attempt to improve the prediction of AKI and duration of AKI. There are various risk factors utilized in the prediction modeling for renal failure and AKI. Major similarities among the models include: age, gender, baseline renal function, heart failure, diabetes, use of intra-aortic balloon pump, and duration on cardiopulmonary bypass (Table 7.3) [48]. Other models to predict renal replacement therapy after cardiac surgery include the Cleveland Clinic score [43], Mehta score [42], and Simplified Renal Index score [44] with external validation [45, 49].

Another approach to predicting the severity of AKI focused on predicting the length of time, or duration, of the acute injury. The duration of AKI was modeled to predict the average projected number of days a patient may sustain AKI and is published as an online risk calculator (http://medicine.yale.edu/intmed/patr/resources/akicalc.aspx). This can be a useful way to determine a patient's risk and length, or duration, or AKI after cardiac surgery. If the duration is projected to be longer than 3 days, a nephrology consult on admission to the ICU may be helpful in preventing the onset of AKI and minimize the duration.

Novel biomarkers have the ability to improve our prediction of AKI events and provide earlier detection. Several biomarkers have been rigorously investigated including plasma cystatin C, urinary neutrophil gelatinase-associated lipocalin (NGAL), urinary interleukin 18 (IL-18), N-acetyl-B-(D)-glucosaminidase (NAG), alpha-1 microglobulin, albuminuria, and urinary kidney injury molecule 1 (KIM-1) [50–53]. The TRIBE-AKI Consortium released evidence that supports the use of serum creatinine and cystatin C in determining risk of AKI prior to cardiac surgery; this was found to be true among all patients and more so for predicting severe AKI [53]. In cardiac surgery, TRIBE also demonstrated the clinical utility of postoperative kidney biomarkers, including plasma NGAL and urinary IL-18 and NGAL. They reported that urinary IL-18 had superior prediction for AKI over plasma or urinary NGAL [51]. A small study of 103 subjects by Liangos and colleagues reported that KIM-1, NAG, NGAL, and IL-18 significantly predicted AKI at 2 h after cardiopulmonary bypass; however, after adjustment for the preoperative Cleveland Clinic Foundation score for acute renal failure and/or cardiopulmonary bypass time, only KIM-1 remained statistically significant [50]. Albuminuria

Table 7.3 Variables included in the models

	Variable	CICSS	Cleveland	STS	SRI	McSPI	AKICS	NNECDSG
Demographics	Age			X		X	X	X
	Gender		X					X
	Race			X				
Clinical	Preoperative renal insufficiency	X	X	X	X	X	X	
	Prior heart surgery	X	X	X	X			X
	Advanced NYHA	X		X			X	
	Congestive heart failure		X			X		X
	Decreased ejection fraction		X		X			
	Cardiomegaly	X						
	Pulse pressure					X		
	Hypertension							X
	PVD/CVD	X						X
	COPD/chronic lung disease		X	X				
	Diabetes mellitus		X	X	X			X
	Preoperative capillary glucose >140						X	
	MI within last 3 weeks			X				
	Prior MI					X		
	Reoperation							
	Preoperative IABP	X	X		X			X
	Emergent surgery		X		X			
	Cardiogenic shock			X				
	Preoperative WBC >12,000							X
Surgery type	Valvular surgery	X	X	X				
	CAPG + valve		X	X			X	
	Other cardiac procedures		X		X			
Inoperative	Increased CPB time					X	X	
	>2 inotropes					X		
	Intraoperative IABP					X		
Postoperative	CVP >14 cm H_2O						X	
	Low cardiac output						X	

Adapted from Huen and Parikh [48]

AKICS acute kidney injury after cardiac surgery, *CAPG* coronary artery bypass graft, *CICSS* Continuous Improvement in Cardiac Surgery Study, *COPD* chronic obstructive pulmonary disease, *CPB* cardiopulmonary bypass, *CVD* cardiovascular disease, *CVP* central venous pressure, *IABP* intra-aortic balloon pump, *McSPI* Multicenter Study of Perioperative Ischemia, *MI* myocardial infarction, *NNECDSG* Northern New England Cardiovascular Disease Study Group, *NYHA* New York Heart Association Functional Classification, *PVD* peripheral vascular disease, *SRI* Simplified Renal Index, *WBC* white blood cell count is a predictive marker for the development of AKI [54–58]. An increase in the ratio between urinary albumin and creatinine has been demonstrated to improve preoperative risk prediction of AKI suggesting the addition of albuminuria to preoperative risk assessment for AKI [57, 59]. KIM-1 and other markers such as L-type fatty acid-binding protein and alpha-1 microglobulin need further large-scale clinical trial investigations.

Prevention and Management of AKI

A systematic review summarized the interventions to prevent AKI that have been evaluated with mixed efficacy in cardiac surgery. Interventions have included anti-inflammatory (N-acetylcysteine, glutathione, fenoldopam, aspirin, dexamethasone, methylprednisolone, and leukodepletion), natriuretics/diuretics (nesiritide, A-type natriuretic peptide [ANP], furosemide, urodilatin, and mannitol), vasodilators (prostaglandin E1 [PGE1], diltiazem, dopexamine, dopamine [DA], mannitol, fenoldopam, angiotensin-converting enzyme (ACE) inhibitor, sodium nitroprusside, theophylline, and prostacyclin), operative techniques (mostly off pump), prophylactic continuous venovenous hemodiafiltration or renal replacement therapy, and other strategies (albumin, insulin, clonidine, and volume expansion) [25]. Park and colleagues concluded that most of the prophylactic strategies conducted prior to cardiac surgery were protective against AKI; these included ANP/nesiritide, fenoldopam, and dopamine [25].

Ischemic preconditioning prior to cardiac surgery may be an alternative prophylactic method to reduce AKI. By preconditioning a remote site in the body (arm or leg) to reduced blood flow, reperfusion injury and AKI may be prevented [60, 61]. Zimmerman and colleagues demonstrated in a small single-center randomized trial that ischemic preconditioning resulting in an absolute risk reduction of 0.27 (12 versus 28 AKI events, $p = 0.004$) and resulted in lower rates of sustained AKI at 2 or more days [61]. It is likely that simple ischemic preconditioning methods could be incorporated at the time of entry to the operating room (OR) and may not only assist in AKI event reduction but also reduce myocardial reperfusion injury.

We have summarized the clinical research that has sought to mitigate AKI in the context of cardiac surgery. Some of these interventions have demonstrated consistency in prevention, while others either need more investigation or the development of new strategies. Most of these efforts have focused around modifying or discontinuing potentially nephrotoxic medication or exposure to nephrotoxins, such as radiocontrast dye. McCoy and colleagues reported on the single-center use of a computerized medication safety tool designed for patients developing AKI. Through the use of this automated intervention tool, 52.6 % of the time potentially nephrotoxic medications were halted or modified within 24 h of an acute increase in serum creatinine qualifying as AKI, a 49 % improvement prior to the intervention [62]. Additional simple and sophisticated process tools should be developed by multidisciplinary teams to study the problem of AKI. When doing so, teams should identify

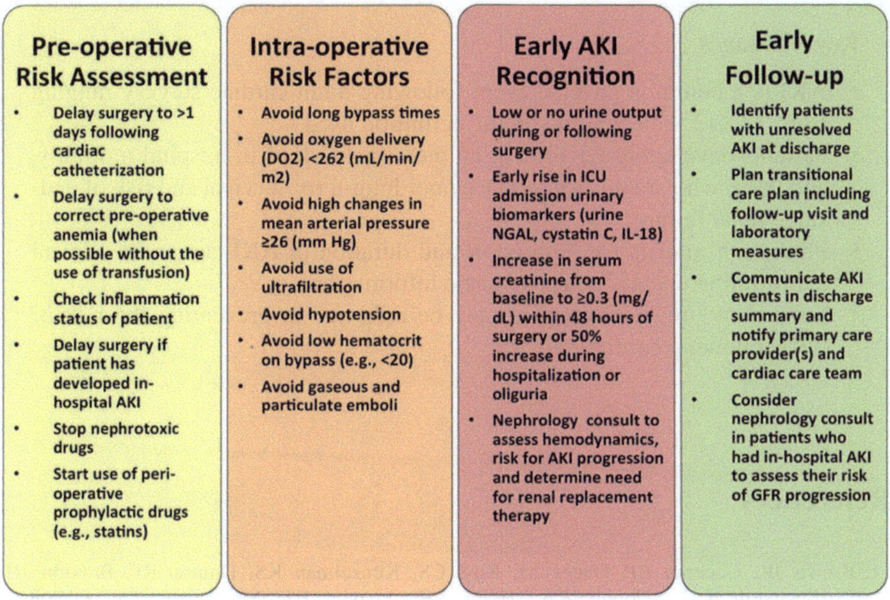

Pre-operative Risk Assessment

- Delay surgery to >1 days following cardiac catheterization
- Delay surgery to correct pre-operative anemia (when possible without the use of transfusion)
- Check inflammation status of patient
- Delay surgery if patient has developed in-hospital AKI
- Stop nephrotoxic drugs
- Start use of peri-operative prophylactic drugs (e.g., statins)

Intra-operative Risk Factors

- Avoid long bypass times
- Avoid oxygen delivery (DO2) <262 (mL/min/m2)
- Avoid high changes in mean arterial pressure ≥26 (mm Hg)
- Avoid use of ultrafiltration
- Avoid hypotension
- Avoid low hematocrit on bypass (e.g., <20)
- Avoid gaseous and particulate emboli

Early AKI Recognition

- Low or no urine output during or following surgery
- Early rise in ICU admission urinary biomarkers (urine NGAL, cystatin C, IL-18)
- Increase in serum creatinine from baseline to ≥0.3 (mg/dL) within 48 hours of surgery or 50% increase during hospitalization or oliguria
- Nephrology consult to assess hemodynamics, risk for AKI progression and determine need for renal replacement therapy

Early Follow-up

- Identify patients with unresolved AKI at discharge
- Plan transitional care plan including follow-up visit and laboratory measures
- Communicate AKI events in discharge summary and notify primary care provider(s) and cardiac care team
- Consider nephrology consult in patients who had in-hospital AKI to assess their risk of GFR progression

Fig. 7.3 AKI risk assessment algorithm

targets for intervention, test those interventions, evaluate their effectiveness, and redesign continually. Such microsystem-level improvement efforts are known as PDSA cycles of change (Plan-Do-Study-Act) [63, 64].

Conclusions

In this chapter, we have discussed the mortality, subsequent health-care costs, utilization, and morbidity that follow subtle changes in serum creatinine known as AKI in the perioperative setting of cardiac surgery. The field has come a long way from 10 years ago where subtle changes in serum creatinine were often ignored to the current volume of research and dedication that has identified and sought solutions for the patient safety issues surrounding cardiac surgery-associated AKI. We provide an algorithm to aid clinical care teams to identify pre- and perioperative modifiable risk factors to minimize the aid in the prevention of cardiac surgery-associated AKI and recommendations for early AKI recognition and follow-up (Fig. 7.3). Majority of the recommendations are based on epidemiologic observations or quality control protocols and require confirmation in interventional trials. In the near future, novel kidney injury biomarkers and risk tools will be available to identify early signs of AKI and acute tubular necrosis and hopefully matched with aggressive tools for medication adjustment and injury-specific interventions to mitigate AKI and its subsequent morbidity and mortality.

Key Messages

- AKI is a common adverse event following adult cardiac surgery ranging from 3 to 42 % depending on the definition used.
- Patients developing AKI are at an increased risk of in-hospital mortality, and those who are discharged face poor long-term survival and risk of end-stage renal failure.
- Prediction models for both onset and duration of AKI can assist clinical teams in therapeutic and prognostic information.
- Several modifiable strategies may be effective in preventing the risk of AKI following cardiac surgery.

References

1. Brown JR, Cochran RP, Dacey LJ, Ross CS, Kunzelman KS, Dunton RF, Braxton JH, Charlesworth DC, Clough RA, Helm RE, Leavitt BJ, Mackenzie TA, O'Connor GT. Perioperative increases in serum creatinine are predictive of increased 90-day mortality after coronary artery bypass graft surgery. Circulation. 2006;114:I409–13.
2. Brown JR, Kramer RS, Coca SG, Parikh CR. Duration of acute kidney injury impacts long-term survival after cardiac surgery. Ann Thorac Surg. 2010;90:1142–8.
3. Hobson CE, Yavas S, Segal MS, Schold JD, Tribble CG, Layon AJ, Bihorac A. Acute kidney injury is associated with increased long-term mortality after cardiothoracic surgery. Circulation. 2009;119:2444–53.
4. Lassnigg A, Schmid ER, Hiesmayr M, Falk C, Druml W, Bauer P, Schmidlin D. Impact of minimal increases in serum creatinine on outcome in patients after cardiothoracic surgery: do we have to revise current definitions of acute renal failure? Crit Care Med. 2008;36:1129–37.
5. Lenihan CR, Montez-Rath ME, Mora Mangano CT, Chertow GM, Winkelmayer WC. Trends in acute kidney injury, associated use of dialysis, and mortality after cardiac surgery, 1999 to 2008. Ann Thorac Surg. 2013;95:20–8.
6. Waikar SS, Liu KD, Chertow GM. Diagnosis, epidemiology and outcomes of acute kidney injury. Clin J Am Soc Nephrol. 2008;3:844–61.
7. Chertow GM, Burdick E, Honour M, Bonventre JV, Bates DW. Acute kidney injury, mortality, length of stay, and costs in hospitalized patients. J Am Soc Nephrol. 2005;16:3365–70.
8. Bellomo R, Ronco C, Kellum JA, Mehta RL, Palevsky P. Acute renal failure – definition, outcome measures, animal models, fluid therapy and information technology needs: the second international consensus conference of the acute dialysis quality initiative (adqi) group. Crit Care (London, England). 2004;8:R204–12.
9. Mehta RL, Kellum JA, Shah SV, Molitoris BA, Ronco C, Warnock DG, Levin A. Acute kidney injury network: report of an initiative to improve outcomes in acute kidney injury. Crit Care (London, England). 2007;11:R31.
10. Coca SG, King Jr JT, Rosenthal RA, Perkal MF, Parikh CR. The duration of postoperative acute kidney injury is an additional parameter predicting long-term survival in diabetic veterans. Kidney Int. 2010;78:926–33.
11. Ishani A, Nelson D, Clothier B, Schult T, Nugent S, Greer N, Slinin Y, Ensrud KE. The magnitude of acute serum creatinine increase after cardiac surgery and the risk of chronic kidney disease, progression of kidney disease, and death. Arch Intern Med. 2011;171:226–33.

12. Amdur RL, Chawla LS, Amodeo S, Kimmel PL, Palant CE. Outcomes following diagnosis of acute renal failure in U.S. Veterans: focus on acute tubular necrosis. Kidney Int. 2009;76:1089–97.
13. Ishani A, Xue JL, Himmelfarb J, Eggers PW, Kimmel PL, Molitoris BA, Collins AJ. Acute kidney injury increases risk of ESRD among elderly. J Am Soc Nephrol. 2009;20:223–8.
14. James MT, Ghali WA, Knudtson ML, Ravani P, Tonelli M, Faris P, Pannu N, Manns BJ, Klarenbach SW, Hemmelgarn BR. Associations between acute kidney injury and cardiovascular and renal outcomes after coronary angiography. Circulation. 2011;123:409–16.
15. Brown JR, O'Connor GT. Coronary heart disease and prevention in the United States. N Engl J Med. 2010;362:2150–3.
16. Karkouti K, Wijeysundera DN, Yau TM, Callum JL, Cheng DC, Crowther M, Dupuis JY, Fremes SE, Kent B, Laflamme C, Lamy A, Legare JF, Mazer CD, McCluskey SA, Rubens FD, Sawchuk C, Beattie WS. Acute kidney injury after cardiac surgery: focus on modifiable risk factors. Circulation. 2009;119:495–502.
17. Brown JR, Robb JF, Block CA, Schoolwerth AC, Kaplan AV, O'Connor GT, Solomon RJ, Malenka DJ. Does safe dosing of iodinated contrast prevent contrast-induced acute kidney injury? Circ Cardiovasc Interv. 2010;3:346–50.
18. Marenzi G, Assanelli E, Campodonico J, Lauri G, Marana I, De Metrio M, Moltrasio M, Grazi M, Rubino M, Veglia F, Fabbiocchi F, Bartorelli AL. Contrast volume during primary percutaneous coronary intervention and subsequent contrast-induced nephropathy and mortality. Ann Intern Med. 2009;150:170–7.
19. Hennessy SA, LaPar DJ, Stukenborg GJ, Stone ML, Mlynarek RA, Kern JA, Ailawadi G, Kron IL. Cardiac catheterization within 24 hours of valve surgery is significantly associated with acute renal failure. J Thorac Cardiovasc Surg. 2010;140:1011–7.
20. Medalion B, Cohen H, Assali A, Vaknin Assa H, Farkash A, Snir E, Sharoni E, Biderman P, Milo G, Battler A, Kornowski R, Porat E. The effect of cardiac angiography timing, contrast media dose, and preoperative renal function on acute renal failure after coronary artery bypass grafting. J Thorac Cardiovasc Surg. 2010;139:1539–44.
21. Ranucci M, Ballotta A, Kunkl A, De Benedetti D, Kandil H, Conti D, Mollichelli N, Bossone E, Mehta RH. Influence of the timing of cardiac catheterization and the amount of contrast media on acute renal failure after cardiac surgery. Am J Cardiol. 2008;101:1112–8.
22. Del Duca D, Iqbal S, Rahme E, Goldberg P, de Varennes B. Renal failure after cardiac surgery: timing of cardiac catheterization and other perioperative risk factors. Ann Thorac Surg. 2007;84:1264–71.
23. Kramer RS, Quinn RD, Groom RC, Braxton JH, Malenka DJ, Kellett MA, Brown JR. Same admission cardiac catheterization and cardiac surgery: is there an increased incidence of acute kidney injury? Ann Thorac Surg. 2010;90:1418–23; discussion 1423–4.
24. Kuss O, von Salviati B, Borgermann J. Off-pump versus on-pump coronary artery bypass grafting: a systematic review and meta-analysis of propensity score analyses. J Thorac Cardiovasc Surg. 2010;140:829–35, 835 e821–3.
25. Park M, Coca SG, Nigwekar SU, Garg AX, Garwood S, Parikh CR. Prevention and treatment of acute kidney injury in patients undergoing cardiac surgery: a systematic review. Am J Nephrol. 2010;31:408–18.
26. Puskas JD, Williams WH, Mahoney EM, Huber PR, Block PC, Duke PG, Staples JR, Glas KE, Marshall JJ, Leimbach ME, McCall SA, Petersen RJ, Bailey DE, Weintraub WS, Guyton RA. Off-pump vs conventional coronary artery bypass grafting: early and 1-year graft patency, cost, and quality-of-life outcomes: a randomized trial. JAMA. 2004;291:1841–9.
27. Kaplan JA, Reich DL, Lake CL, Konstadt SN. Organ protection during cardiopulmonary bypass. In: Kaplan's cardiac anesthesia. 5th ed. Philadelphia: Saunders; 2006. p. 996–1033.
28. Ranucci M, Romitti F, Isgro G, Cotza M, Brozzi S, Boncilli A, Ditta A. Oxygen delivery during cardiopulmonary bypass and acute renal failure after coronary operations. Ann Thorac Surg. 2005;80:2213–20.
29. Ranucci M. Perioperative renal failure: hypoperfusion during cardiopulmonary bypass? Semin Cardiothorac Vasc Anesth. 2007;11:265–8.

30. Ranucci M, Isgro G, Carlucci C, De La Torre T, Enginoli S, Frigiola A. Central venous oxygen saturation and blood lactate levels during cardiopulmonary bypass are associated with outcome after pediatric cardiac surgery. Crit Care. 2010;14:R149.
31. Walter R, Mark M, Gaudenz R, Harris LG, Reinhart WH. Influence of nitrovasodilators and endothelin-1 on rheology of human blood in vitro. Br J Pharmacol. 1999;128:744–50.
32. Koch CG, Li L, Sessler DI, Figueroa P, Hoeltge GA, Mihaljevic T, Blackstone EH. Duration of red-cell storage and complications after cardiac surgery. N Engl J Med. 2008;358:1229–39.
33. Benedetto U, Angeloni E, Luciani R, Refice S, Stefanelli M, Comito C, Roscitano A, Sinatra R. Acute kidney injury after coronary artery bypass grafting: does rhabdomyolysis play a role? J Thorac Cardiovasc Surg. 2010;140:464–70.
34. Brown JR, Cochran RP, Leavitt BJ, Dacey LJ, Ross CS, MacKenzie TA, Kunzelman KS, Kramer RS, Hernandez Jr F, Helm RE, Westbrook BM, Dunton RF, Malenka DJ, O'Connor GT. Multivariable prediction of renal insufficiency developing after cardiac surgery. Circulation. 2007;116:I139–43.
35. Brown JR, Kramer RS, MacKenzie TA, Coca SG, Sint K, Parikh CR. Determinants of acute kidney injury duration after cardiac surgery: an externally validated tool. Ann Thorac Surg. 2012;93:570–6.
36. de Somer F, Mulholland JW, Bryan MR, Aloisio T, Van Nooten GJ, Ranucci M. O2 delivery and co2 production during cardiopulmonary bypass as determinants of acute kidney injury: time for a goal-directed perfusion management? Crit Care (London, England). 2011;15:R192.
37. Kanji HD, Schulze CJ, Hervas-Malo M, Wang P, Ross DB, Zibdawi M, Bagshaw SM. Difference between pre-operative and cardiopulmonary bypass mean arterial pressure is independently associated with early cardiac surgery-associated acute kidney injury. J Cardiothorac Surg. 2010;5:71.
38. Lima RS, da Silva Junior GB, Liborio AB, Daher EF. Acute kidney injury due to rhabdomyolysis. Saudi J Kidney Dis Transpl. 2008;19:721–9.
39. Mao H, Katz N, Ariyanon W, Blanca-Martos L, Adybelli Z, Giuliani A, Danesi TH, Kim JC, Nayak A, Neri M, Virzi GM, Brocca A, Scalzotto E, Salvador L, Ronco C. Cardiac surgery-associated acute kidney injury. Cardiorenal Med. 2013;3:178–99.
40. Rosner MH, Okusa MD. Acute kidney injury associated with cardiac surgery. Clin J Am Soc Nephrol. 2006;1:19–32.
41. Chertow GM, Lazarus JM, Christiansen CL, Cook EF, Hammermeister KE, Grover F, Daley J. Preoperative renal risk stratification. Circulation. 1997;95:878–84.
42. Mehta RH, Grab JD, O'Brien SM, Bridges CR, Gammie JS, Haan CK, Ferguson TB, Peterson ED. Bedside tool for predicting the risk of postoperative dialysis in patients undergoing cardiac surgery. Circulation. 2006;114:2208–16; quiz 2208.
43. Thakar CV, Arrigain S, Worley S, Yared JP, Paganini EP. A clinical score to predict acute renal failure after cardiac surgery. J Am Soc Nephrol. 2005;16:162–8.
44. Wijeysundera DN, Karkouti K, Dupuis JY, Rao V, Chan CT, Granton JT, Beattie WS. Derivation and validation of a simplified predictive index for renal replacement therapy after cardiac surgery. JAMA. 2007;297:1801–9.
45. Englberger L, Suri RM, Li Z, Dearani JA, Park SJ, Sundt 3rd TM, Schaff HV. Validation of clinical scores predicting severe acute kidney injury after cardiac surgery. Am J Kidney Dis. 2010;56:623–31.
46. Aronson S, Fontes ML, Miao Y, Mangano DT. Risk index for perioperative renal dysfunction/failure: critical dependence on pulse pressure hypertension. Circulation. 2007;115:733–42.
47. Palomba H, de Castro I, Neto AL, Lage S, Yu L. Acute kidney injury prediction following elective cardiac surgery: AKICS score. Kidney Int. 2007;72:624–31.
48. Huen SC, Parikh CR. Predicting acute kidney injury after cardiac surgery: a systematic review. Ann Thorac Surg. 2012;93:337–47.

49. Kiers HD, van den Boogaard M, Schoenmakers MC, van der Hoeven JG, van Swieten HA, Heemskerk S, Pickkers P. Comparison and clinical suitability of eight prediction models for cardiac surgery-related acute kidney injury. Nephrol Dial Transplant. 2013;28:345–51.
50. Liangos O, Tighiouart H, Perianayagam MC, Kolyada A, Han WK, Wald R, Bonventre JV, Jaber BL. Comparative analysis of urinary biomarkers for early detection of acute kidney injury following cardiopulmonary bypass. Biomarkers. 2009;14:423–31.
51. Parikh CR, Coca SG, Thiessen-Philbrook H, Shlipak MG, Koyner JL, Wang Z, Edelstein CL, Devarajan P, Patel UD, Zappitelli M, Krawczeski CD, Passik CS, Swaminathan M, Garg AX. Postoperative biomarkers predict acute kidney injury and poor outcomes after adult cardiac surgery. J Am Soc Nephrol: JASN. 2011;22:1748–57.
52. Parikh CR, Devarajan P, Zappitelli M, Sint K, Thiessen-Philbrook H, Li S, Kim RW, Koyner JL, Coca SG, Edelstein CL, Shlipak MG, Garg AX, Krawczeski CD. Postoperative biomarkers predict acute kidney injury and poor outcomes after pediatric cardiac surgery. J Am Soc Nephrol. 2011;22:1737–47.
53. Shlipak MG, Coca SG, Wang Z, Devarajan P, Koyner JL, Patel UD, Thiessen-Philbrook H, Garg AX, Parikh CR. Presurgical serum cystatin c and risk of acute kidney injury after cardiac surgery. Am J Kidney Dis. 2011;58:366–73.
54. Grams ME, Astor BC, Bash LD, Matsushita K, Wang Y, Coresh J. Albuminuria and estimated glomerular filtration rate independently associate with acute kidney injury. J Am Soc Nephrol. 2010;21:1757–64.
55. Hsu CY, Ordonez JD, Chertow GM, Fan D, McCulloch CE, Go AS. The risk of acute renal failure in patients with chronic kidney disease. Kidney Int. 2008;74:101–7.
56. James MT, Hemmelgarn BR, Wiebe N, Pannu N, Manns BJ, Klarenbach SW, Tonelli M. Glomerular filtration rate, proteinuria, and the incidence and consequences of acute kidney injury: a cohort study. Lancet. 2010;376:2096–103.
57. Huang TM, Wu VC, Young GH, Lin YF, Shiao CC, Wu PC, Li WY, Yu HY, Hu FC, Lin JW, Chen YS, Lin YH, Wang SS, Hsu RB, Chang FC, Chou NK, Chu TS, Yeh YC, Tsai PR, Huang JW, Lin SL, Chen YM, Ko WJ, Wu KD. Preoperative proteinuria predicts adverse renal outcomes after coronary artery bypass grafting. J Am Soc Nephrol. 2011;22:156–63.
58. Tonelli M, Muntner P, Lloyd A, Manns BJ, James MT, Klarenbach S, Quinn RR, Wiebe N, Hemmelgarn BR. Using proteinuria and estimated glomerular filtration rate to classify risk in patients with chronic kidney disease: a cohort study. Ann Intern Med. 2011;154:12–21.
59. Coca SG, Jammalamadaka D, Sint K, Thiessen-Philbrook H, Shlipak MG, Zappitelli M, Devarajan P, Hashim S, Garg AX, Parikh CR. Preoperative proteinuria predicts acute kidney injury in patients undergoing cardiac surgery. J Thorac Cardiovasc Surg. 2012;143: 495–502.
60. Ali ZA, Callaghan CJ, Lim E, Ali AA, Nouraei SA, Akthar AM, Boyle JR, Varty K, Kharbanda RK, Dutka DP, Gaunt ME. Remote ischemic preconditioning reduces myocardial and renal injury after elective abdominal aortic aneurysm repair: a randomized controlled trial. Circulation. 2007;116:I98–105.
61. Zimmerman RF, Ezeanuna PU, Kane JC, Cleland CD, Kempananjappa TJ, Lucas FL, Kramer RS. Ischemic preconditioning at a remote site prevents acute kidney injury in patients following cardiac surgery. Kidney Int. 2011;80:861–7.
62. McCoy AB, Waitman LR, Gadd CS, Danciu I, Smith JP, Lewis JB, Schildcrout JS, Peterson JF. A computerized provider order entry intervention for medication safety during acute kidney injury: a quality improvement report. Am J Kidney Dis. 2010;56:832–41.
63. Batalden PB, Nelson EC, Edwards WH, Godfrey MM, Mohr JJ. Microsystems in health care: part 9. Developing small clinical units to attain peak performance. Jt Comm J Qual Saf. 2003;29:575–85.

64. Nelson EC, Godfrey MM, Batalden PB, Berry SA, Bothe Jr AE, McKinley KE, Melin CN, Muething SE, Moore LG, Wasson JH, Nolan TW. Clinical microsystems, part 1. The building blocks of health systems. Jt Comm J Qual Patient Saf. 2008;34:367–78.
65. Conlon PJ, Stafford-Smith M, White WD, Newman MF, King S, Winn MP, Landolfo K. Acute renal failure following cardiac surgery. Nephrol Dial Transplant. 1999;14:1158–62.
66. Andersson LG, Ekroth R, Bratteby LE, Hallhagen S, Wesslen O. Acute renal failure after coronary surgery–a study of incidence and risk factors in 2009 consecutive patients. Thorac Cardiovasc Surg. 1993;41:237–41.
67. Thakar CV, Liangos O, Yared JP, Nelson DA, Hariachar S, Paganini EP. Predicting acute renal failure after cardiac surgery: validation and re-definition of a risk-stratification algorithm. Hemodial Int. 2003;7:143–7.
68. Brown JR, Parikh CR. Cardiovascular surgery and acute kidney injury. In: Turner N, editor. Textbook of clinical nephrology. London: Oxford University Press; 2014 (in press).

Chapter 8
Acute Kidney Injury After Cardiovascular Surgery in Children

David M. Kwiatkowski and Catherine D. Krawczeski

Objectives

- To understand the etiology and epidemiology of acute kidney injury after pediatric cardiovascular surgery.
- To learn the current methods used to diagnose acute kidney injury and their limitations, as well as potential biomarker diagnostic tools.
- To apply the current management and novel treatment strategies of acute kidney injury in the pediatric patient after cardiac surgery.

Introduction

Acute kidney injury (AKI) is a frequent and serious complication after pediatric cardiovascular surgery, affecting up to 60 % of patients [1, 2]. Multiple studies have demonstrated that even minor degrees of AKI are associated with worse clinical outcomes, including mortality [1–5]. Infants are particularly vulnerable to AKI given the immaturity of their nephron system and the complexity of their cardiac repairs, often necessitating long durations of cardiopulmonary bypass (CPB). Within the neonatal cohort, surgery for congenital heart disease comprises the leading cause of AKI and has been the subject of considerable research [6].

D.M. Kwiatkowski, MD (✉)
The Heart Institute, Cincinnati Children's Hospital Medical Center,
3333 Burnet Avenue, Cincinnati, OH 45229, USA
e-mail: david.kwiatkowski@cchmc.org

C.D. Krawczeski, MD
Department of Cardiology, Lucile Packard Children's Hospital,
750 Welch Road, Suite 325, Palo Alto, CA 94304-5731, USA
e-mail: ckraw@stanford.edu

C.V. Thakar, C.R. Parikh (eds.), *Perioperative Kidney Injury: Principles of Risk Assessment, Diagnosis and Treatment*, DOI 10.1007/978-1-4939-1273-5_8

Table 8.1 Pediatric-modified RIFLE (pRIFLE) criteria

	GFR criteria	Urine output criteria
Risk	eCCl decrease by 25 %	<0.5 ml/kg/h for 8 h
Injury	eCCl decrease by 50 %	<0.5 ml/kg/h for 16 h
Failure	eCCl decrease by 75 % or eCCl <35 ml/min/1.73 m^2	<0.3 ml/kg/h for 24 h or anuric for 12 h
Loss	Persistent failure >4 weeks	
End-stage	End-stage renal disease (persistent failure >3 months)	

Reprinted by permission from Macmillan Publishers Ltd: [7], copyright 2007
Abbreviations: *eCCl* estimated creatinine clearance using the Schwartz formula (eCCl = k*ht/Scr), *pRIFLE* pediatric risk, injury, failure, loss, and end-stage renal disease

The most commonly used definition for pediatric AKI is the pRIFLE criteria (pediatric risk, injury, failure, loss, and end-stage renal disease), which is a modification of the adult RIFLE system. This validated classification system differs by having decreased diagnostic thresholds to account for lower normal pediatric creatinine ranges and urine outputs (Table 8.1) [7]. The AKI Network (AKIN) created a similar definition with three numerical categories corresponding to risk, injury, and failure [8]. Both definitions use a lower creatinine threshold to define risk (1.5-fold increase or 0.3 mg/dl) and incorporate urine output.

Pathophysiology

The mechanism of AKI after CPB has many contributing factors, including renal ischemia and reperfusion injury, oxidative stress, a maladaptive inflammatory response, and microemboli (Table 8.2). In periods of low cardiac output, the renal medulla is at particularly high risk of ischemic injury. Despite being a small organ, the kidney depends on a large portion of the body's cardiac output, and the ion transport channels within the nephron require a significant amount of energy via ATP. Periods of decreased oxygen delivery can be detrimental to the kidney and cause generation of reactive oxidation molecules and increases in intracellular calcium levels, which are both deleterious processes [9]. The dependence of the kidney on oxygen delivery has been demonstrated in an adult study post-CPB which associated lower urinary partial pressure of oxygen (PO_2) levels with the development of AKI [10].

As with any other organ, the kidney has the ability to maintain consistent perfusion during a period of diminished blood flow through a process called autoregulation. With changes in cardiac output or increased metabolic demand, afferent and efferent arterioles within the nephron dilate or constrict to modify vascular resistance and ensure a relatively constant perfusion pressure. However, the ability to adapt for significant decreases in blood flow is not known, especially in pediatric and neonatal physiologies.

Table 8.2 Causes of AKI in the pediatric population

Pathophysiology of AKI
Ischemia and reperfusion injury (vasoconstriction and low cardiac output)
Inflammation
Oxidative stress
ATP depletion
Microemboli
Apoptosis

This table lists multiple factors involved in the complex pathophysiology involved in AKI after cardiopulmonary bypass in the pediatric setting

Inflammation is thought to have a major role in all ischemic and reperfusion renal injury and is exacerbated by extracorporeal circulation. The complex interactions between injured endothelial cells and inflammatory cells in the milieu of cytokine and chemokine upregulation likely worsen AKI. Inflammatory cascades implicit in renal injury include the proinflammatory cytokines of tumor necrosis factor-α (TNF-α), interleukin-6 (IL-6), interleukin-1β (IL-1β), and transforming growth factor β (TGF-β) which may ultimately serve as targets for diagnosis or treatment.

Lastly, CPB exposes blood cells to nonphysiologic surfaces and shear forces, leading to cell lysis and the release of plasma free hemoglobin into the circulation. This, and other microemboli that may occur with CPB, may contribute to further tubular damage.

Epidemiology and Risk Factors

AKI rates after CPB in children continue to be exceedingly high affecting up to 60 % of high-risk patients [1, 2]. Among children, palliative surgery for congenital heart disease is the most common cause for AKI [6] and associated with a worse outcome. Postoperative pediatric patients may have multiple risk factors contributing to the development of AKI. The TRIBE-AKI group, a large multicenter consortium sponsored by the National Institutes of Health/National Heart, Lung, and Blood Institute (NIH/NHLBI) designed to study AKI in adults and children after heart surgery, reported that 87 % of patients with AKI had intraoperative hypotension, 15 % were exposed to gentamicin, 56 % were exposed to nonsteroidal antiinflammatory drugs (NSAIDs), and 6 % experienced low cardiac output syndrome [1]. Unlike other models of kidney injury, sepsis and urinary tract obstruction are rare, presenting in less than 5 % of this population [1]. Unlike adult populations who often are exposed to multiple comorbidities including diabetes mellitus, tobacco use, and coronary artery disease, pediatric cohorts are generally without chronic kidney disease or factors which may predispose AKI [3].

Identified risk factors for development of AKI are generally unavoidable and relate to patient size and complexity of required repair. Smaller patients, both by age and body surface area, have been demonstrated to be more likely to develop AKI [1, 2, 4, 5, 11, 12], and children older than 2 years are 70 % less likely to develop AKI when compared to those younger than 2 [1]. Higher surgical complexity, by Risk Adjustment for Congenital Heart Surgery (RACHS-1) surgical severity score, has been demonstrated to be independently associated with AKI in multiple studies [1, 2, 4, 5, 11, 12]. The TRIBE-AKI group reported that when stratified by RACHS-1 score, AKI was present 0, 42, 43, and 75 % for categories 1–4, respectively. Surprisingly, preoperative lactate elevation and inotropic medication demands did not correlate with later AKI, although there was a correlation with elevated preoperative serum creatinine level [2].

The primary intraoperative risk factors for AKI development are the duration of CPB [1, 2, 4, 5, 11, 12] and use of deep hypothermic circulatory arrest [2, 11]. There is a suggestion that longer aortic cross-clamp time is associated with AKI [1, 2], although a statistical association has not been demonstrated. The TRIBE-AKI group compared the incidence of AKI to a standard duration of CPB less than 60 min and found that bypass of 90–120 min had an odds ratio of 2.5 (95 % CI: 1.08, 5.65) and >180 min had an odds ratio of 7.6 for the development of AKI (95 % CI: 2.62, 21.92) [1].

Outcomes After AKI

AKI after CPB is most commonly a self-limited state which typically occurs within the first 24–48 postoperative hours. In the TRIBE-AKI consortium, 47 % of patients met AKI diagnostic criteria for 1 day, and only 11 % of patients still met the AKI definition by the fourth postoperative day [1]. Only 2/130 patients studied required dialysis within the first week [1].

AKI-related morbidity is most commonly related to fluid overload and has been considered a biomarker for worse outcomes. As the degree of fluid overload increases, the likelihood of mortality increases, irrespective of illness severity scores [13, 14]. Fluid overload is associated with worsening oxygenation indices and prolonged durations of mechanical ventilation [15].

AKI is an independent risk factor for prolonged duration of mechanical ventilation [1, 2]. In the TRIBE-AKI consortium, 30 % of patients with AKI were mechanically ventilated after 48 h as opposed to 8 % of patients without AKI [1]. Intensive care unit stay and hospital stay were demonstrated to be longer for patients with AKI [1]. Mortality is higher in patients with AKI after CPB in adult studies, even with mild degrees of injury [3]. Mortality in pediatric heart surgery is low, and institutional volumes are relatively small, making an association between AKI and mortality difficult to discern. However, within a large Canadian cohort, patients with severe AKI were shown to have an increase in mortality and neonates who required postoperative dialysis were 6.4 times more likely to die in the hospital [2].

Postoperative AKI portends worse long-term outcomes, and there is growing evidence that after laboratory and functional markers of injury improve, patients often suffer from subclinical kidney injury. Even when controlling for gestational age, age at surgery, surgical group, preoperative ventilation, the highest lactate value, and extracorporeal membrane oxygenation (ECMO) use, a Canadian group demonstrated that as AKI status worsened, 2-year follow-up weight percentile decreased and more specialists were seen, with more cardiac-related hospitalizations [2]. There is evidence that these children remain affected by subclinical kidney disease years after CPB. This was demonstrated in a cohort of children who had a persistent elevation of kidney injury biomarkers despite a lack of clinical evidence of chronic kidney disease 7 years after bypass [16]. It is as yet unknown if these children will go on to develop clinical signs of chronic kidney disease.

Diagnosis of AKI

One of the key challenges to management of AKI after CPB is the difficulty achieving prompt diagnosis. Laboratory evidence of AKI relies upon serum creatinine elevation which is insensitive for damage, because creatinine elevations are not seen until 50 % of kidney function is lost. AKI-related creatinine elevation is secondary to functional changes in glomerular filtration rate, which is delayed from the initial structural damage that occurs with the operative and postoperative renal injury [17]. Waiting for creatinine elevation for management decisions is analogous to waiting for cardiac output to decrease before treating a myocardial infarction.

The concept of "renal angina" is often used to illustrate the challenges associated with delayed diagnosis of AKI [18]. Unlike the chest pain and dyspnea experienced by a patient with a myocardial infarction, kidney injury is painless, with low urine output as the only symptom. At current time, unlike myocardial infarctions, there are no commercially available troponin-like biomarkers to diagnose AKI early enough to direct therapy. Fortunately, there are many promising novel biomarkers being investigated, with some likely to be commercially available soon. Infants with AKI after CPB are often chosen as the population to study these biomarkers because they have a planned, finite exposure of renal ischemia and lack comorbidities which affect other populations. The most promising candidate biomarkers are neutrophil gelatinase-associated lipocalin (NGAL), interleukin-18 (IL-18), liver-type fatty acid-binding protein (L-FABP), kidney injury molecule-1 (KIM-1), and cystatin C (CyC). For a full description of these biomarkers, see Chap. 3. A brief review of these biomarkers in the pediatric cardiac setting is included here.

NGAL may be the most promising biomarker of AKI in pediatric settings, reliably showing elevation as early as 2 h after bypass [4, 19], and has been shown to predict clinical outcomes such as hospital and intensive care unit (ICU) stay, duration of AKI, duration of mechanical ventilation, dialysis requirement, and mortality [19–21]. NGAL may also have AKI treatment applications for renal tubule survival and recovery through its role of iron transportation [22]. IL-18 is also a sensitive early (4–6 h post-bypass) biomarker for AKI and correlates well with severity of AKI and associated outcomes [23]. In limited pediatric studies, later elevation (12–24 h post-bypass) of KIM-1 has been shown to be predictive of worsening degrees of AKI and associated sequelae [4]. Serum level of cystatin C is a commonly used clinical tool to estimate kidney function; however, pediatric studies have shown that urine cystatin can be used as a sensitive and specific predictor of the duration and severity of AKI, with an odds ratio of 17 of predicting AKI when compared to creatinine elevation [24, 25].

Pediatric models have shown these biomarkers have different temporal elevations and their individual specificity and sensitivity can be increased when used as part of biomarker "panels" [4]. They may help distinguish between various etiologies causing AKI and help direct optimal treatment. Many of these biomarkers are still in research phases, and large-scale post-clinical research will be helpful after they arrive to the market.

Prevention and Treatment of AKI During the Perioperative Period

Intraoperative Prevention

Since longer bypass times and the use of circulatory arrest are associated with higher incidence of AKI, both should be limited whenever possible. The use of modified ultrafiltration after separation from CPB has been shown to reduce the accumulation of total body water, decrease postoperative blood loss, decrease the need for postoperative blood product need, and improve postoperative ventricular systolic function and is often used in surgery for congenital heart disease [26–28].

Postoperative AKI Management

The natural history of postoperative AKI is generally self-limited, and therefore the management of AKI is typically directed toward managing the sequelae of AKI, namely, fluid overload. Fluid overload has been shown to be an independent predictor of hospital stay, and severity of fluid overload is associated with worsening outcomes in children [15, 29]. The quintessential step for limiting fluid overload is controlling the volume given to patients; however, nutritional demands, blood products, medications, and resuscitation fluids often exceed outputs, especially in the face of AKI-related oliguria.

Diuretics are the mainstay of treatment for postoperative oliguria, most commonly with loop diuretics, such as furosemide and bumetanide. These are often used in synergy with thiazide diuretics, such as chlorothiazide and metolazone.

The timing of initiation of renal replacement therapy (RRT) and specific indications for intervention is somewhat controversial with recent research arguing for earlier initiation. There are two commonly used modalities of RRT in children after cardiac surgery: continuous renal replacement therapy [30] and peritoneal dialysis

(PD) [11, 12, 31]. In the United States, PD is the most commonly used method [11, 12, 31, 32]. Although some centers insert PD catheters after they have developed AKI, many postulate that inserting PD catheters at the time of surgery is less likely to cause adverse events including bowel injury and peritonitis [31, 33]. The benefits of PD use in early AKI are demonstrated in a retrospective study which showed that initiation of PD within the first 24 h of surgery is associated with lower mortality [11]. The concept of prophylactic PD has also been proposed, with retrospective data demonstrating that this practice is associated with shorter time to extubation and negative fluid balance when compared to peritoneal drain [12]. Although center variation exists, a common PD prescription consists of 1.5 % dextrose diasylate with 10 ml/kg dwell volumes with continuous 1-h cycles [11, 12, 31].

There is a saying that the "best diuretic is a good cardiac output." Although often said in jest, without adequate renal perfusion, no treatment will be adequate. A case-control study of AKI post-CPB for patients receiving PD showed arterial hypotension and poor cardiac performance-related venous hypertension were independent risk factors for AKI development and stronger risk factors than preexisting renal failure [34]. In the postoperative period, inotropic and vasoactive medications are often essential for adequate renal perfusion and constitute primary prevention of AKI.

Novel Treatments

Rather than managing the effects of AKI, there has been recent research focused on preventative measures. Some of the most promising representatives are discussed below (Table 8.3):

Fenoldopam is a selective dopamine-1 receptor agonist which causes systemic vasodilation, increasing renal and splanchnic blood flow, thus augmenting tubular sodium excretion. It has been used for short-term management of adult hypertension and to increase renal perfusion as an adjunct to conventional diuretic therapy [35], although its use is limited by the potential complication of systemic hypotension. There has been recent interest in fenoldopam to prevent AKI, and a recent prospective randomized study among neonates demonstrated the addition of fenoldopam was associated with less need for diuretics, lower NGAL and CyC values, and trends toward less AKI [36]. Although individual studies have mixed data, a meta-analysis of 440 patients from 6 studies showed a pooled odds ratio of 0.41 for developing AKI in adult patients, suggesting reno-protective properties [37].

By a similar mechanism, it is thought that natriuretic peptides may help prevent AKI. Among other actions, natriuretic peptides are antagonists of the renin-angiotensin system and induce selective dilation of the afferent arterioles and constriction of efferent arterioles causing an increase in glomerular filtration rate (GFR). Nesiritide is a commercially available recombinant brain natriuretic peptide which is used for the diuresis of acutely decompensated adult congestive heart failure. Adult studies of the prophylactic use of nesiritide have demonstrated a decrease in AKI

Table 8.3 Novel therapies for AKI

Timing	Earlier	→						Later
Pathology of injury	Ischemia (vasoconstriction)	Ischemia (low cardiac output)	ATP depletion	Oxidative stress	Inflammatory response	Apoptosis	Ongoing injury	Regeneration
Mechanism of treatment	Vasodilation	Improving cardiac output	ATP donors	Antioxidants	Antiinflammatory	Antiapoptotic	Renal replacement therapy	Nephron repair
Potential therapies	Fenoldopam	Inotropic medications		N-acetylcysteine	Glucocorticoids		Peritoneal dialysis	Growth factor (NGAL)
	Nesiritide							
	Aminophylline			Rasburicase	Peritoneal dialysis		CRRT	Stem cells

This table lists various mechanisms of acute kidney injury and proposed mechanisms of intervention with potential candidate therapies, where available. Notably, a majority of these interventions are experimental and not used in clinical practice incidence, but no change in hospital length of stay, mortality, or need for dialysis [38]. At present, there are no pediatric studies for CPB-related AKI, although there are limited data supporting its use in children with congestive heart failure [39].

Since the mechanism of AKI is multifactorial with some component of injury likely due to oxidative stress, there is a growing body of literature to investigate the use of N-acetylcysteine (NAC) to prevent AKI by free radical scavenging and prevention of oxidative stress. There are several large randomized adult studies which show no clear improvement in outcomes with NAC as prophylaxis for AKI after CPB [40]. However, NAC continues to be commonly used especially in patients with chronic kidney disease as it is generally considered a benign medication. A recent randomized trial among neonates undergoing the arterial switch operation demonstrated the use of perioperative NAC was associated with reduced AKI, reduced need for RRT, shorter ICU stays, and less time to negative fluid balance [41]. By a similar mechanism, there is growing literature that the antioxidant uric acid may have a detrimental association with AKI after CPB. Adult studies have demonstrated that elevated postoperative uric acid levels were associated with a 40-fold risk in AKI [42], while treatment with rasburicase to lower uric acid levels was associated with a decrease in NGAL levels [43].

A more thorough understanding of the mechanism of CPB-associated AKI, plus earlier diagnosis through the use of biomarkers, should allow continued investigation of potential therapies directed at the prevention of AKI.

Conclusion

AKI is a frequent and serious complication of cardiac surgery in children and is independently associated with negative outcomes. Currently, practitioners are challenged by delays in diagnosis and poor treatment options. However, a recent increase in research will likely expedite the advent of novel biomarkers to improve diagnosis and guide thoughtful management.

Key Messages

- Acute kidney injury (AKI) is a frequent and serious complication after pediatric cardiovascular surgery. Infants are particularly vulnerable to AKI.
- Even minor degrees of AKI are associated with worse clinical outcomes.
- Limitations of serum creatinine prevent timely diagnosis. New biomarkers in research development promise to facilitate earlier diagnosis with higher sensitivity and specificity.
- Current treatment strategies are focused on managing AKI-related fluid overload.
- Early renal replacement therapy, often with institution of peritoneal dialysis, is becoming increasingly common in these patients.

References

1. Li S, et al. Incidence, risk factors, and outcomes of acute kidney injury after pediatric cardiac surgery: a prospective multicenter study. Crit Care Med. 2011;39(6):1493–9.
2. Morgan CJ, et al. Risk factors for and outcomes of acute kidney injury in neonates undergoing complex cardiac surgery. J Pediatr. 2013;162(1):120–127.e1.
3. Karkouti K, et al. Acute kidney injury after cardiac surgery: focus on modifiable risk factors. Circulation. 2009;119(4):495–502.
4. Krawczeski CD, et al. Temporal relationship and predictive value of urinary acute kidney injury biomarkers after pediatric cardiopulmonary bypass. J Am Coll Cardiol. 2011;58(22): 2301–9.
5. Blinder JJ, et al. Congenital heart surgery in infants: effects of acute kidney injury on outcomes. J Thorac Cardiovasc Surg. 2012;143(2):368–74.
6. Williams DM, et al. Acute kidney failure: a pediatric experience over 20 years. Arch Pediatr Adolesc Med. 2002;156(9):893–900.
7. Akcan-Arikan A, et al. Modified RIFLE criteria in critically ill children with acute kidney injury. Kidney Int. 2007;71(10):1028–35.
8. Mehta RL, et al. Acute Kidney Injury Network: report of an initiative to improve outcomes in acute kidney injury. Crit Care. 2007;11(2):R31.
9. Devarajan P. Update on mechanisms of ischemic acute kidney injury. J Am Soc Nephrol. 2006;17(6):1503–20.
10. Kainuma M, Yamada M, Miyake T. Continuous urine oxygen tension monitoring in patients undergoing cardiac surgery. J Cardiothorac Vasc Anesth. 1996;10(5):603–8.
11. Bojan M, et al. Early initiation of peritoneal dialysis in neonates and infants with acute kidney injury following cardiac surgery is associated with a significant decrease in mortality. Kidney Int. 2012;82(4):474–81.
12. Sasser WC, et al. Prophylactic peritoneal dialysis following cardiopulmonary bypass in children is associated with decreased inflammation and improved clinical outcomes. Congenit Heart Dis. 2013. doi:10.1111/chd.12072. [epub ahead of print].
13. Goldstein SL, et al. Outcome in children receiving continuous venovenous hemofiltration. Pediatrics. 2001;107(6):1309–12.
14. Goldstein SL, et al. Pediatric patients with multi-organ dysfunction syndrome receiving continuous renal replacement therapy. Kidney Int. 2005;67(2):653–8.
15. Arikan AA, et al. Fluid overload is associated with impaired oxygenation and morbidity in critically ill children. Pediatr Crit Care Med. 2012;13(3):253–8.
16. Cooper DS, et al. Novel urinary biomarkers remain elevated years after acute kidney injury following cardiac surgery in children. J Am Coll Cardiol. 2013;61(10):E438.
17. Murray PT, et al. A framework and key research questions in AKI diagnosis and staging in different environments. Clin J Am Soc Nephrol. 2008;3(3):864–8.
18. Goldstein SL, Chawla LS. Renal angina. Clin J Am Soc Nephrol. 2010;5(5):943–9.
19. Mishra J, et al. Neutrophil gelatinase-associated lipocalin (NGAL) as a biomarker for acute renal injury after cardiac surgery. Lancet. 2005;365(9466):1231–8.
20. Dent CL, et al. Plasma neutrophil gelatinase-associated lipocalin predicts acute kidney injury, morbidity and mortality after pediatric cardiac surgery: a prospective uncontrolled cohort study. Crit Care. 2007;11(6):R127.
21. Bennett M, et al. Urine NGAL predicts severity of acute kidney injury after cardiac surgery: a prospective study. Clin J Am Soc Nephrol. 2008;3(3):665–73.
22. Mishra J, et al. Amelioration of ischemic acute renal injury by neutrophil gelatinase-associated lipocalin. J Am Soc Nephrol. 2004;15(12):3073–82.
23. Parikh CR, et al. Urine IL-18 is an early diagnostic marker for acute kidney injury and predicts mortality in the intensive care unit. J Am Soc Nephrol. 2005;16(10):3046–52.
24. Krawczeski CD, et al. Serum cystatin C is an early predictive biomarker of acute kidney injury after pediatric cardiopulmonary bypass. Clin J Am Soc Nephrol. 2010;5(9):1552–7.

25. Zappitelli M, et al. Early postoperative serum cystatin C predicts severe acute kidney injury following pediatric cardiac surgery. Kidney Int. 2011;80(6):655–62.
26. Naik SK, Knight A, Elliott M. A prospective randomized study of a modified technique of ultrafiltration during pediatric open-heart surgery. Circulation. 1991;84(5 Suppl):III422–31.
27. Chaturvedi RR, et al. Modified ultrafiltration improves global left ventricular systolic function after open-heart surgery in infants and children. Eur J Cardiothorac Surg. 1999;15(6):742–6.
28. Davies MJ, et al. Modified ultrafiltration improves left ventricular systolic function in infants after cardiopulmonary bypass. J Thorac Cardiovasc Surg. 1998;115(2):361–9; discussion 369–70.
29. Sutherland SM, et al. Fluid overload and mortality in children receiving continuous renal replacement therapy: the prospective pediatric continuous renal replacement therapy registry. Am J Kidney Dis. 2010;55(2):316–25.
30. Jander A, et al. Continuous veno-venous hemodiafiltration in children after cardiac surgery. Eur J Cardiothorac Surg. 2007;31(6):1022–8.
31. Sorof JM, et al. Early initiation of peritoneal dialysis after surgical repair of congenital heart disease. Pediatr Nephrol. 1999;13(8):641–5.
32. Picca S, Ricci Z, Picardo S. Acute kidney injury in an infant after cardiopulmonary bypass. Semin Nephrol. 2008;28(5):470–6.
33. Swan P, et al. The safety of peritoneal drainage and dialysis after cardiopulmonary bypass in children. J Thorac Cardiovasc Surg. 1997;114(4):688–9.
34. Picca S, et al. Risks of acute renal failure after cardiopulmonary bypass surgery in children: a retrospective 10-year case-control study. Nephrol Dial Transplant. 1995;10(5):630–6.
35. Costello JM, et al. Initial experience with fenoldopam after cardiac surgery in neonates with an insufficient response to conventional diuretics. Pediatr Crit Care Med. 2006;7(1):28–33.
36. Ricci Z, et al. High-dose fenoldopam reduces postoperative neutrophil gelatinase-associated lipocaline and cystatin C levels in pediatric cardiac surgery. Crit Care. 2011;15(3):R160.
37. Zangrillo A, et al. Fenoldopam and acute renal failure in cardiac surgery: a meta-analysis of randomized placebo-controlled trials. J Cardiothorac Vasc Anesth. 2012;26(3):407–13.
38. Ejaz AA, et al. Prophylactic nesiritide does not prevent dialysis or all-cause mortality in patients undergoing high-risk cardiac surgery. J Thorac Cardiovasc Surg. 2009;138(4):959–64.
39. Simsic JM, et al. Hemodynamic effects and safety of nesiritide in neonates with heart failure. J Intensive Care Med. 2008;23(6):389–95.
40. Adabag AS, et al. Efficacy of N-acetylcysteine in preventing renal injury after heart surgery: a systematic review of randomized trials. Eur Heart J. 2009;30(15):1910–7.
41. Aiyagari R, et al. Effects of N-acetylcysteine on renal dysfunction in neonates undergoing the arterial switch operation. J Thorac Cardiovasc Surg. 2010;139(4):956–61.
42. Lapsia V, et al. Elevated uric acid increases the risk for acute kidney injury. Am J Med. 2012;125(3):302. e9–17.
43. Ejaz AA, et al. Effect of uric acid lowering therapy on the prevention of acute kidney injury in cardiovascular surgery. Int Urol Nephrol. 2013;45(2):449–58.

Chapter 9
Acute Kidney Injury in the Era of Ventricular Assist Devices

Meredith A. Brisco and Jeffrey M. Testani

Objectives

- To outline changes in renal function after ventricular assist device (VAD) placement
- To describe the relationship between changes in post-VAD renal function and mortality
- To examine the impact of VAD flow on renal outcomes

Introduction

With improved treatment of coronary artery disease and life-threatening arrhythmias, more and more patients are surviving long enough to develop advanced heart failure. Although heart transplantation is a therapeutic option, limited organ availability necessitated development of other therapies, the mainstay of which is the ventricular assist device (VAD).

Over the last decade, VADs have become a vital treatment in the advanced heart failure cardiologist's armamentarium [1]. The nearly exponential increase in successful VAD implants with marked mortality benefit has led to a shift in clinical

M.A. Brisco, MD, MSCE (✉)
Division of Cardiology, Section of Advanced Heart Failure and Cardiac Transplantation, Medical University of South Carolina, 25 Courtenay Drive, ART 7061, MSC 592, Charleston, SC 29425-5920, USA
e-mail: brisco@musc.edu

J.M. Testani, MD, MTR
Program of Applied Translational Research, Yale University, 60 Temple Street, Suite 6C, New Haven, CT 06510, USA
e-mail: jeffrey.testani@yale.edu

C.V. Thakar, C.R. Parikh (eds.), *Perioperative Kidney Injury: Principles of Risk Assessment, Diagnosis and Treatment*, DOI 10.1007/978-1-4939-1273-5_9

focus from surviving device implant to decreasing morbidity and improving/maintaining end-organ function, with specific focus on kidney function [2–4]. Unfortunately, renal dysfunction (RD) is particularly common in advanced heart failure (HF) and is one of the most powerful predictors of prognosis [5, 6]. Patients with concomitant renal and cardiac dysfunction undergoing VAD placement have the potential to achieve marked improvements in renal function with normalization of circulatory function but are likewise at risk for acute kidney injury (AKI) following major cardiac surgery. This chapter will provide a brief overview of VAD mechanics and their potential effect on renal function while focusing on renal outcomes following mechanical support and their relationship with mortality.

Indications for VAD Placement

As per the Heart Failure Society of America HF practice guidelines, there are three major indications for VAD placement: (1) as a bridge to cardiac transplantation in patients who have become refractory to medical management, (2) as permanent mechanical assistance in patients who are refractory to medical management and otherwise transplant ineligible as a destination therapy, or (3) as a bridge to myocardial recovery in those patients expected to improve with time or aggressive medical therapy [7]. With a rapidly growing elderly population and a fixed number of donor organs available, destination therapy is becoming the most common reason for VAD placement [8]. Absolute contraindications include irreversible hepatic, neurologic, or renal disease, including chronic dialysis, medical nonadherence, severe psychosocial limitations, or insurmountable operative risk [1, 9]. The difficulty in candidacy determination lies in establishing what percentage of end-organ dysfunction, particularly RD, is likely to improve with restoration of a normal cardiac output such that the benefit of a VAD outweighs the estimated risk.

VAD Structure and Mechanical Function

The first-generation left ventricular assist devices (LVADs) (Thoratec Paracorporeal VAD, HeartMate XVE, Novacor) were volume displacement pumps that filled and ejected blood with a systole and diastole similar to normal physiology with resulting pulsatile flow. Despite their ability to provide full cardiac support as well as improve survival and end-organ function, they had many disadvantages, which limited their use and longevity. The devices were large, limiting their use in smaller individuals and women; they required an extensive surgical dissection; and their multiple moving parts, including mechanical bearings and valves, were prone to failure after 1 year of support [10, 11]. Although the HeartMate XVE and Novacor are no longer used, the Thoratec Paracorporeal VAD is still utilized for biventricular support as bridge to transplantation.

The second generation of LVADs that are currently implanted employ rotary technology that provides continuous flow (CF) to the body with a reduced or absent pulse. Advantages of CF-LVADs include the lack of valves, smaller size, and fewer moving parts which translate into improved durability and quality of life with less adverse events (strokes, infection, death, etc.) than had plagued the first-generation LVADs [2, 3, 12, 13]. The HeartMate II (Thoratec, Pleasanton, CA), an axial-flow device, is currently the most implanted LVAD in the United States and is Food and Drug Administration (FDA) approved for both bridge to transplantation and destination therapy indications (Fig. 9.1). The HeartWare (HeartWare International, Inc., Framingham, MA) is a centrifugal-flow pump that is FDA approved currently for bridge to transplantation only [4]. Pump flow in *both* types of CF-LVADs is determined by the pump speed (set in rotations per minute) but is sensitive

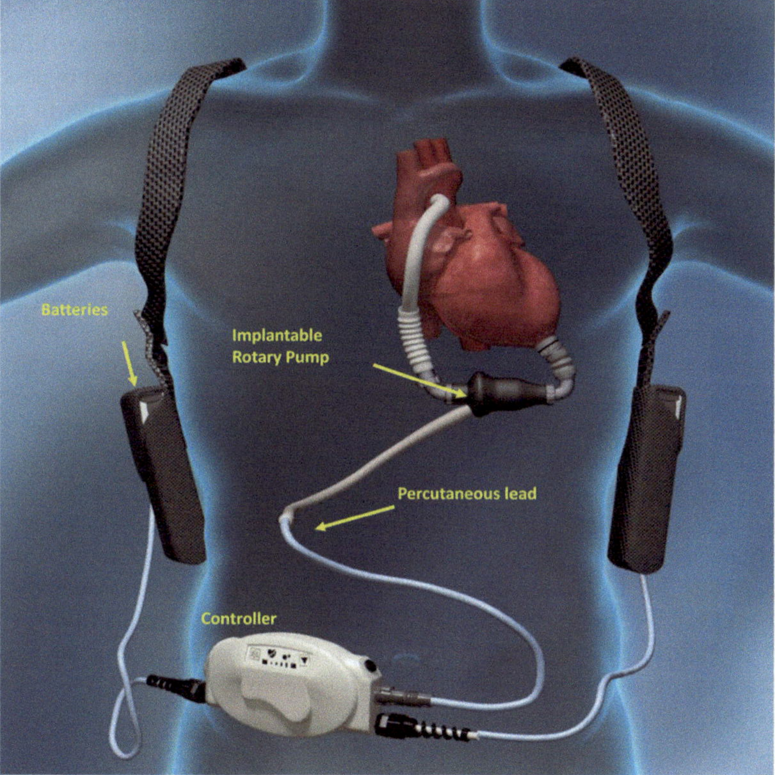

Fig. 9.1 The HeartMate II continuous-flow left ventricular assist device. The HeartMate II is comprised of three basic parts: the pump, the system controller, and the power source. The pump is connected to the heart via an inflow cannula placed in the left ventricular apex that diverts blood from the heart into the pump and an outflow cannula that directs blood from the pump into the ascending aorta. The system controller programs and runs the pump and is connected to the pump via a percutaneous lead or driveline. Pump power is provided by either battery packs (as pictured here) or a power base unit (Reprinted with the permission of Thoratec Corporation)

and inversely proportional to the pressure differential between the aortic and left ventricular pressures [14]. Importantly, inherent myocardial contractility can alter VAD flow producing pulsatility in some patients with CF devices.

AKI After VAD Placement

As most patients who require a VAD exhibit many of the most powerful risk factors for AKI after cardiovascular surgery, including reduced ejection fraction (EF), cardiogenic shock, and presence of an intra-aortic balloon pump, it is not surprising that the incidence of AKI post-VAD ranges anywhere between as little as 5 % to as much as 56 % depending on the study population, AKI definition used, and type of device implanted [4, 11, 15–30]. From a surgical perspective, the majority of durable VADs require a median sternotomy and partial or total support with cardiopulmonary bypass. The older pulsatile devices were larger and much more difficult to implant and as a result, lengthened both total surgical procedural and bypass time. The newer CF-LVADs require less surgical dissection and bypass time. In general, the average reported risk of AKI following pulsatile VADs exceeds that of CF-VADs (Table 9.1) and is supported by data from the HeartMate II Destination Therapy clinical trial which revealed 0.34 RD events/patient year in the pulsatile group compared to 0.10 RD events/patient year in CF group ($p<0.001$) [2]. Still, AKI incidence in the CF-VAD population is far from negligible, and therefore, the primary driver of the increased risk of AKI after VAD is likely a combination of patient-related factors and the complexity of the surgery itself.

Although all patients considered for VAD are by definition critically ill, older age and markers of increased disease severity have been associated with postoperative AKI, including the presence of right ventricular (RV) dysfunction, shock, ventilator-dependent respiratory failure, and coagulopathy [17, 19, 28]. Perhaps the most widely used disease severity indicators are the Interagency Registry for Mechanically Assisted Circulatory Support (INTERMACS) profiles, where profile 1 represents a critical cardiogenic shock/"crashing and burning patient" to the least severe, profile 7, which represents an advanced New York Heart Association class III patient [31]. Not only are INTERMACS profile 1 patients at the highest risk for 30-day mortality (29.4 % compared to 5 % in less ill patients), their incidence of AKI requiring renal replacement therapy (RRT) can reach 30 % [8, 18, 32]. These studies and others are partially responsible for the paradigm shift away from implanting INTERMACS 1 patients.

Another commonly reported patient-related risk factor for AKI after VAD placement is baseline RD, which in the VAD literature is often defined as an estimated glomerular filtration rate (eGFR) less than 60 mL/kg/1.73 m^2 [24, 27]. With the extension of VAD implants to non-transplant candidates under the destination therapy indication, the presence of pre-implant RD has only further increased, as has the severity of other comorbid conditions associated with renal damage, most notably diabetes (36.5 % in INTERMACS) [8]. This only creates more difficulty as not all RD is created equally and RD that is HF induced is thought to improve after

Table 9.1 Incidence of acute kidney injury and renal replacement therapy after CF-VAD implantation

Acute kidney injury

Author	*N*	Flow type	AKI incidence (%)	AKI definition
Aaronson [4]	140	Centrifugal	5.7	Cr increase ≥3 times baseline or Cr >5.0 for 48 h or RRT; HeartWare BTT clinical trial
Alba [17]	12	Axial	33.3	Injury or greater RIFLE criteria
Brisco [29]	2,476	Axial	7.4	Greater than or equal to 25 % worsening in eGFR at 1 month
Borgi [19]	100	Axial, centrifugal	28.0	Injury or greater RIFLE criteria
Slaughter [30]	332	Centrifugal	5.1	Cr increase ≥3 times baseline or Cr >5.0 for 48 h or RRT

Renal replacement therapy

Author	*N*	Flow type	RRT incidence (%)	Comment
Demirozu [21]	107	Axial	14.0	RRT temporary in 10 out of 15 patients
Feller [23]	13	Axial	15.3	
Hasin [24]	83	Axial	10.0	RRT permanent in 50 % of patients
Miller [3]	133	Axial	13.3	Incidence in first 30 days; HeartMate II BTT clinical trial
Sandner [26]	63	Axial	38.1	
Sandner [27]	86	Axial, centrifugal	34.8	
Slaughter [2]	134	Axial	16.0	HeartMate II DT clinical trial
Starling [20]	169	Axial	10.1	

CF-LVAD continuous-flow left ventricular assist device, *AKI* acute kidney injury, *Cr* serum creatinine, *RRT* renal replacement therapy, *BTT* bridge to transplant, *eGFR* estimated glomerular filtration rate, *DT* destination therapy

VAD implantation. So although patients with RD are certainly at higher risk for postoperative AKI, they also have the potential for improvement in renal function depending on the mechanism of their RD. To date, no study has attempted to further categorize RD at time of VAD implant and the subsequent risk for morbidity and mortality. As a result, despite the accepted risks associated with RD, there is no current consensus on an eGFR below which a VAD should not at least be considered [1, 9].

Perioperative AKI and Post-VAD Mortality

In accordance with the extensive epidemiologic literature linking postsurgical AKI and mortality, patients who develop AKI following VAD placement also have a marked survival disadvantage, particularly if the injury is significant enough to warrant RRT. In a European study of over 200 pulsatile VAD patients, only 38 % of patients with AKI leading to RRT were alive at 30 days compared to 61 % of patients without AKI ($p<0.01$) [25]. Although the incidence of AKI may have improved since that study with advancements in devices and surgical techniques, the magnitude of the detrimental association between VAD-related AKI on survival persists with nearly twice as many patients with AKI dying within 30 days compared to those without renal injury in the current era of predominantly CF-VADs [17, 27, 28]. Patients with AKI requiring RRT are also less likely to go on to transplantation, 52.4 % vs. 83.5 % without AKI in one study, further impairing survival as transplantation is still regarded as the best therapy for end-stage HF [28]. As RD itself negatively impacts survival and is a powerful part of the currently used HeartMate II survival score for therapy consideration, one might argue that baseline RD is primarily responsible for the increased risk [8, 33]. Sandner et al. demonstrated in a small cohort of CF-LVAD patients that although an eGFR <60 was associated with more post-VAD AKI, the resultant decreased post-LVAD survival did not vary according to baseline renal function [27]. It is difficult to determine whether the AKI itself accounts for the survival disadvantage or if it is merely a marker of disease severity, especially given most data generated is single center, limited by small patient numbers. However, a study of 3,363 adult patients in INTERMACS further supported the mortality risk associated with post-VAD AKI given that patients with any worsening in their renal function experienced increased mortality [29]. Importantly, patients with significant improvement in renal function suffered a similarly increased risk for mortality. It appears from this study that factors driving the change in eGFR are potentially responsible for the observed risk.

Early Post-VAD Improvement in Renal Function

Although the first part of this chapter focused on post-VAD injury, the majority of patients actually experience improvement in renal function (IRF) following VAD implantation [17, 21, 24, 26, 27, 29, 34–38]. These improvements were apparent in the earlier studies of pulsatile devices: Frazier et al. reported decreases in mean creatinine from 1.5 (0.4–8.9) to 1.1 (0.1–6.2) following HeartMate XVE LVAD in 271 patients ($p<0.001$), and Butler et al. showed a mean increase in creatinine clearance of 77 ± 46 to 107 ± 51 mL/min at 1-month post-implant in 220 pulsatile bridge to transplantation patients [11, 39]. With the advent of CF technology, many were concerned about the effect that reduced arterial pulsatility would have on kidney function, but clinical trial data from both the HeartMate II and HeartWare devices showed no difference in early renal function between CF and pulsatile flow [2, 4]. Subsequent single-center studies confirmed the marked early IRF after CF-LVADs with an average serum creatinine decrease of 0.5 mg/dL and an average eGFR increase of 25 mL/min/1.73 m^2 [24, 26, 34, 37, 40]. In the INTERMACS population, we found that in the first few weeks following implantation, a $\geq$25 % improvement in eGFR occurred in 69 % of patients and $\geq$100 % improvement was found in 22.3 % of patients regardless of VAD indication (Fig. 9.2a) [29].

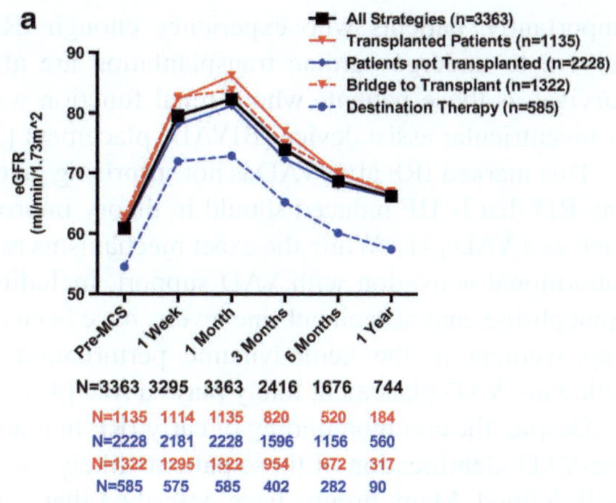

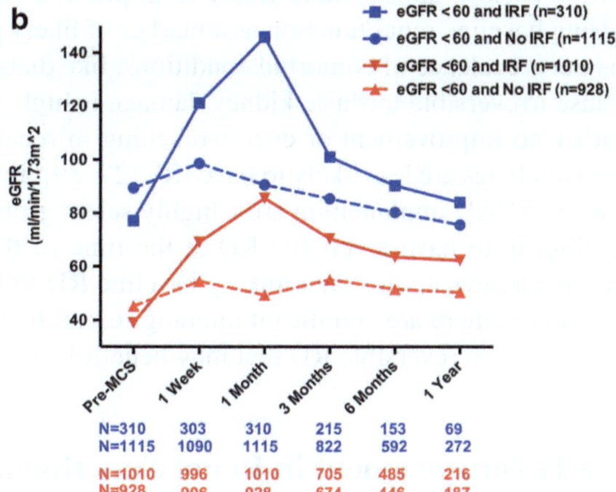

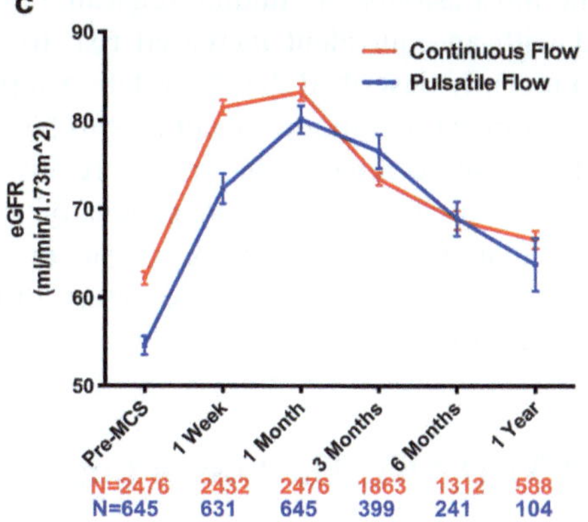

Fig. 9.2 Mean eGFR over time grouped by device strategy, baseline renal function, and presence of post-VAD improvement in renal function and device flow. (**a**) Mean eGFR over time by baseline device strategy or transplant status at end of follow-up. (**b**) Mean eGFR over time by baseline INTERMACS profile. (**c**) The slope of the lines reflects the rate of change in eGFR over time. Sample sizes (*n*) refer to the number of patients in each group through 1 month and sample sizes (*N*) refer to the number of patients with data available at each of the subsequent time points. *eGFR* estimated glomerular filtration rate, *MCS* mechanical circularity support. Bridge to transplant defined as patients listed for transplantation or those deemed likely by the treating physician to be listed at the time of implantation (Reprinted with permission from Brisco et al. [29])

Importantly, patients who experience enough IRF to attain an eGFR >60 and survive to undergo cardiac transplantation are afforded the same posttransplant survival as those patients whose renal function was normal prior to either LVAD or biventricular assist device (BIVAD) placement [37].

This marked IRF after VAD is not surprising given that HF is a cause for RD, and any RD that is HF induced should in theory improve with definitive HF treatment such as a VAD [41]. While the exact mechanisms remain unclear, reductions in neurohormonal activation with VAD support, including plasma renin, angiotensin II, epinephrine, and norepinephrine levels, have been demonstrated [42]. Additionally, improvement in the hemodynamic perturbations that are characteristic of HF following VAD placement likely plays a role [43].

Despite the common finding of early IRF in many patients after VAD placement, pre-VAD identification of those patients likely to experience post-VAD IRF is less well defined. Many groups have described that patients with more significant RD pre-VAD also appear more likely to improve their eGFR post-VAD [24, 37, 39]. Using baseline renal function as a marker of likely post-VAD benefit is problematic as the prevalence of comorbid conditions, like diabetes and hypertension, known to cause irreversible intrinsic kidney damage is high, placing these patients at risk for either no improvement or even worsening in renal function. Incidentally, patients with diabetes are less likely to have IRF [27, 39]. Importantly, patients with RD who undergo VAD implantation are a highly select group who are believed by their cardiologists to have reversible RD at the time of the evaluation or they would not receive a device, thus data linking baseline RD to IRF is potentially highly biased. Currently, there are significant ongoing research efforts aimed at better identifying patients with reversible RD that may benefit from VAD implantation.

Early Improvement in Renal Function and Mortality

Perhaps the most astonishing finding regarding post-VAD IRF is that it is actually associated with an equivalent increased risk for mortality as perioperative AKI. Our group recently described that the relationship between changes in eGFR from pre- to post-implant and mortality appears to be U shaped, such that patients with the largest relative decrements and largest relative improvements in renal function experience the worst survival, independent of patient and device characteristics [29]. Given that it is highly unlikely that an improvement in GFR itself can worsen survival, further research is necessary to better understand this seemingly paradoxical relationship.

Late Post-VAD AKI: The Loss of Improvement in Renal Function

Against the backdrop of CF-VAD dominance and the resulting climb in patient survival to 80 % at 1 year and 70 % at 2 years post-implant, research and clinical attention have shifted toward decreasing morbidity and the durability of noncardiac function [8]. To that end, two small single-center studies in patients with CF-VADs recently described a late progressive decrement in renal function with longer-term support, a signal which appeared to be present in several previous studies [21, 24, 30, 36]. This finding was further supported by a study of 3,363 adult patients in INTERMACS which also indicated a worsening in renal function relative to an initial peak at 1 month such that the median improvement in eGFR was only 2.6 mL/min/1.73 m^2 above the pre-VAD value at 1 year [29]. This pattern of improvement then decline was consistent across subgroups regardless of device strategy (Fig. 9.2a) or INTERMACS profile. Importantly, the majority of the late AKI occurred in those patients who had significant IRF at 1 month first, regardless of the presence of pre-implant RD (Fig. 9.2b). It appears that patients who experience significant post-VAD IRF are unable to maintain the initial improvement in eGFR [29]. The transient nature of the recovery of renal function may in part explain the worsened survival associated with early IRF. With over 10,000 implants since 2006 in the United States alone, further research into understanding these changes in eGFR during VAD support is imperative [8].

The Continuous vs. Pulsatile Flow Debate

Although the smaller size, increased durability, and prolonged patient survival with CF pumps served to prove their superiority, questions remained about the longer-term safety of a circulatory system with reduced pulsatility [44]. These theoretical concerns were not unfounded as animal data revealed that CF-VAD support caused abnormalities in the kidney such as smooth muscle cell hypertrophy, periarteritis, and upregulation of the local renal renin-angiotensin-aldosterone system [45–47]. Human data followed showing that plasma renin and aldosterone levels fell twice as much in ten patients supported with pulsatile devices compared to CF-VADs after 70 days of support [42]. Real-world experience from INTERMACS examined changes in renal function in 645 pulsatile-device patients and 2,476 CF-VAD patients and found that both groups experienced a qualitatively similar pattern of early improvement and late decline (Fig. 9.2c) [29]. While there may be plausible mechanisms that raise concern for a detrimental renal effect of CF-VADs, the similar renal outcomes with pulsatile devices in INTERMACS and the substantially superior survival continue to quiet the device flow debate.

Dialysis in VAD Patients

Much of the driving force for moderate to severe renal dysfunction serving as a significant relative contraindication for VAD placement stems from the challenges inherent in providing long-term RRT to VAD patients. First and foremost, as driveline and device-related infections remain a substantial cause of morbidity and mortality, the increased risk of bacteremia associated with dialysis could be disastrous in this population. As a result, placement of more permanent long-term access to mitigate some of the infection risk is reasonable; however, there are currently no studies to support one form of vascular access over another [48]. Given the continuous-flow circulatory environment created by current VADs, arteriovenous fistulas are not recommended, particularly in light of the necessity of pulsatile flow for adequate fistula maturation [48]. Regarding RRT modality, in addition to intermittent hemodialysis, peritoneal dialysis has been successfully employed in VAD patients given the pre-peritoneal location of the HeartMate II and the intrapericardial location of the HeartWare VAD. Theoretical benefits of peritoneal dialysis include lower rates of bacteremia and sustained daily ultrafiltration potentially providing more hemodynamic stability [49]. Further research is necessary to determine which dialysis method is superior in VAD patients.

Another difficulty with long-term RRT in VAD patients stems from the intricacies involved in monitoring blood pressure. Due to the decreased pulse pressure in CF-VAD patients, automated blood pressure monitors, while accurate, are less than 50 % successful [50]. As a result, Doppler ultrasound is commonly used which closely approximates systolic blood pressure as opposed to mean arterial pressure. To more precisely determine systolic and diastolic blood pressures, monitors with oscillometric slow-deflation technology like the Terumo Elemano (Somerset, NJ) have been shown to correlate with invasive arterial line measurements in VAD patients [50]. Current clinical guidelines recommend maintaining the mean arterial pressure between 70 and 80 mmHg; pressures above 90 mmHg should be avoided given that high afterload may decrease flow through the pump [51]. For this reason, blood pressure monitoring during hemodialysis is imperative and can be challenging in the outpatient setting. For successful delivery of RRT to VAD patients, close communication between VAD cardiologists, VAD coordinators, and nephrologists is of paramount importance.

Conclusion

With the advent of CF technology, VAD implantation for the treatment of advanced heart failure has increased exponentially. Although the high percentage of concomitant baseline RD in these patients translates into an increased risk of post-VAD AKI, early improvement in kidney function is far more common, albeit transient. However, both worsening *and* improvement in renal function appear to identify patients at a high risk of death, and recurrence of baseline renal dysfunction with longer duration of support is very common. Additional research to better understand the mechanism, prognostic importance, and potential treatment strategies for these large changes in renal function will be critical.

Key Messages

- Renal dysfunction is common in heart failure patients referred for VAD placement and is a major risk factor for post-VAD acute kidney injury.
- Although the majority of patients experience improvement in renal function following VAD placement, this improvement is largely transient, with subsequent resurgence of renal dysfunction with prolonged VAD support.
- Both post-VAD worsening in renal function and post-VAD improvement in renal function identify patients at an increased risk of death.

References

1. Peura JL, Colvin-Adams M, Francis GS, Grady KL, Hoffman TM, Jessup M, John R, Kiernan MS, Mitchell JE, Connell JB, Pagani FD, Petty M, Ravichandran P, Rogers JG, Semigran MJ, Toole JM, American Heart Association Heart Failure and Transplantation Committee of the Council on Clinical Cardiology; Council on Cardiopulmonary, Critical Care, Perioperative and Resuscitation; Council on Cardiovascular Disease in the Young; Council on Cardiovascular Nursing; Council on Cardiovascular Radiology and Intervention, and Council on Cardiovascular Surgery and Anesthesia. Recommendations for the use of mechanical circulatory support: device strategies and patient selection: a scientific statement from the American Heart Association. Circulation. 2012;126:2648–67.
2. Slaughter MS, Rogers JG, Milano CA, Russell SD, Conte JV, Feldman D, Sun B, Tatooles AJ, Delgado RM, Long JW, Wozniak TC, Ghumman W, Farrar DJ, Frazier OH, Investigators HI. Advanced heart failure treated with continuous-flow left ventricular assist device. N Engl J Med. 2009;361:2241–51.
3. Miller LW, Pagani FD, Russell SD, John R, Boyle AJ, Aaronson KD, Conte JV, Naka Y, Mancini D, Delgado RM, MacGillivray TE, Farrar DJ, Frazier OH, Investigators HIC. Use of a continuous-flow device in patients awaiting heart transplantation. N Engl J Med. 2007;357:885–96.
4. Aaronson KD, Slaughter MS, Miller LW, McGee EC, Cotts WG, Acker MA, Jessup ML, Gregoric ID, Loyalka P, Frazier OH, Jeevanandam V, Anderson AS, Kormos RL, Teuteberg JJ, Levy WC, Naftel DC, Bittman RM, Pagani FD, Hathaway DR, Boyce SW, Investigators HVADHBtTAT. Use of an intrapericardial, continuous-flow, centrifugal pump in patients awaiting heart transplantation. Circulation. 2012;125:3191–200.
5. Bock JS, Gottlieb SS. Cardiorenal syndrome: new perspectives. Circulation. 2010;121:2592–600.
6. Ronco C, Haapio M, House A, Anavekar N, Bellomo R. Cardiorenal syndrome. J Am Coll Cardiol. 2008;52:1527–39.
7. America HFSo. Executive summary: HFSA 2010 comprehensive heart failure practice guideline. J Card Fail. 2010;16:475–539.
8. Kirklin JK, Naftel DC, Kormos RL, Stevenson LW, Pagani FD, Miller MA, Timothy Baldwin J, Young JB. Fifth INTERMACS annual report: risk factor analysis from more than 6,000 mechanical circulatory support patients. J Heart Lung Transplant. 2013;32:141–56.
9. Feldman D, Pamboukian SV, Teuteberg JJ, Birks E, Lietz K, Moore SA, Morgan JA, Arabia F, Bauman ME, Buchholz HW, Deng M, Dickstein ML, El-Banayosy A, Elliot T, Goldstein DJ, Grady KL, Jones K, Hryniewicz K, John R, Kaan A, Kusne S, Loebe M, Massicotte MP, Moazami N, Mohacsi P, Mooney M, Nelson T, Pagani F, Perry W, Potapov EV, Rame JE, Russell SD, Sorensen EN, Sun B, Strueber M, Mangi AA, Petty MG, Rogers J. The 2013

international society for heart and lung transplantation guidelines for mechanical circulatory support executive summary. J Heart Lung Transplant. 2013;32:157–87.

10. Rose EA, Gelijns AC, Moskowitz AJ, Heitjan DF, Stevenson LW, Dembitsky W, Long JW, Ascheim DD, Tierney AR, Levitan RG, Watson JT, Meier P, Ronan NS, Shapiro PA, Lazar RM, Miller LW, Gupta L, Frazier OH, Desvigne-Nickens P, Oz MC, Poirier VL, Group REoMAftToCHFRS. Long-term use of a left ventricular assist device for end-stage heart failure. N Engl J Med. 2001;345:1435–43.
11. Frazier OH, Rose EA, Oz MC, Dembitsky W, McCarthy P, Radovancevic B, Poirier VL, Dasse KA. Multicenter clinical evaluation of the heartmate vented electric left ventricular assist system in patients awaiting heart transplantation. J Thorac Cardiovasc Surg. 2001;122: 1186–95.
12. Rogers JG, Aaronson KD, Boyle AJ, Russell SD, Milano CA, Pagani FD, Edwards BS, Park S, John R, Conte JV, Farrar DJ, Slaughter MS, Investigators HI. Continuous flow left ventricular assist device improves functional capacity and quality of life of advanced heart failure patients. J Am Coll Cardiol. 2010;55:1826–34.
13. Park SJ, Milano CA, Tatooles AJ, Rogers JG, Adamson RM, Steidley DE, Ewald GA, Sundareswaran KS, Farrar DJ, Slaughter MS, Investigators HIC. Outcomes in advanced heart failure patients with left ventricular assist devices for destination therapy. Circ Heart Fail. 2012;5:241–8.
14. Moazami N, Fukamachi K, Kobayashi M, Smedira NG, Hoercher KJ, Massiello A, Lee S, Horvath DJ, Starling RC. Axial and centrifugal continuous-flow rotary pumps: a translation from pump mechanics to clinical practice. J Heart Lung Transplant. 2013;32:1–11.
15. Thakar CV, Arrigain S, Worley S, Yared J-P, Paganini EP. A clinical score to predict acute renal failure after cardiac surgery. J Am Soc Nephrol. 2005;16:162–8.
16. Rosner MH, Okusa MD. Acute kidney injury associated with cardiac surgery. Clin J Am Soc Nephrol. 2006;1:19–32.
17. Alba AC, Rao V, Ivanov J, Ross HJ, Delgado DH. Predictors of acute renal dysfunction after ventricular assist device placement. J Card Fail. 2009;15:874–81.
18. Yoshioka D, Sakaguchi T, Saito S, Miyagawa S, Nishi H, Yoshikawa Y, et al. Predictor of early mortality for severe heart failure patients with left ventricular assist device implantation: significance of INTERMACS level and renal function. Circ J. 2012;76(7):1631–8.
19. Borgi J, Tsiouris A, Hodari A, Cogan CM, Paone G, Morgan JA. Significance of postoperative acute renal failure after continuous-flow left ventricular assist device implantation. Ann Thorac Surg. 2013;95:163–9.
20. Starling RC, Naka Y, Boyle AJ, Gonzalez-Stawinski G, John R, Jorde U, Russell SD, Conte JV, Aaronson KD, McGee EC, Cotts WG, DeNofrio D, Pham DT, Farrar DJ, Pagani FD. Results of the post-U.S. Food and Drug Administration-approval study with a continuous flow left ventricular assist device as a bridge to heart transplantation: a prospective study using the INTERMACS (interagency registry for mechanically assisted circulatory support). J Am Coll Cardiol. 2011;57:1890–8.
21. Demirozu ZT, Etheridge WB, Radovancevic R, Frazier OH. Results of heartmate ii left ventricular assist device implantation on renal function in patients requiring post-implant renal replacement therapy. Healun. 2011;30:182–7.
22. Genovese EA, Dew MA, Teuteberg JJ, Simon MA, Kay J, Siegenthaler MP, Bhama JK, Bermudez CA, Lockard KL, Winowich S, Kormos RL. Incidence and patterns of adverse event onset during the first 60 days after ventricular assist device implantation. Ann Thorac Surg. 2009;88:1162–70.
23. Feller ED, Sorensen EN, Haddad M, Pierson RN, Johnson FL, Brown JM, Griffith BP. Clinical outcomes are similar in pulsatile and nonpulsatile left ventricular assist device recipients. Ann Thorac Surg. 2007;83:1082–8.
24. Hasin T, Topilsky Y, Schirger JA, Li Z, Zhao Y, Boilson BA, Clavell AL, Rodeheffer RJ, Frantz RP, Edwards BS, Pereira NL, Joyce L, Daly R, Park SJ, Kushwaha SS. Changes in renal function after implantation of continuous-flow left ventricular assist devices. J Am Coll Cardiol. 2012;59:26–36.

25. Kaltenmaier B, Pommer W, Kaufmann F, Hennig E, Molzahn M, Hetzer R. Outcome of patients with ventricular assist devices and acute renal failure requiring renal replacement therapy. ASAIO J. 2000;46:330–3.
26. Sandner SE, Zimpfer D, Zrunek P, Dunkler D, Schima H, Rajek A, Grimm M, Wolner E, Wieselthaler GM. Renal function after implantation of continuous versus pulsatile flow left ventricular assist devices. J Heart Lung Transplant. 2008;27:469–73.
27. Sandner SE, Zimpfer D, Zrunek P, Rajek A, Schima H, Dunkler D, Grimm M, Wolner E, Wieselthaler GM. Renal function and outcome after continuous flow left ventricular assist device implantation. Ann Thorac Surg. 2009;87:1072–8.
28. Topkara VK, Dang NC, Barili F, Cheema FH, Martens TP, George I, Bardakci H, Oz MC, Naka Y. Predictors and outcomes of continuous veno-venous hemodialysis use after implantation of a left ventricular assist device. J Heart Lung Transplant. 2006;25:404–8.
29. Brisco MA, Kimmel SE, Coca SG, Putt ME, Jessup M, Tang W, Parikh CR. Prevalence and prognostic importance of changes in renal function following mechanical circulatory support. Circ Heart Fail. 2014;7:68–75.
30. Slaughter MS, Pagani FD, McGee EC, Birks EJ, Cotts WG, Gregoric I, Howard Frazier O, Icenogle T, Najjar SS, Boyce SW, Acker MA, John R, Hathaway DR, Najarian KB, Aaronson KD, Investigators HBtTAT. Heartware ventricular assist system for bridge to transplant: combined results of the bridge to transplant and continued access protocol trial. J Heart Lung Transplant. 2013;32:675–83.
31. Stevenson LW, Pagani FD, Young JB, Jessup M, Miller L, Kormos RL, Naftel DC, Ulisney K, Desvigne-Nickens P, Kirklin JK. INTERMACS profiles of advanced heart failure: The current picture. J Heart Lung Transplant. 2011;28:535–41.
32. Boyle AJ, Ascheim DD, Russo MJ, Kormos RL, John R, Naka Y, Gelijns AC, Hong KN, Teuteberg JJ. Clinical outcomes for continuous-flow left ventricular assist device patients stratified by pre-operative INTERMACS classification. J Heart Lung Transplant. 2011;30:402–7.
33. Cowger J, Sundareswaran K, Rogers JG, Park SJ, Pagani FD, Bhat G, Jaski B, Farrar DJ, Slaughter MS. Predicting survival in patients receiving continuous flow left ventricular assist devices: the HeartMate II risk score. J Am Coll Cardiol. 2013;61(3):313–21. Epub 2012 Dec 19.
34. Kamdar F, Boyle A, Liao K, Colvin-Adams M, Joyce L, John R. Effects of centrifugal, axial, and pulsatile left ventricular assist device support on end-organ function in heart failure patients. J Heart Lung Transplant. 2009;28:352–9.
35. Iwashima Y, Yanase M, Horio T, Seguchi O, Murata Y, Fujita T, Toda K, Kawano Y, Nakatani T. Serial changes in renal function as a prognostic indicator in advanced heart failure patients with left ventricular assist system. Ann Thorac Surg. 2012;93:816–23.
36. Radovancevic B, Vrtovec B, de Kort E, Radovancevic R, Gregoric ID, Frazier OH. End-organ function in patients on long-term circulatory support with continuous- or pulsatile-flow assist devices. J Heart Lung Transplant. 2007;26:815–8.
37. Singh M, Shullo M, Kormos R, Lockard K, Zomak R, Simon M, Bermudez C, Bhama J, McNamara D, Toyoda Y, Teuteberg J. Impact of renal function before mechanical circulatory support on posttransplant renal outcomes. Ann Thorac Surg. 2011;91:1348–54.
38. Russell SD, Rogers JG, Milano CA, Dyke DB, Pagani FD, Aranda JM, Klodell CT, Boyle AJ, John R, Chen L, Massey HT, Farrar DJ, Conte JV, Investigators HIC. Renal and hepatic function improve in advanced heart failure patients during continuous-flow support with the heartmate ii left ventricular assist device. Circulation. 2009;120:2352–7.
39. Butler J, Geisberg C, Howser R, Portner PM, Rogers JG, Deng MC, Pierson RN. Relationship between renal function and left ventricular assist device use. Ann Thorac Surg. 2006;81:1745–51.
40. Letsou GV, Myers TJ, Gregoric ID, Delgado R, Shah N, Robertson K, Radovancevic B, Frazier OH. Continuous axial-flow left ventricular assist device (Jarvik 2000) maintains kidney and liver perfusion for up to 6 months. Ann Thorac Surg. 2003;76:1167–70.
41. Heywood J, Fonarow G, Costanzo M, Mathur V, Wigneswaran J, Wynne J, Committee A, Investigators. High prevalence of renal dysfunction and its impact on outcome in 118,465 patients hospitalized with acute decompensated heart failure: a report from the adhere database. J Card Fail. 2007;13:422–30.

42. Welp H, Rukosujew A, Tjan TDT, Hoffmeier A, Kösek V, Scheld HH, Drees G. Effect of pulsatile and non-pulsatile left ventricular assist devices on the renin-angiotensin system in patients with end-stage heart failure. Thorac Cardiovasc Surg. 2010;58 Suppl 2:S185–8.
43. Drakos SG, Wever-Pinzon O, Selzman CH, Gilbert EM, Alharethi R, Reid BB, Saidi A, Diakos NA, Stoker S, Davis ES, Movsesian M, Li DY, Stehlik J, Kfoury AG, Investigators UUCRP. Magnitude and time course of changes induced by continuous-flow left ventricular assist device unloading in chronic heart failure: insights into cardiac recovery. J Am Coll Cardiol. 2013;61:1985–94.
44. Saito S, Nishinaka T, Westaby S. Hemodynamics of chronic nonpulsatile flow: implications for lvad development. Surg Clin N Am. 2004;84:61–74.
45. Kihara S, Litwak KN, Nichols L, Litwak P, Kameneva MV, Wu Z, Kormos RL, Griffith BP. Smooth muscle cell hypertrophy of renal cortex arteries with chronic continuous flow left ventricular assist. Ann Thorac Surg. 2003;75:178–83; discussion 183.
46. Ootaki C, Yamashita M, Ootaki Y, Kamohara K, Weber S, Klatte RS, Smith WA, Massiello AL, Emancipator SN, Golding LA. Reduced pulsatility induces periarteritis in kidney: role of the local renin–angiotensin system. J Thorac Cardiovasc Surg. 2008;136:150–8.
47. Saito S, Westaby S, Piggot D, Dudnikov S, Robson D, Catarino PA, Clelland C, Nojiri C. End-organ function during chronic nonpulsatile circulation. Ann Thorac Surg. 2002;74:1080–5.
48. Patel AM, Adeseun GA, Ahmed I, Mitter N, Rame JE, Rudnick MR. Renal failure in patients with left ventricular assist devices. Clin J Am Soc Nephrol. 2013;8:484–96.
49. Guglielmi AA, Guglielmi KE, Bhat G, Siemeck R, Tatooles AJ. Peritoneal dialysis after left ventricular assist device placement. ASAIO J. 2014;60:127–8.
50. Lanier GM, Orlanes K, Hayashi Y, Murphy J, Flannery M, Te-Frey R, Uriel N, Yuzefpolskaya M, Mancini DM, Naka Y, Takayama H, Jorde UP, Demmer RT, Colombo PC. Validity and reliability of a novel slow cuff-deflation system for noninvasive blood pressure monitoring in patients with continuous-flow left ventricular assist device. Circ Heart fail. 2013;6:1005–12.
51. Slaughter MS, Pagani FD, Rogers JG, Miller LW, Sun B, Russell SD, Starling RC, Chen L, Boyle AJ, Chillcott S, Adamson RM, Blood MS, Camacho MT, Idrissi KA, Petty M, Sobieski M, Wright S, Myers TJ, Farrar DJ, Investigators HIC. Clinical management of continuous-flow left ventricular assist devices in advanced heart failure. J Heart Lung Transplant. 2010;29: S1–39.

Chapter 10
Kidney Injury After Vascular Surgery

Shamsuddin Akhtar

Objectives

- To discuss the incidence of AKI after vascular surgery and its impact on subsequent clinical outcomes.
- To evaluate the risk factors (patient-related factors, surgery-related factors, and management-related factors) that predispose patients to AKI after vascular surgery.
- To understand pre-, intra-, and postoperative management strategies and goals of care that should be considered in patients at risk for AKI after vascular surgery.

Introduction

Peripheral vascular disease (PAD) affects approximately 8.5 million Americans over 40 years of age [1]. It is associated with significant morbidity and mortality. PAD is more prevalent in older individuals, and it disproportionally affects African Americans. As with other atherosclerotic conditions, it is associated with hypertension, diabetes mellitus, chronic kidney disease, and smoking. However, diabetes mellitus and cigarette smoking are stronger risk factors for PAD than for atherosclerotic heart disease. Presence of PAD (defined by ankle-brachial index of <0.9) is a marker for systemic atherosclerosis [2]. In one recent trial involving patients presenting for abdominal aortic aneurysm repair (AAA), the incidence of concomitant coronary artery disease, diabetes mellitus, and hypertension was 39, 22, and 78 %,

S. Akhtar, MD (✉)
Department of Anesthesiology, Yale University School of Medicine,
333 Cedar Street, TMP #3, New Haven, CT 06520, USA
e-mail: shamsuddin.akhtar@yale.edu

C.V. Thakar, C.R. Parikh (eds.), *Perioperative Kidney Injury: Principles of Risk Assessment, Diagnosis and Treatment*, DOI 10.1007/978-1-4939-1273-5_10

respectively. A third of the patients enrolled in the randomized trial had glomerular filtration rate (GFR) <60 ml/min per 1.73 m^2 [3]. As the patients have significant comorbidities, any significant physiological perturbation and major systemic inflammatory response in the perioperative period can lead to worsening of cardio-pulmonary function, worsening of renal function, and possible new acute kidney injury (AKI). This chapter will discuss incidence and risk factors that predispose patients to AKI after vascular surgery. As in patients who undergo cardiac surgery, timely and clinically relevant diagnosis of AKI is challenging. Current prophylactic and management strategies that may protect the kidney in patients who undergo vascular procedures will be also discussed.

With the advent of cardiovascular stents, the field of vascular surgery has undergone significant changes in the past 15 years and continues to evolve very rapidly. As endovascular technology improves exponentially, the outcomes after endovascular interventions have improved dramatically. Three major trials EVAR (UK endovascular aneurysm repair), DREAM (Dutch randomized endovascular aneurysm repair), and OVER (open surgery vs. endovascular repair Veterans Affairs Cooperative Study) have confirmed early benefits of endovascular aneurysm repair [2]. In the EVAR trial, the procedural mortality was 4.3 % compared to 1.8 % with endovascular repair. In the OVER trial, patients in the endovascular repair group had reduced median procedure time (2.9 vs. 3.7 h), blood loss (200 vs. 1,000 ml), transfusion requirement (0 vs. 1.0 units), duration of mechanical ventilation (3.6 vs. 5.0 h), intensive care unit stay (1 vs. 4 days), and hospital stay (3 vs. 7 days), but required substantial exposure to fluoroscopy and contrast [3]. However, long-term mortality (after 2 years) has not been shown to be much different between the two groups. As expected, major open aortic procedures are decreasing in frequency. Endovascular repair of abdominal aortic aneurysm (AAA) and thoracic aortic aneurysm (TAA) is well established in many centers. Hybrid procedures which involve both endovascular repair and open repairs are being performed for complex vascular pathologies and will continue to increase in foreseeable future.

Incidence of Acute Kidney Injury

AKI has always been a significant concern in patients undergoing aortic vascular surgery, especially ruptured or emergency procedures. In many patients, AKI is transient but in some patients the renal injury is significant requiring either short-term renal replacement therapy or lifelong dialysis. Suprarenal and juxtarenal interventions are likely to cause more renal dysfunction. Even though mild to moderate degrees of AKI are common, 2–8 % of the patients after aortic surgery require renal replacement therapy (RRT) which is associated with elevated short-term mortality of up to 64 %. AKI also affects long-term mortality, even for patients with partial and complete recovery. The incidence of AKI after thoracic aortic surgery ranges from 18 to 55 %. The reported incidence varies according to the definition of AKI and aortic pathology used by the investigators [4].

With elective open AAA repair, the incidence of AKI has been reported to be 1–13 %. Vascular procedures that do not directly impact renal blood flow or procedures with minimal or transient hemodynamic perturbations are less likely to cause AKI. Predictably higher incidence has been reported for surgeries requiring supraceliac clamp and suprarenal clamps than for infrarenal clamps. However, infrarenal clamping is not totally benign. Infrarenal aortic clamping is associated with changes in renal blood flow and plaque embolization (due to aortic manipulation), which can cause perioperative AKI.

In the case of endovascular aneurysm repair (EVAR), the incidence of AKI ranges from 1 to 23 % and is lower compared to open repair [5]. Initial reports suggested significant decrease in renal function after EVAR; however, subsequently reports have not supported this observation. Despite the use of contrast, typically 130–260 ml during EVAR, lower incidence of renal dysfunction has been reported, when compared to open repairs. With ever improving stent technology and procedural expertise, the future incidence of AKI after vascular procedures is likely to decrease, especially endovascular procedures.

Risk Factors of AKI

The pathogenesis of AKI in the context of any major systemic insult is a result of complex interaction between baseline comorbidity, hemodynamic disturbances, nephrotoxic drugs, and inflammatory responses. Many risk factors that can lead to AKI in patients after vascular surgery have been identified. Rather than a single characteristic, patients often have multiple risk factors that result in a cumulative risk of developing AKI. They can be grouped into three broad categories: patient-related factors, surgery-related factors, and management-related factors (Table 10.1).

Patient-Related Factors

These include patient's age, chronic kidney disease (pre-procedure or baseline renal function), and proteinuria [6]. In cardiac surgery patients, anemia has been associated with risk of developing AKI; however, its role in vascular surgery patients has not been investigated. Chronic kidney disease (CKD) is the most common risk factor for AKI. Even though creatinine may remain within normal limits, renal function declines progressively with aging. Older patients are at increased risk of developing renal dysfunction or AKI. A recent meta-analysis shows a strong relationship with low preoperative estimated glomerular filtration rate (eGFR) and postoperative outcomes. Within 30 days of surgery, eGFR less than 60 ml/min/1.73 m [2] was associated with a threefold increased risk of death and AKI. An eGFR less than 60 ml/min/1.73 m [2] was also associated with an increased risk of all-cause mortality and major adverse cardiovascular events during long-term follow-up. This analysis included both cardiac and noncardiac surgery patients [7].

Table 10.1 Risk factors that contribute to AKI in vascular surgery patients

Patient-related risk factors	Older age
	Decreased preoperative eGFR
	Limb ischemia prior to surgery
	Preoperative anemia?
Surgery-related risk factors	Location of surgery: thoracic aorta, abdominal aorta, juxtarenal, peripheral vascular surgery, or carotid surgery
	Complexity of surgery
	Total surgical trauma
	Specific surgical technique: open vs. endovascular vs. hybrid
	Specifics of endograft
	Hemodynamic changes during surgery
	Emergency surgery
Management-related risk factors	Hypovolemia
	Hypervolemia
	Cardiac output
	Starch-containing IV fluids
	IV contrast agents
	Use of nephrotoxic drugs: e.g., aminoglycosides, NSAIDs
	High chloride-containing fluids?

Specifically, patients with GFR <45 ml/min are an increased risk of AKI and requiring temporary or long-term renal replacement therapy after vascular surgery. End-stage renal disease (ESRD) patients undergoing elective major vascular surgery were significantly more likely than non-ESRD patients to develop surgical site infection, unplanned intubation, ventilator dependence, combined pulmonary outcome, and a need for reoperation within 30 days of surgery. The death rate in ESRD patients after elective vascular surgery was fourfold higher for all operations [8].

Surgery-Related Factors

These include the type of vascular surgery, emergency surgery, complexity of surgery, hemodynamic and inflammatory perturbations resulting from the surgery, and specific surgical techniques or maneuvers that may affect renal function. Surgeries involving the aorta have a higher incidence of AKI. Hypoperfusion of the kidneys either due to direct interruption of blood flow (supraceliac, supra-mesenteric, suprarenal, or juxtarenal clamping) or systemic hypotension (due to blood loss, myocardial dysfunction) can lead to AKI. In one recent study involving 169 patients, postoperative transient renal dysfunction occurred in 37.3 % of patients after open juxtarenal AAA repair. Technical factors including total renal ischemia time, aortic clamp position, and left renal vein division were the strongest predictors of renal dysfunction [9]. Duration of interruption of blood flow is also well correlated to AKI.

Healthy kidneys can typically tolerate 30–60 min of ischemia [10]. Keeping the total ischemic time to less than 30 min has been a standard recommendation based on retrospective and animal studies [11]. Malpositioning of the surgical clamps can lead to suboptimal blood flow to the kidney. Furthermore, increased atherosclerotic burden and plaques near the renal vessels can lead to atheroembolic ischemia of the kidney. More proximal clamping also causes more pronounced inflammatory response and reperfusion injury, not only involving the kidneys but also other mesenteric organs which can indirectly contribute to changes in intrarenal renal blood flow and lead to AKI. Furthermore, extensive dissection, significant blood loss, and significant fluid shifts cause profound neuroendocrine-inflammatory stress response, which will then predispose the patients to AKI. The ultimate consequence will depend on the overall involvement of the kidney and its baseline function.

EVAR are less likely to cause AKI compared to open procedures; however, they are not innocuous and renal function can decline in some patients. The pathophysiology of AKI in EVAR is complex: contrast-induced nephropathy, renal microembolization, and acute tubular necrosis are all implicated. EVAR has the intrinsic potential effect to cause adverse events on renal function due to endoluminal manipulations and contrast administration during endograft deployment and secondary endovascular procedures, as well as for contrast nephropathy from repetitive serial computed tomography (CT) scans [12]. Type of endovascular grafts also affects the frequency of AKI. Deterioration in renal function after fenestrated EVAR has been reported to be as high as 10–30 % [13].

Management-Related Factors

Predictably presence of nephrotoxic drugs, choice of intravenous fluids, and use of colloids can impact on AKI. Aminoglycosides and contrast media (ionic and nonionic) can cause AKI. The use of contrast media should be kept to the minimum, especially, in patients with baseline CKD. There is some evidence that hyperchloremic solutions (like normal saline) can affect renal function in intensive care unit (ICU) patients [14]. Its detrimental role in patients undergoing major vascular surgery has not been well elucidated. However, it is not uncommon for patients undergoing aortic surgery or complex vascular surgery to receive significant amount of cell-saver blood. Since salvaged blood is washed in normal saline, many patients develop hyperchloremic metabolic acidosis, perioperatively. As for colloids, starch-containing colloids have been associated with poor outcomes, especially in ICU patients with sepsis [15]. Since many major vascular surgery patients are admitted to ICU, have significant hemodynamic perturbations, and experience significant systemic inflammatory response, it may be prudent to avoid starch-containing fluids. The role of starch-containing fluids, specifically in patients undergoing major vascular surgery, has not been well elucidated, and this recommendation is based on extrapolation of data from ICU patients and risk factors that are usually present in patients who present for vascular surgery.

Approaches for Management of Kidney Injury

Identifying patients who are at risk of developing perioperative AKI is very essential. Optimizing renal function preoperatively is important. Prevention strategies include hydration, avoidance of nephrotoxic drugs (e.g., nonsteroidal antiinflammatory drugs [NSAIDs]), and pharmacological agents to prevent contrast-induced nephropathy. However, no pharmacological agents have been proven to be efficacious in preventing perioperative AKI, especially in patients with normal renal function. Intraoperatively, the use of mannitol has been advocated in open AAA repairs; however, the key is to maintain stable hemodynamics, keeping renal ischemic time to the minimum. If the patient develops AKI, the use of early renal replacement therapy may be indicated. There is no level I evidence regarding the prevention of AKI in patients undergoing vascular surgery.

Preoperative Strategies

Prior to scheduled vascular surgery many patient have had angiography or other radiological procedures to better delineate vascular anatomy. The use of contrast agents during those procedures can affect renal function that may become apparent 48–72 h after the diagnostic procedure. If AKI develops after diagnostic procedure, elective vascular surgery should be postponed until renal function returns back to baseline or stabilizes. Nephrotoxic agents should be avoided perioperatively, especially NSAIDs and aminoglycosides. Angiotensin-converting enzyme inhibitors and angiotensin-receptor blockers are typically held 24 h prior to elective surgery. Prevention of contrast-induced AKI (CIAKI) is a key preoperative consideration.

Contrast-Induced AKI (CIAKI)

Endovascular procedures and open peripheral vascular procedures typically require use of contrast media to establish success of the procedure. However, contrast media can have significant detrimental effect on renal function. Detailed discussion of this topic is beyond the scope of this chapter, and only important concepts are discussed below.

Many strategies for prevention of CIAKI have been tried. Drugs that have been evaluated include calcium antagonists, adenosine antagonists, N-acetylcysteine, prostaglandin analogs, L-arginine, statins, atrial natriuretic peptide, endothelin antagonists, dopamine, fenoldopam, hypertonic mannitol, and furosemide. With the possible exception of high-dose N-acetylcysteine, no treatment has been unequivocally proven in reducing CIAKI risk, while endothelin antagonists may even have detrimental effects [16]. Elective vascular surgery patients are at a unique advantage as preventative strategies like hydration with isotonic fluids can be started preoperatively. A meta-analysis of 19 studies of patients who underwent coronary angiography or peripheral angiographic or interventional procedures showed decreased incidence of AKI with sodium bicarbonate than normal saline [17]. Most of the studies comparing the two fluids used the "Merten protocol," which consists of administration of 3 ml/kg/h of sodium bicarbonate in a glucose solution containing 154 mmol/l of sodium bicarbonate during the first hour preceding the contrast procedure, followed by infusion at a rate of 1 ml/kg/h for 6 h after the procedure.

Intraoperative Strategies

Hemodynamic Optimization

Reduction in renal blood flow and renal ischemia has been regarded as central to pathogenesis of AKI. Thus, maintaining adequate cardiac output, renal perfusion, and oxygen delivery have been key goals in preventing perioperative AKI. This was conventionally achieved by optimal fluid therapy and keeping the patient euvolumic. On the one hand, failure to prescribe adequate intravenous fluid can place a patient at risk of hypovolemia and AKI; on the other hand, excessive fluid infusion may promote third-space loss and intra-abdominal hypertension (IAH), which can lead to decreased renal perfusion. Thus, in the context of the kidney, both hyper- and hypovolemia are deleterious. Practitioners should recognize the limitations of frequently used pressure monitors (central venous pressure [CVP], pulmonary artery occlusion pressure [PAOP]) as measure of volume status. Flow-related indices and devices that monitor cardiac output and stroke volume variations have their own limitations. However, at the moment, an individualized, timely fluid "replacement" therapy, by titration of volume to physiologic flow-related end points with appropriate monitoring, seems a rational choice [18]. In a recent meta-analysis, goal-directed fluid therapy (GDT), where treatment and control groups received similar volumes of fluids, found that GDT was associated with improved renal outcomes compared to controls [19]. Results of an ongoing randomized control trial (OPTIMISE, Optimization of Perioperative Cardiovascular Management to Improve Surgical Outcome) will help in guiding hemodynamic therapy in patients undergoing noncardiac surgery.

Mannitol

Mannitol has been used in open aortic aneurysm surgery since the early 1960s. It improves perioperative urine output. Mannitol not only acts as an osmotic diuretic, but also attenuates the reduction in cortical blood flow that occurs during and immediately after aortic cross-clamping. It scavenges oxygen-derived free radicals decreases subclinical glomerular and renal tubular damage. However, objective improvement in renal function has not been consistently demonstrated in randomized control trials [20]. Currently, use of mannitol is practitioner dependent.

Fenoldopam

Fenoldopam mesylate is a selective dopamine-1 (DA-1) agonist, with no effects on dopamine-2 (DA-2) and alpha-1 receptors, that increases both medullary and cortical blood flows and reduces the oxygen demand. A meta-analysis including 1,290 patients found that fenoldopam significantly reduced the need for RRT and in-hospital mortality. This study involved only 328 noncardiac surgery patients (kidney and liver transplant, vascular surgery). A later review confirmed a beneficial effect in cardiac surgical patients, but no conclusion can be drawn regarding noncardiac surgery, and further adequately powered studies are needed prior to recommending its use [18].

Hypothermia

Regional renal hypothermia has been used occasionally for many years to protect the kidney, especially in patients undergoing AAA repair, on a valid premise that cooling the kidney would decrease its metabolic rate. The technique typically involves infusion of 500 to 1 l of cold (4–5 °C) crystalloid solution into an isolated aortic segment or directly into the renal artery. The strategy has shown some benefit and is practiced by some centers, especially when significant renal ischemia is expected, for example, procedures involving complex repair of thoracoabdominal aorta [21].

Postoperative Strategies

Though the insult to the kidney will occur in the intraoperative period, with the current diagnostic markers, the true extent of injury only becomes apparent in the postoperative period. Consequences of neurohumoral-inflammatory stress become more evident within the first 24 h after major vascular surgery. Surgical trauma leads to fluid redistribution into extravascular space, and fluid requirements continue to be high after open aortic procedures. Myoglobinuria may develop especially if total ischemic time was significant and/or ischemic limbs get vascularized. The effects of intravenous (IV) contrast after diagnostic or endovascular procedures also become apparent during this time. The goals of management in the postoperative period are based on the same principles as in the pre- and intraoperative period: maintain renal perfusion by optimizing cardiac output and avoiding hypovolemia, avoid nephrotoxic drugs, keep the renal tubules flushed, and prevent volume overload. If the patient develops acute renal failure, early renal replacement therapy may be preferable; however, outcome benefits of early dialysis in postsurgical vascular patients have not been studied. Hence, at this time, the role of dialysis is viewed to be supportive. Specific modalities of dialysis and other postoperative complications are discussed elsewhere.

Conclusion

Patients who undergo vascular surgery have significant comorbidities, and AKI after vascular surgery is not uncommon. The incidence of AKI after vascular surgery is dependent on various modifiable (e.g., surgical technique, total ischemic time, optimization of preoperative renal function) and nonmodifiable perioperative factors (age, diabetes, preoperative renal function). No pharmacological agents have been proven to be efficacious in preventing perioperative AKI, especially in patients with normal renal function. Early recognition and supportive intervention may decrease the overall renal damage and improve patient outcomes in vascular surgery setting.

Key Messages

- In patients with baseline vascular disease, any significant physiological perturbations and major systemic inflammatory response in the perioperative period can lead to worsening of renal function and possible new acute kidney injury (AKI).
- Although the incidence of AKI after vascular surgery varies significantly, it is of particular concern in patients undergoing aortic vascular surgery, especially for ruptured or emergency procedures.
- Surgical types/techniques (e.g., thoracic, abdominal, open, endovascular, etc.), in concert with other factors, do impact the risk of postoperative AKI.
- The pathogenesis of AKI in this setting is a result of complex interaction between patient-related factors (baseline predispositions), surgery-related factors (techniques and intraoperative events), and management-related factors (nephrotoxic injury).

References

1. Go AS, Mozaffarian D, Roger VL, Benjamin EJ, Berry JD, Borden WB, Bravata DM, Dai S, Ford ES, Fox CS, Franco S, Fullerton HJ, Gillespie C, Hailpern SM, Heit JA, Howard VJ, Huffman MD, Kissela BM, Kittner SJ, Lackland DT, Lichtman JH, Lisabeth LD, Magid D, Marcus GM, Marelli A, Matchar DB, McGuire DK, Mohler ER, Moy CS, Mussolino ME, Nichol G, Paynter NP, Schreiner PJ, Sorlie PD, Stein J, Turan TN, Virani SS, Wong ND, Woo D, Turner MB, American Heart Association Statistics Committee and Stroke Statistics Subcommittee. Heart disease and stroke statistics–2013 update: a report from the American Heart Association. Circulation. 2013;127:e6–245.
2. Rooke TW, Hirsch AT, Misra S, Sidawy AN, Beckman JA, Findeiss LK, Golzarian J, Gornik HL, Halperin JL, Jaff MR, Moneta GL, Olin JW, Stanley JC, White CJ, White JV, Zierler RE, Society for Cardiovascular Angiography and Interventions; Society of Interventional Radiology; Society for Vascular Medicine; Society for Vascular Surgery. 2011 ACCF/AHA focused update of the guideline for the management of patients with peripheral artery disease (updating the 2005 guideline): a report of the American College of Cardiology Foundation/American Heart Association Task Force on Practice Guidelines. J Am Coll Cardiol. 2011;58:2020–45.

3. Lederle FA, Freischlag JA, Kyriakides TC, Padberg Jr FT, Matsumura JS, Kohler TR, Lin PH, Jean-Claude JM, Cikrit DF, Swanson KM, Peduzzi PN. Outcomes following endovascular vs open repair of abdominal aortic aneurysm: a randomized trial. JAMA. 2009;302:1535–42. doi:10.1001/jama.2009.1426.
4. Roh GU, Lee JW, Nam SB, Lee J, Choi JR, Shim YH. Incidence and risk factors of acute kidney injury after thoracic aortic surgery for acute dissection. Ann Thorac Surg. 2012;94:766–71. doi:10.1016/j.athoracsur.2012.04.057. Epub 2012 Jun 21.
5. Saratzis AN, Goodyear S, Sur H, Saedon M, Imray C, Mahmood A. Acute kidney injury after endovascular repair of abdominal aortic aneurysm. J Endovasc Ther. 2013;20:315–30.
6. Sharfuddin AA, Molitoris BA. Pathophysiology of ischemic acute kidney injury. Nat Rev Nephrol. 2011;7:189–200.
7. Mooney JF, Ranasinghe I, Chow CK, Perkovic V, Barzi F, Zoungas S, Holzmann MJ, Welten GM, Biancari F, Wu VC, Tan TC, Cass A, Hillis GS. Preoperative estimates of glomerular filtration rate as predictors of outcome after surgery: a systematic review and meta-analysis. Anesthesiology. 2013;118:809–24. doi:10.1097/ALN.0b013e318287b72c.
8. Gajdos C, Hawn MT, Kile D, Henderson WG, Robinson T, McCarter M, Nehler M. The risk of major elective vascular surgical procedures in patients with end-stage renal disease. Ann Surg. 2013;257:766–73. doi:10.1097/SLA.0b013e3182686b87.
9. Dubois L, Durant C, Harrington DM, Forbes TL, Derose G, Harris JR. Technical factors are strongest predictors of postoperative renal dysfunction after open transperitoneal juxtarenal abdominal aortic aneurysm repair. J Vasc Surg. 2013;57:648–54. doi:10.1016/j.jvs.2012.09.043. Epub 2013 Jan 9.
10. Parekh DJ, Weinberg JM, Ercole B, Torkko KC, Hilton W, Bennett M, Devarajan P, Venkatachalam MA. Tolerance of the human kidney to isolated controlled ischemia. J Am Soc Nephrol. 2013;24:506–17. doi:10.1681/ASN.2012080786. Epub 2013 Feb 14.
11. Thompson RH, Lane BR, Lohse CM, Leibovich BC, Fergany A, Frank I, Gill IS, Blute ML, Campbell SC. Every minute counts when the renal hilum is clamped during partial nephrectomy. Eur Urol. 2010;58:340–5.
12. Antonello M, Menegolo M, Piazza M, Bonfante L, Grego F, Frigatti P. Outcomes of endovascular aneurysm repair on renal function compared with open repair. J Vasc Surg. 2013;17:00706–4.
13. Abdelhamid MF, Davies RS, Vohra RK, Adam DJ, Bradbury AW. Assessment of renal function by means of cystatin C following standard and fenestrated endovascular aneurysm repair. Ann Vasc Surg. 2013;27:708–13. doi:10.1016/j.avsg.2012.06.016. Epub 2013 Mar 31.
14. Yunos NM, Bellomo R, Hegarty C, Story D, Ho L, Bailey M. Association between a chloride-liberal vs chloride-restrictive intravenous fluid administration strategy and kidney injury in critically ill adults. JAMA. 2012;308:1566–72.
15. Myburgh JA, Finfer S, Bellomo R, Billot L, Cass A, Gattas D, Glass P, Lipman J, Liu B, McArthur C, McGuinness S, Rajbhandari D, Taylor CB, Webb SA, CHEST Investigators; Australian and New Zealand Intensive Care Society Clinical Trials Group. Hydroxyethyl starch or saline for fluid resuscitation in intensive care. N Engl J Med. 2012;367:1901–11.
16. Seeliger E, Sendeski M, Rihal CS, Persson PB. Contrast-induced kidney injury: mechanisms, risk factors, and prevention. Eur Heart J. 2012;33:2007–15.
17. Jang JS, Jin HY, Seo JS, Yang TH, Kim DK, Kim TH, Urm SH, Kim DS, Kim DK, Seol SH, Kim DI, Cho KI, Kim BH, Park YH, Je HG, Ahn JM, Kim WJ, Lee JY, Lee SW. Sodium bicarbonate therapy for the prevention of contrast-induced acute kidney injury – a systematic review and meta-analysis. Circ J. 2012;76:2255–65.
18. Brienza N, Giglio MT, Marucci M. Preventing acute kidney injury after noncardiac surgery. Curr Opin Crit Care. 2010;16:353–8.
19. Prowle JR, Chua HR, Bagshaw SM, Bellomo R. Clinical review: volume of fluid resuscitation and the incidence of acute kidney injury – a systematic review. Crit Care. 2012;16:230.
20. Herseya P, Poullisb M. Does the administration of mannitol prevent renal failure in open abdominal aortic aneurysm surgery? Interact Cardiovasc Thorac Surg. 2008;7:906–9.
21. Coselli JS. Strategies for renal and visceral protection in thoracoabdominal aortic surgery. J Thorac Cardiovasc Surg. 2010;140:S147–9; discussion S185–90.

Part III
Abdominal and Urologic Surgery

Chapter 11
Acute Kidney Injury After Major Abdominal Surgery: Epidemiology and Management Challenges

Sherif Awad and Dileep N. Lobo

Objectives

- To describe the definition, epidemiology, and clinical importance of developing perioperative acute kidney injury (AKI) in patients undergoing major abdominal surgery.
- To highlight the commonly encountered predisposing factors and etiologies underlying development of AKI.
- To discuss the management of perioperative AKI with an emphasis on initial assessment and parenteral fluid management in these patients.

Introduction

This chapter discusses the development of acute kidney injury (AKI) in patients undergoing major abdominal surgery in both the elective and emergency settings. AKI epidemiology and its effects on perioperative outcomes as well as acute management options will be considered. Finally, a best-practice algorithm will be suggested with the aim of reducing development of and improving outcomes of perioperative AKI.

S. Awad, FRCS, PhD
Division of Gastrointestinal Surgery, Nottingham Digestive Diseases Centre NIHR Biomedical Research Unit, Queen's Medical Centre, E-Floor, West Block, Nottingham NG7 2UH, UK
e-mail: drsherifawad@yahoo.co.uk

D.N. Lobo, MS, DM, FRCS, FACS, FRCPE (✉)
Division of Gastrointestinal Surgery, Nottingham Digestive Diseases Centre NIHR Biomedical Research Unit, Nottingham University Hospitals, Queen's Medical Centre, Nottingham NG7 2UH, UK
e-mail: dileep.lobo@nottingham.ac.uk

C.V. Thakar, C.R. Parikh (eds.), *Perioperative Kidney Injury: Principles of Risk Assessment, Diagnosis and Treatment*, DOI 10.1007/978-1-4939-1273-5_11

Epidemiology of AKI and Relevance to Perioperative Practice

The incidence of AKI is estimated at 7.5 % of all acute hospitalizations, and approximately 40 % of all cases of AKI are observed in the perioperative setting [1]. Most data on the effects of postoperative AKI originate from patients undergoing cardiac surgery; however, AKI has also been associated with adverse outcomes in patients undergoing noncardiac surgery. Among 1,227 patients who underwent bariatric surgery over a 6-year period, 5.8 % developed AKI resulting in higher rates of blood transfusions, postoperative complications, and longer hospital stay [2]. Analysis of prospectively collected data from the UK Intensive Care National Audit and Research Centre (ICNARC) Case Mix Programme found that surgical admissions accounted for 16.4 % patients admitted with severe AKI during the first 24 h of stay in an intensive care unit, of whom 5.6 % followed elective and 10.8 % emergency surgery [3], and AKI accounted for nearly 10 % of all intensive care unit (ICU) bed days. A retrospective study of 1,200 noncardiac surgery patients demonstrated AKI to be an independent predictor of hospital mortality (odds ratio 3.12, 95 % confidence interval 1.41–6.93, $p=0.005$) leading to a hospital mortality rate of 26 % *vs.* 3 % in patients without AKI [4]. The association of postoperative AKI also leads to dysfunction of other organs, electrolyte and acid-base disturbance, fluid overload, impaired mobility, and wound healing, all of which increases length of hospital stay [1, 5]. The incidence of AKI requiring renal replacement therapy (RRT) has reportedly been as high as 203 patients per million per year [6]. Furthermore, development of AKI increases the risk of incident and progressive chronic kidney disease [1]. Finally, in patients with normal baseline renal function, development of postoperative AKI was independently associated with increased risk of long-term mortality, as demonstrated in a retrospective study of 10,518 patients, 70 % of whom underwent noncardiac surgery [7]. Management of AKI in hospitals has been poor. Data from the 2009 UK National Confidential Enquiry into Patient Outcome and Death (NCEPOD) found that only 50 % of AKI care was considered good, there was an unacceptable delay in recognizing post-admission AKI in 43 %, 20 % of post-admission AKI was predictable and avoidable, and finally, complications of AKI were missed in 13 %, were avoidable in 17 %, and were mismanaged in 22 % of cases [8].

Predisposing Factors and Pathophysiology of AKI

A number of patient-related, intraoperative and postoperative factors have been shown to increase in the risk of developing AKI. In a recently reported matched case-control study of patients aged over 65 years undergoing orthopedic, colonic, or thoracic surgery, obese patients (body mass index [BMI] ≥ 35 kg/m^2) had an increased risk of development of postoperative AKI (odds ratio = 1.68, $p=0.01$) [9]. Prospectively collected data from over 76,000 operations in the USA was used to

Table 11.1 Drugs and agents that may adversely affect renal function perioperatively

Class of drug/agent	Mechanism(s) of action
Analgesics	
NSAIDs and COX2i	Reduced glomerular perfusion due to inhibition of prostaglandin-mediated dilatation of glomerular arterioles. Also may cause interstitial nephritis
Antihypertensives	
ACE inhibitors and ARB	Impair renal autoregulation by reducing ability of efferent arteriole to constrict
Antimicrobials	
Aminoglycosides, bacterial cell wall inhibitors (e.g., penicillin, cephalosporin), fluoroquinolones (e.g., ciprofloxacin)	At high concentrations cause tubular toxicity or interstitial nephritis
Intravenous contrast agents	Cause pathological vasoconstriction in an at-risk kidney
Intraoperative agents	
Vasopressors, diuretics, mannitol	Alter renal perfusion pressures and electrolyte and fluid balance and cause vasoconstriction of renal arterioles

Abbreviations: *NSAIDs* nonsteroidal anti-inflammatory drugs, *COX 2i* cyclooxygenase-2 inhibitors, *ACE* angiotensin converting enzyme, *ARB* angiotensin receptor blockers

devise a risk index for AKI in patients undergoing general surgery [10]. Risk factors in the latter study included: age ≥56 years, male sex, active congestive cardiac failure, presence of ascites, hypertension, emergency surgery, intraperitoneal surgery, preoperative creatinine 106 μmol/L, and diabetes mellitus. Patients with six or more risk factors had a 9 % incidence of developing AKI (hazard ratio 46.3 [95 % confidence interval 34.2–62.6]) compared with those with 0–2 risk factors. Medications commonly in use during the perioperative period may also affect renal function adversely and cause AKI (Table 11.1). Factors that increase the risk of contrast-induced AKI include: advanced age, chronic kidney disease, diabetes mellitus, high doses of contrast media, intra-arterial contrast, hypertension, congestive cardiac failure, hypotension, anemia, nonsteroidal anti-inflammatory drugs, and hypovolemia [5]. In such patients, Kidney Disease Improving Global Outcomes (KDIGO) guidelines recommend using oral N-acetyl cysteine (NAC) together with intravenous volume expansion with isotonic crystalloids [11]. Certain specialist abdominal procedures may be associated with increased risk of developing AKI. Liver transplantation carries reported AKI incidence rates between 17 and 95 %, while over 50 % of those undergoing open abdominal aortic aneurysm repair will have elevated creatinine concentrations from baseline [5]. Finally, any abdominal surgical procedure that results in elevated intra-abdominal pressure and development of abdominal compartment syndrome (reviewed in Chap. 12) may be associated with development of AKI.

Management of the Surgical Patient with AKI

While detailed review of present international guidelines on the management of AKI [11] is beyond the scope of this chapter, the forthcoming discussion will pay emphasis to the initial assessment of AKI in patients following major abdominal surgery and discuss fluid management strategies in these patients.

Initial Assessment and Treatment

In common with other surgical emergencies, assessment of the patients at risk of or with AKI should initially comprise detailed history taking and clinical examination. The aims of the former are to elicit risk factors and determine the etiology of AKI (Table 11.1), while that of the latter is to determine the volume status of the patient, thereby guiding initial parenteral fluid resuscitation. Baseline investigations should include urinalysis and a renal ultrasound within 24 h (if obstruction of the collecting system is suspected). Further general supportive measures include the optimization of hemodynamic status by appropriate parenteral fluid therapy (*vide infra*), transfer of the patient to a higher care setting if necessary, administration of vasopressors and/or inotropes, and elimination of any underlying sources of sepsis. Additionally, nephrotoxic medication should be stopped and therapeutic drug dosing adjusted in line with the stages of AKI. Nutrition should be preferentially provided by the enteral route and should aim to provide a total energy intake of 20–30 kcal/kg/day with a protein content of 0.8–1.0 g/kg/day in non-catabolic AKI patients without need for dialysis [11]. KDIGO guidelines recommend not using diuretics to prevent or treat AKI (except in cases of volume overload) and not using any of low-dose dopamine, fenoldopam, atrial natriuretic peptide (ANP), and recombinant human insulin-like growth factor I (IGF-I) to prevent or treat AKI, due to an inadequate evidence base providing support for the aforementioned agents [11]. Finally, NAC is not recommended for prevention of postsurgical AKI.

Perioperative Parenteral Fluids in Patients with AKI

Development of perioperative AKI should alarm clinicians as a predisposing factor for multiorgan dysfunction, which, if inappropriately managed, could worsen surgical outcomes. Critical in the management of these patients is the choice of parenteral fluids administered, specifically the avoidance of salt and water overload. Unfortunately, assessing parenteral fluid requirements and subsequent prescribing is often left to the most junior members of the clinical team. Numerous surveys over the past decade have highlighted an inadequate knowledge base among junior residents, often resulting in inappropriate fluid prescribing habits leading to salt and water overload [12, 13]. The latter is also resultant from misconceptions about the composition of parenteral solutions such as 0.9 % sodium chloride, which is commonly termed "normal" or "physiological" saline. Yet as previously reviewed [14], there is nothing chemically normal or physiological about 0.9 % sodium chloride solution, 1 l of which contained almost 150 % of daily maintenance requirements of chloride and sodium. Infusion of excessive quantities of the 0.9 % saline results in hyperchloremic acidosis and salt overload. The vulnerable postoperative kidney, which may have already been subjected to insults secondary to dehydration, hypovolemia, sepsis, nephrotoxic antibiotics, and contrast media, is unable to excrete the increased sodium and chloride load, resulting in fluid retention, weight gain, and interstitial edema that may persist for up to 3 weeks. A recently published study provides support for chloride-restrictive fluid strategies in critically ill patients with AKI [15]. In an open-label prospective sequential manner, 760 patients consecutively admitted to intensive care (30 % of whom were admitted after elective surgery) received either traditional chloride-rich solutions (0.9 % sodium chloride, 4 % succinylated gelatin solution, or 4 % albumin solution) or chloride-restricted (Hartmann's solution, Plasma-Lyte 148, or chloride-poor 20 % albumin). After adjusting for confounding variables, the chloride-restricted group had decreased incidence of AKI and use of RRT. However, there were no differences in hospital mortality and hospital or ICU length of stay [15]. Another study of almost 32,000 patients examined the effects of infusion of either 0.9 % sodium chloride or balanced crystalloid solution on the day of surgery [16]. Use of a calcium-free balanced crystalloid solution for replacement of fluid losses on the day of major surgery was associated with fewer postoperative complications (odds ratio [OR] 0.79, $p<0.001$), postoperative infection ($p<0.001$), renal failure requiring dialysis ($p<0.001$), blood transfusion ($p<0.001$), and electrolyte disturbance ($p<0.005$) [16]. Finally, nationally approved best-practice guidelines have been developed with the aim of guiding clinicians in perioperative parenteral fluid therapy [17]. Experimentally, high chloride loads have been shown to cause renal vasoconstriction and reduce both renal blood flow and glomerular filtration in animals [18, 19]. Recent healthy human volunteer work using magnetic resonance imaging has also shown that 0.9 % saline produces interstitial space and renal edema and reduces renal artery flow velocity and renal cortical tissue perfusion, a phenomenon that does not occur after infusion of a balanced crystalloid [20, 21]. Proposed mechanisms for this phenomenon include intrarenal tissue hypertension caused by edema in an organ surrounded by a capsule and the fact that when the renal tubule is presented with fluid with a high chloride concentration, there is entry of chloride into the macula densa, causing depolarization of the basement membrane and release of adenosine which, in turn, leads to afferent arteriolar vasoconstriction, reduced renal blood flow, and reduced glomerular filtration rate [20, 21]. These changes are also manifest by a reduction in urinary output [20, 21].

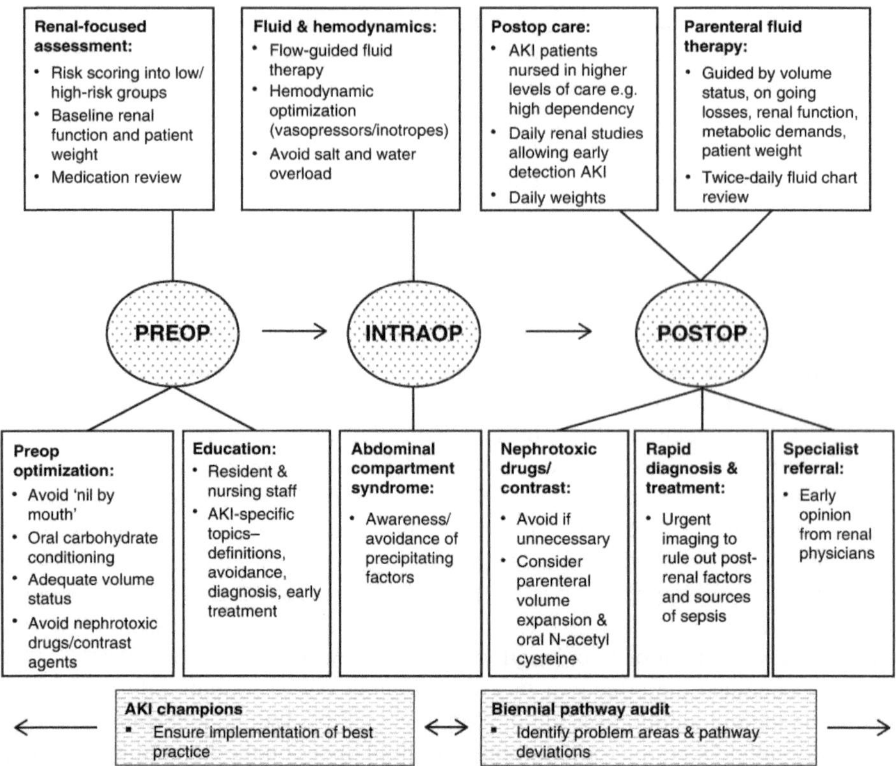

Fig. 11.1 A best-practice, multimodal perioperative pathway to reduce the occurrence and consequences of AKI in patients undergoing major abdominal surgery

Prevention of AKI and Utilization of a Best-Practice Multimodal Perioperative Pathway

Given the high attendant morbidity and mortality associated with development of perioperative AKI, attention should be focused to implementing multimodal interventions to aid prevention, early identification, and treatment of AKI in surgical patients. Educational programs to raise awareness of the newly accepted definitions, clinical relevance, and initial assessment and management of AKI are one strategy to reduce development of and improve outcomes of postoperative AKI [8]. In present times of competing clinical interests, providing financial incentives for hospitals to reduce occurrence of AKI perioperatively may be a means by which adherence to international best-practice guidelines may be achieved. An evidence-based, best-practice, multimodal perioperative pathway to reduce occurrence and consequences of AKI in patients undergoing major abdominal surgery is suggested and shown in Fig. 11.1.

Key Messages

- AKI after major abdominal surgery, including bariatric surgery, carries the same morbidity and mortality as in other clinical settings.
- Several patient- and provider-related risk factors, unique to this surgical setting, are associated with postoperative AKI.
- Following development of AKI in patients after major abdominal surgery, a chloride-restrictive parenteral fluid strategy should be considered for volume management.
- Modern AKI care needs to be streamlined to a multidisciplinary management algorithm, encompassing perioperative risk scoring, early detection of AKI, elimination of precipitating factors, and early involvement of nephrologists.

Competing Interests SA has received educational support and travel bursaries from Baxter Healthcare and Fresenius Kabi. DNL has received research funding and speaker's honoraria from BBraun, Fresenius Kabi, and Baxter Healthcare.

Funding No external funding was received for this article.

References

1. Thakar CV. Perioperative acute kidney injury. Adv Chronic Kidney Dis. 2013;20:67–75.
2. Weingarten TN, Gurrieri C, McCaffrey JM, et al. Acute kidney injury following bariatric surgery. Obes Surg. 2013;23:64–70.
3. Kolhe NV, Stevens PE, Crowe AV, et al. Case mix, outcome and activity for patients with severe acute kidney injury during the first 24 hours after admission to an adult, general critical care unit: application of predictive models from a secondary analysis of the ICNARC Case Mix Programme database. Crit Care. 2008;12 Suppl 1:S2.
4. Abelha FJ, Botelho M, Fernandes V, Barros H. Outcome and quality of life of patients with acute kidney injury after major surgery. Nefrologia. 2009;29:404–14.
5. Borthwick E, Ferguson A. Perioperative acute kidney injury: risk factors, recognition, management, and outcomes. BMJ. 2010;341:c3365.
6. Metcalfe W, Simpson M, Khan IH, et al. Acute renal failure requiring renal replacement therapy: incidence and outcome. QJM. 2002;95:579–83.
7. Bihorac A, Yavas S, Subbiah S, et al. Long-term risk of mortality and acute kidney injury during hospitalization after major surgery. Ann Surg. 2009;249:851–8.
8. National Confidential Enquiry into Patient Outcome and Death (NCEPOD). Adding insult to injury: a review of the care of patients who died in hospital with a primary diagnosis of acute kidney injury (acute renal failure). Available at. http://www.ncepod.org.uk/2009report1/Downloads/AKI_report.pdf. Accessed 3 Aug 2013
9. Kelz RR, Reinke CE, Zubizarreta JR, et al. Acute kidney injury, renal function, and the elderly obese surgical patient: a matched case-control study. Ann Surg. 2013;258:359–63.

10. Kheterpal S, Tremper KK, Heung M, et al. Development and validation of an acute kidney injury risk index for patients undergoing general surgery: results from a national data set. Anesthesiology. 2009;110:505–15.
11. Kidney Disease: Improving Global Outcomes (KDIGO) Acute Kidney Injury Work Group. KDIGO clinical practice guideline for acute kidney injury. Kidney Int Suppl. 2012;2:1–138.
12. Lobo DN, Dube MG, Neal KR, et al. Problems with solutions: drowning in the brine of an inadequate knowledge base. Clin Nutr. 2001;20:125–30.
13. Awad S, Allison SP, Lobo DN. Fluid and electrolyte balance: the impact of goal directed teaching. Clin Nutr. 2008;27:473–8.
14. Awad S, Allison SP, Lobo DN. The history of 0.9 % saline. Clin Nutr. 2008;27:179–88.
15. Yunos NM, Bellomo R, Hegarty C, et al. Association between a chloride-liberal vs chloride-restrictive intravenous fluid administration strategy and kidney injury in critically ill adults. JAMA. 2012;308:1566–72.
16. Shaw AD, Bagshaw SM, Goldstein SL, et al. Major complications, mortality, and resource utilization after open abdominal surgery: 0.9 % saline compared to Plasma-Lyte. Ann Surg. 2012;255:821–9.
17. Powell-Tuck J, Gosling P, Lobo DN et al. British Consensus Guidelines on Intravenous Fluid Therapy for Adult Surgical Patients (GIFTASUP). The British Association for Parenteral and Enteral Nutrition (BAPEN). 2008. http://www.bapen.org.uk/pdfs/bapen_pubs/giftasup.pdf. Accessed 21 Feb 2014
18. Hansen PB, Jensen BL, Skott O. Chloride regulates afferent arteriolar contraction in response to depolarization. Hypertension. 1998;32:1066–70.
19. Wilcox CS. Regulation of renal blood flow by plasma chloride. J Clin Invest. 1983;71: 726–35.
20. Chowdhury AH, Cox EF, Francis ST, Lobo DN. A randomized, controlled, double-blind crossover study on the effects of 2-L infusions of 0.9 % saline and plasma-lyte® 148 on renal blood flow velocity and renal cortical tissue perfusion in healthy volunteers. Ann Surg. 2012;256: 18–24.
21. Lobo DN, Awad S. Should chloride-rich crystalloids remain the main stay of fluid resuscitation to prevent "pre-renal" acute kidney injury? Con. Kidney Int. 2014, Apr 9. doi: 10.1038/ki.2014.105. [Epub ahead of print].

Chapter 12
Kidney Injury in Abdominal Compartment Syndrome

Anna Parker Sattah and Lakhmir S. Chawla

Objectives

- To review the definition and diagnosis of intra-abdominal hypertension (IAH) and abdominal compartment syndrome (ACS)
- To review the systemic manifestations of IAH and ACS with a focus on renal manifestations of the syndrome
- To review the medical and surgical management of patient with IAH and ACS

Introduction

Elevated intra-abdominal pressures have become increasingly well-recognized phenomena in acute care setting, with a large range of interrelated clinical manifestations. Although descriptions of abdominal compartment syndrome date back to the early nineteenth century [1], intra-abdominal hypertension (IAH) was described as a specific clinical entity in 1984 by Kron et al. when they reported four cases of abdominal compartment syndrome (ACS) following abdominal aortic aneurysm repair [2]. He subsequently went on to describe a method of noninvasive monitoring of intra-abdominal pressure (IAP) using a Foley catheter [3] opened this field up to a broad array of clinical research.

A.P. Sattah, MD
Department of Anesthesiology and Critical Care Medicine, George Washington University Medical Center, 900 23rd Street, NW, Washington, DC 20037, USA

L.S. Chawla, MD (✉)
Department of Anesthesiology and Critical Care Medicine, George Washington University, 900 23rd Street, NW, Washington, DC 20037, USA
e-mail: minkchawla@gmail.com

C.V. Thakar, C.R. Parikh (eds.), *Perioperative Kidney Injury: Principles of Risk Assessment, Diagnosis and Treatment*, DOI 10.1007/978-1-4939-1273-5_12

Normal intra-abdominal pressure is considered less than 7 mmHg in a spontaneously breathing animal [4]. Intra-abdominal pathology, ranging from acute pancreatitis [5] to ruptured aortic aneurysms [2] to traumatic injury [6], is frequently associated with massive fluid resuscitation. The associated inflammatory response can lead to profound intra- and retroperitoneal tissue edema as well as accumulation of intraluminal and interstitial fluid within the bowel and to extraperitoneal fluid in the form of ascites or hemorrhage. All of this occurs within the relatively rigid abdominal compartment and may lead to increased pressure.

Conceptually, the abdominal cavity can be thought of as the lower half of a relatively fixed thoracoabdominal cavity. Pressures on either side of the diaphragm communicate and affect blood flow through the vessels, which traverse them. To that end, it is hard to separate out the effects of increased pressures on any single organ system, without discussing the interplay between them. This review is intended to focus on the clinical effects of IAH and ACS as they apply to the kidney. We will also briefly outline some of the concurrent physiology that will likely be at play in other organ systems in a patient developing renal dysfunction alongside IAH/ACS.

Definition, Incidence, and Etiology

In 2004, the World Society of the Abdominal Compartment Syndrome (WSACS) was convened, and an international consensus statement was published establishing a precise definition for ACS. The most recent consensus guidelines, updated in 2013, defined IAH as sustained IAP of ≥12 mmHg. In the more severe form, ACS was defined as IAPs that rose to levels ≥20 mmHg and were associated with new organ dysfunction/failure [7]. IAH is classified into 4 grades of severity-based IAP [7] (Table 12.1) and three basic types (Table 12.2). Primary ACS occurs in the setting of abdominal pathology, as a consequence of surgery, intestinal ischemia/edema, or traumatic insult. Secondary ACS is the development of ACS in the absence of primary abdominal pathology, usually due to capillary leak, fluid resuscitation, or sepsis. Recurrent ACS is one that recurs after the initially successful treatment of either primary or secondary ACS (Table 12.2) [7].

The factors associated with the development of ACS are heterogeneous and are broken down into several categories by the WSACS: diminished abdominal wall compliance, increased intraluminal contents, increased intra-abdominal contents, capillary leak/fluid resuscitation, and other risk factors [7] (Table 12.3).

Table 12.1 World Society of the Abdominal Compartment Syndrome grading scheme for IAH

Grade	IAP (mmHg)
I	12–15
II	16–20
III	21–25
IV	25

Reprinted from Al-Mufarrej et al. [15]
Abbreviations: *IAH* intra-abdominal hypertension, *IAP* intra-abdominal pressure

Table 12.2 Types of abdominal compartment syndrome

Type	Definition	Causes
Primary	Occurs in the setting of abdominal pathology	Surgery/trauma
		Intestinal edema
		Pancreatitis
		Retroperitoneal bleed
Secondary	Develops in the absence of primary abdominal pathology	Fluid resuscitation
		Capillary leak/sepsis
Recurrent	Redevelops after the treatment of either primary or secondary ACS	Tightly placed silo

Reprinted from Al-Mufarrej et al. [15]
Abbreviations: *ACS* abdominal compartment syndrome

Table 12.3 Risk factors for intra-abdominal hypertension and abdominal compartment syndrome

Risk factor
Diminished abdominal wall compliance
Abdominal surgery
Major trauma
Major burns
Prone positioning
Increased intraluminal contents
Gastroparesis/gastric distention/ileus
Ileus
Colonic pseudo-obstruction
Volvulus
Increased intra-abdominal contents
Acute pancreatitis
Distended abdomen
Hemoperitoneum/pneumoperitoneum or intraperitoneal fluid collections
Intra-abdominal infection/abscess
Intra-abdominal or retroperitoneal tumors
Laparoscopy with excessive insufflation pressures
Liver dysfunction/cirrhosis with ascites
Peritoneal dialysis
Capillary leak/fluid resuscitation
Acidosis
Damage control laparotomy
Hypothermia
Increased APACHE II or SOFA score
Massive fluid resuscitation or positive fluid balance
Polytransfusion

(continued)

Table 12.3 (continued)

Risk factor
Others/miscellaneous
Age
Bacteremia
Coagulopathy
Increased head of bed angle
Massive incisional hernia repair
Mechanical ventilation
Obesity or increased body mass index
PEEP
Peritonitis
Pneumonia
Sepsis
Shock or hypotension

Adapted from Kirkpatrick et al. [7]

The incidence of IAH and ACS varies with the patient population studied with ranges as high as 40.7 % of admissions to a surgical intensive care unit [8] and between 4 and 8 % among general medical-surgical patients [9]. The incidence of associated multiorgan failure (MOF) and mortality is also high. Among trauma patients with ACS, the rate of MOF is 32–55 % and the mortality rate is 43–64 % [10]. By comparison, trauma patients matched for injury severity score who do not develop ACS have much lower rates of MOF and mortality, 8–12 % and 12–17 %, respectively [10].

Diagnosis

Physical exam has not been shown to be effective at diagnosing the presence or absence of IAH [11]. Multiple modalities for the measurement of ACS have been described ranging from intragastric to transrectal approaches [12]. The WSACS however continues to recommend the use of a transvesicular technique for measurement of IAP [7]. The pressure is obtained using a transducer connected to a Foley catheter instilled of no more than 25 ml of sterile saline. It is measured at end expiration in the supine position after ensuring that abdominal muscle contractions are absent and with the transducer zeroed at the level of the midaxillary line [7]. Changes in patient positioning can affect intra-abdominal pressures. Hence, supine positioning, particularly in obese patients, is necessary to achieve the greatest accuracy.

Abdominal perfusion pressure (APP) is defined as the mean abdominal pressure (MAP) minus the intra-abdominal pressure (APP=MAP – IAP) [7]. In patients with ACS, maintaining APP at 50 mmHg has been correlated with better survival. APP has been demonstrated to be a better marker than MAP, IAP, arterial pH, base deficit, arterial lactate, and urine output in predicting survival from IAH and ACS [13].

While relative perfusion pressure remains an interesting and potentially useful measure, in most literature as well as the WSACS guidelines, IAP and ACS continue to be defined by absolute IAP [7].

Traditional methods of monitoring IAP rely on intermittent IAP (IIAP) measurements using indwelling bladder catheters. These, however, are only "snap shots" of a dynamic parameter; thus, they may not reflect the patient's true clinical status and may delay the recognition of IAH. Continuous monitoring of IAP, like other pressures, provides the clinician with the greatest insight into the patient's evolving condition [12]. From a nursing standpoint, continuous monitors tend to be less labor intensive than IAPs. Also, continuous pressure monitoring eliminates the many variables that affect IAP measurements described above. Recently, several methods of continuous IAP (CIAP) monitoring have been developed. One method is continuous urinary bladder pressure measurement using a three-way catheter [14]. While continuous monitoring may allow us to more closely follow trends in IAP, it also presents new challenges such as compensating for non-supine positioning and has yet to become mainstream.

Extrarenal Manifestations of IAH

IAH is a systemic condition and cannot be fully understood without an appreciation for its global effects on a patient. We therefore briefly review some of the extrarenal manifestations, which are likely to be at play in any patient at risk for renal dysfunction secondary to IAP.

Cellular and Biochemical

IAH has been linked to derangements at the cellular level including release of proinflammatory cytokines and the development of neutrophil priming. This priming effect predisposes a patient to a subsequent exaggerated neutrophil response and has been linked to organ dysfunction [15]. Shah et al. reviewed substantial evidence suggesting the systemic reabsorption of mesenteric-derived lymphatic fluid leads to neutrophil priming and is associated with distant organ failure. They went on to describe a potential ischemia-reperfusion injury, which occurred when progressively increasing IAP leads to mesenteric ischemia followed by rapid reperfusion with surgical decompression [16]. Several studies have shown that IAH, even when occult, promotes significant mesenteric ischemia [17]. In the setting of such ischemic injury, the gastrointestinal tract produces high levels of pro-inflammatory lipids [18]. Levels of interleukin-6 (IL-6) and tumor necrosis factor-α (TNF-α) are also elevated following gut ischemia and reperfusion [19]. These cellular and inflammatory changes persist following surgical decompression and may explain the refractory organ dysfunction seen despite resolution of the inciting pressures [20].

Neurologic

One of the less recognized organ systems affected by IAH is the central nervous system. Multiple animal models have shown that IAH leads to a functional obstruction of the cerebral venous outflow by increasing the intrathoracic and central venous pressures (CVP). This venous obstruction is believed to lead to elevated intracranial pressure (ICP) [21]. More recent studies have demonstrated a strong correlation between IAP and ICP that is independent of cardiopulmonary function [22]. This association has been dramatically demonstrated in a case series by Scalea et al. in which abdominal laparotomy was used in patients with concurrent intra-abdominal hypertension and refractory ICPs. Rapid normalization of ICPs was seen following abdominal decompression [23]. While a full discussion of the interplay between and management of IAH and refractory ICH is outside the scope of this chapter, we present this idea to emphasize the wide-reaching and interconnected effects that IAP can have.

Cardiovascular

IAH causes decreased venous return to the heart by direct compression on the inferior vena cava (IVC). In a canine model, resistance to venous return is highest at the subdiaphragmatic, suprahepatic IVC [24]. Impairment of venous return can occur at pressures of 15 mmHg or above [25] resulting in a decrease in cardiac output (CO). In order to maintain stroke volume, a compensatory tachycardia is typically seen. Substantial diaphragmatic elevation due to IAH causes further decreases in CO by increasing intrathoracic and pleural pressures [26]. Increased intrathoracic pressure (ITP) adversely affects CO. First, the elevated ITP increases systemic vascular resistance (SVR) and afterload [27]. Second, the increased ITP decreases the transmural filling pressure for a given ventricular end-diastolic pressure, thus decreasing the corresponding ventricular end-diastolic volume. Ventricular compliance is also decreased as ITP increases (>30 mmHg) due to direct compression on the heart [25].

Decreases in CO in the setting of IAH can be further exacerbated by hypovolemia, inhalational anesthesia, elevated positive end-expiratory pressures (PEEP), and myocardial dysfunction [25]. The administration of intravenous fluids tends to mitigate this drop in CO, but can worsen tissue edema and exacerbate rising IAP. High PEEP further exacerbates the CO reduction in the setting of IAH by further increasing the ITP and impairing left ventricular function [26].

Respiratory

IAH causes increased ITP, lower lobe compression atelectasis, increased intrapulmonary shunting, dead space ventilation, and impaired oxygenation [28]. Moreover, increased ITP results in increased pleural and airway pressures (peak, plateau, and mean) and decreased functional residual capacity (FRC) [29]. The high pleural and intra-abdominal pressures also reduce static and dynamic lung and chest wall compliance, promoting hypercarbia and ventilatory compromise [29]. Furthermore, pulmonary vascular resistance increases with IAH [30] due to increased ITP, decreased FRC, and increased alveolar to arterial O2 difference [29].

IAH also increases the risk for ventilator-associated barotraumas due to the elevate PEEP levels often used in an attempt to recruit collapsed alveoli. The increased propensity for pulmonary edema, likely multifactorial, may be due to increased intrathoracic pressure and subsequent increase in intra-alveolar and interstitial fluid formation. IAH may also promote acute lung injury and capillary leakage by promoting the release of pro-inflammatory cytokines (e.g., IL-6, IL-1, TNFα) [20]. Frequently, it is a combination of a patient's worsening pulmonary function, rising peak pressures, and declining renal function, which indicate progression from IAH to ACS and the need for surgical decompression.

Gastrointestinal and Hepatic

IAH has multiple hepatic and gastrointestinal effects. While it can cause intestinal edema by impairing lymphatic flow [31], IAH imparts its most substantial effect on the gastrointestinal tract and liver by causing mesenteric hypoperfusion likely analogous to but more well described than renal hypoperfusion discussed below. Animal studies suggest that mesenteric arterial (MAF), intestinal mucosal (IMF), hepatic arterial (HAF), hepatic microcirculatory (HMF), and portal venous blood flow (PVF) all decrease in the setting of raised IAP [32]. The deleterious effects of raised IAP on intestinal perfusion have been reflected in at least six case reports of fatal intestinal infarction following laparoscopic cholecystectomies [33]. Intestinal and hepatic ischemia is also known to lead to sepsis and MOF due to cytokine release and bacterial translocation [34]. Mucosal hypoperfusion and acidosis may occur with IAH long before the onset of clinically recognizable ACS, and if left uncorrected, it may lead to intestinal ischemia, ACS, and MOF [30, 32].

Renal Manifestations of IAH

Physiologic Effects

In 1923, Thorington et al. described an association between elevated IAP and renal failure [35]. Using instillation of intraperitoneal fluid in a dog, they generated increasing IAPs noting a progressive decline in urine output with the development of complete anuria at 30 mmHg. They suggested that the drop in UOP was likely due to partial occlusion of the renal veins and that a fall in systemic blood pressure was secondary to a temporary collapse of the IVC [35].

Nearly 60 years later, a more familiar study was published looking at the effects of elevated intra-abdominal pressure on renal function in dogs [36]. They demonstrated decreases in renal blood flow, glomerular filtration rate (GFR), and CO in association with IAP. Subsequent volume expansion was able to correct the decrease in CO, but the renal effects remained with both renal blood flow and GFR less than 25 % of the normal values. The calculated renal vascular resistance rose by 555 %, which represented a 15-fold increase relative to the modest (30.4 %) rise seen in the systemic vascular resistance when exposed to IAH [36]. The results of this initial animal study have since been validated in animal models [37].

Further study has attempted to dissect out what factors lead to the decline in renal function, with ureteral occlusion, and renal parenchymal pressure having been largely ruled out. The effects of renal venous hypertension, however, seem to be involved. Isolated renal venous hypertension was evaluated by Doty et al. in pigs by placement of an adjustable band around the renal vein to create a partial venous obstruction in pigs [38]. This model generated elevated renal vein pressure with a subsequent decrease in renal artery blood flow and direct measures of GFR. They also found increases in renin and aldosterone levels as well as urinary protein leak [38]. A similar study has shown elevation in antidiuretic hormone (ADH) with IAH in a canine model [39]. In combination, this evidence suggests a significant hormonal component to the renal effects seen with rises in IAP. Elevated levels of ADH and aldosterone lead to sodium and water retention, while elevated renin and angiotensin levels as well as ET-1 expression augment renal vascular resistance. The hormonal effects in conjunction with hydrostatic effects associated with increasing renal venous pressure appear to combine generating progressive renal dysfunction.

Clinical Evidence

Numerous case reports have reported IAH and ACS in association with renal failure [40]. Sugrue et al. examined this in more detail in a prospective study of 263 patients in a surgical intensive care unit. He found IAH in 40.7 % of patients and identified it as an independent risk factor for the development of acute renal failure [8].

Cardiorenal Syndrome

Acute decompensated heart failure often presents with fluid overload and progressive renal failure. The use of diuretics, the mainstay in therapy, can present challenges in patients in whom renal dysfunction has already begun. Mullens et al. began an observational study of all patients admitted to the intensive care unit (ICU) for acute decompensated heart failure [41]. They measured IAP on admission and found elevated IAPs in 60 % of patients (IAP $\geq$8 mmHg). This was associated with worsening renal function ($p=0.009$). Subsequent pressure monitoring identified a strong correlation between decrease in IAP and improvement in renal function [41]. In a comprehensive review of renal venous hypertension, Ross proposed that heart failure led to increased right atrial pressures and renal venous congestion. Numerous downstream effects ranging from increases in renin-angiotensin-aldosterone system and atrial natriuretic peptide, tissue hypoxia, vasoconstriction, and increased transglomerular pressure ultimately led to decreased GFR and glomerular sclerosis [42]. Given the common pathway from both heart failure and IAH to renal venous hypertension and renal dysfunction, it may be useful to consider renal failure associated with IAP as similar to that seen in cardiorenal syndrome.

Treatment

Monitoring

The best approach to ACS is prevention. In a review by De Waele et al., they recommend all ICU patients with acute kidney injury (AKI) be evaluated for IAH [40]. This involves frequent IAP monitoring, determining accurate goal-directed resuscitation end points, and avoiding over-resuscitation [43]. In the setting of IAH, lactate levels, base deficit, and central venous oxygen saturations are all variables that may be used in guiding resuscitation. Commonly used hemodynamic variables such as CVP, pulmonary artery pressure (PAP), and pulmonary capillary wedge pressure (PCWP), however, are unreliable in patients with IAP [44]. Typically, these pressures are elevated due to the increased thoracoabdominal pressures which can fool the clinician into believing that the patient is intravascularly replete when in fact just the opposite is true [27]. Urine output is also a poor measure of intravascular volume given the direct effects of IAP on renal function discussed above. As a result, resuscitation in this patient population should be directed by more precise measures of ventricular preload, such as right ventricular end-diastolic volume index (RVEDVI), global end-diastolic volume index (GEDVI), cardiac index (CI), and intrathoracic blood volume (ITBV) [45, 46].

Medical Management

ACS is frequently thought of as a surgical disease; however, there are a number of medical interventions that can be utilized in the setting of early IAH in an attempt to prevent the development of ACS and its associated organ dysfunction [7]. Treatment of IAH $\geq$12 mmHg must be considered in high-risk patients prior to the clinical onset of ACS.

There are a myriad of nonsurgical treatments for IAH (Fig. 12.1), which can be utilized in an attempt to prevent progression to ACS. This is similar to the medical

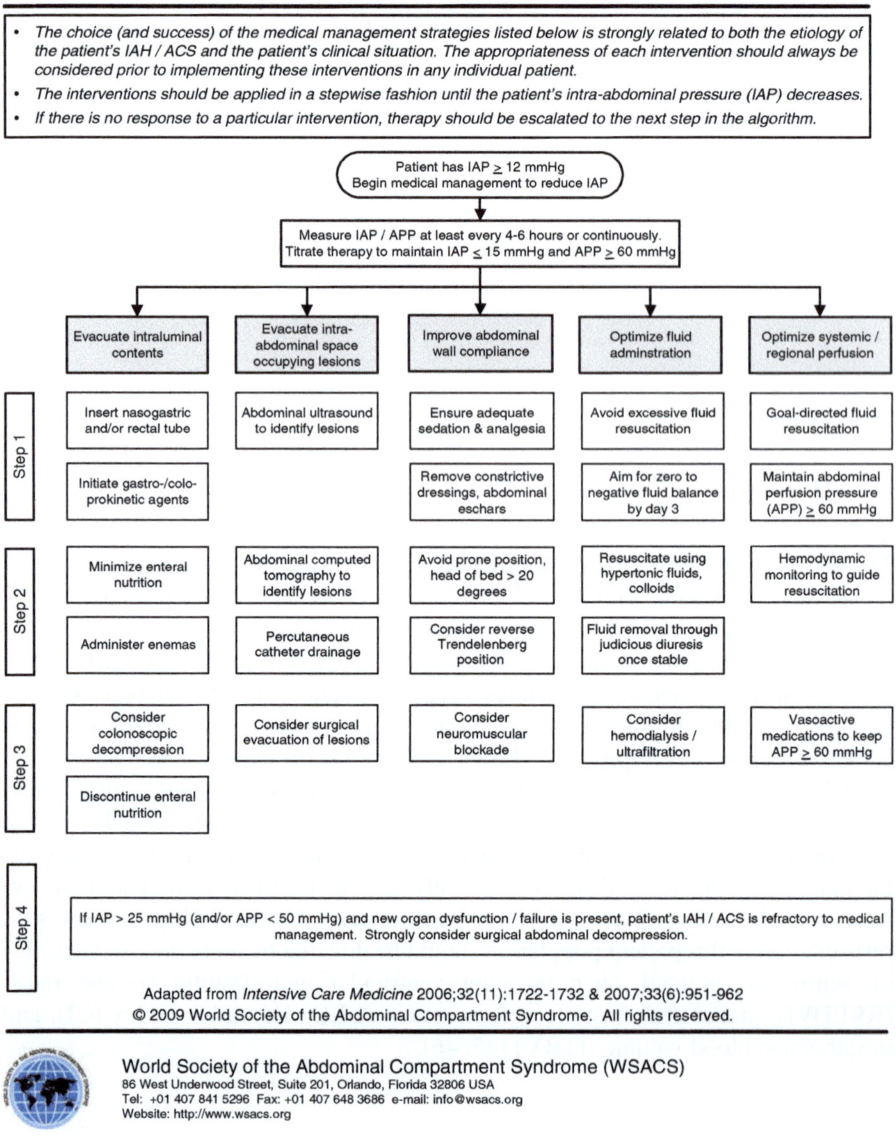

- *The choice (and success) of the medical management strategies listed below is strongly related to both the etiology of the patient's IAH / ACS and the patient's clinical situation. The appropriateness of each intervention should always be considered prior to implementing these interventions in any individual patient.*
- *The interventions should be applied in a stepwise fashion until the patient's intra-abdominal pressure (IAP) decreases.*
- *If there is no response to a particular intervention, therapy should be escalated to the next step in the algorithm.*

Patient has IAP ≥ 12 mmHg
Begin medical management to reduce IAP

Measure IAP / APP at least every 4-6 hours or continuously.
Titrate therapy to maintain IAP ≤ 15 mmHg and APP ≥ 60 mmHg

	Evacuate intraluminal contents	Evacuate intra-abdominal space occupying lesions	Improve abdominal wall compliance	Optimize fluid adminstration	Optimize systemic / regional perfusion
Step 1	Insert nasogastric and/or rectal tube	Abdominal ultrasound to identify lesions	Ensure adequate sedation & analgesia	Avoid excessive fluid resuscitation	Goal-directed fluid resuscitation
	Initiate gastro-/colo-prokinetic agents		Remove constrictive dressings, abdominal eschars	Aim for zero to negative fluid balance by day 3	Maintain abdominal perfusion pressure (APP) ≥ 60 mmHg
Step 2	Minimize enteral nutrition	Abdominal computed tomography to identify lesions	Avoid prone position, head of bed > 20 degrees	Resuscitate using hypertonic fluids, colloids	Hemodynamic monitoring to guide resuscitation
	Administer enemas	Percutaneous catheter drainage	Consider reverse Trendelenberg position	Fluid removal through judicious diuresis once stable	
Step 3	Consider colonoscopic decompression	Consider surgical evacuation of lesions	Consider neuromuscular blockade	Consider hemodialysis / ultrafiltration	Vasoactive medications to keep APP ≥ 60 mmHg
	Discontinue enteral nutrition				

Step 4: If IAP > 25 mmHg (and/or APP < 50 mmHg) and new organ dysfunction / failure is present, patient's IAH / ACS is refractory to medical management. Strongly consider surgical abdominal decompression.

Adapted from *Intensive Care Medicine* 2006;32(11):1722-1732 & 2007;33(6):951-962

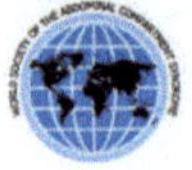

World Society of the Abdominal Compartment Syndrome (WSACS)
86 West Underwood Street, Suite 201, Orlando, Florida 32806 USA
Tel: +01 407 841 5296 Fax: +01 407 648 3686 e-mail: info@wsacs.org
Website: http://www.wsacs.org

Fig. 12.1 IAH/ACS medical management algorithm

management strategies taken in patients with elevated ICPs prior to decompressive craniectomy. The most direct of which may be the use of strategies aimed at reducing excessive crystalloid resuscitation. This, however, is subject to significant interpretation. In the updated 2013 guidelines, the WSACS suggested using a resuscitation protocol that attempted to avoid a positive cumulative fluid balance in critically ill or injured patients at risk for IAH/ACS once initial resuscitation had been achieved and the inciting issues addressed (grade 2c recommendation) [7]. They were, however, unable to recommend for or against the use of albumin or diuretic therapy, and clinical judgment will remain a key determinant in the extent and composition of resuscitation [7].

Sedation and neuromuscular blockade provide additional tools for the medical management of IAH by increasing abdominal wall compliance [47]. Opioids, on the other hand, may acutely raise IAP by promoting active phasic expiration. Removal of excessive fluids by drainage, diuresis, hemofiltration, and ultrafiltration are alternative potentially effective medical treatments for IAH [7]. In patients with significant gaseous bowel distension, the use of prokinetics, nasogastric decompression, rectal drainage, and enemas may sustain minor reductions in IAP [7]. Avoiding reverse Trendelenburg positioning or proning may prevent further increases in IAP [7].

Surgical Decompression

IAH that has progressed to the point of ACS, i.e., organ failure, must be treated surgically [48]. This typically presents clinically with IAP ≥20–25 mmHg in association with hypotension, raised airway pressures, impaired ventilation, or oliguria. Decompressive laparotomy (DL) is almost always effective and is associated with a rapid improvement in airway pressures, PaO2/FIO2 ratio, and urine output [49]. When necessary, it can be performed at bedside for those too unstable to travel [50].

Elevated renin and angiotensin levels have been found to normalize in an animal model of acute ACS after surgical decompression with intravascular volume expansion [51]. The preemptive volume expansion used in that study is likely necessary to counteract the sudden drop in vascular resistance which immediately follows fascial release [52]. Similarly, many trauma surgeons, when faced with IAP secondary to tense hemoperitoneum, advocate volume expansion prior to surgical decompression in order to counteract the hypotension that accompanies the drop in SVR seen when opening the abdomen. Some authors have also suggested using mannitol and/or sodium bicarbonate prior to decompression. Unfortunately, the improvements in end organ dysfunction are less reliable particularly in advanced cases, and mortality remains as high as 50 % [48].

In patients that are recognized to be at high risk of developing ACS, such as those with significant stool spillage or mesenteric ischemia, temporary abdominal closures may be used at the time of their initial operation to allow more room for the abdominal contents to expand postoperatively [53]. This is analogous to releasing a belt buckle a few notches before it gets too tight. It is important to note that the use of the term "open abdomen" does not imply a completely unrestricted abdominal cavity. It simple means the fascial edges were not reapproximated.

In patients with an "open abdomen" or "temporary abdominal closure," a number of approaches can be used in the operating room. The fascial edges can be sutured to a temporary bridge ranging from a piece of mesh or a towel or a sterile sheet of plastic (Bogota bag) [54]. Alternatively, a number of vacuum closure techniques can be used similar to the negative-pressure wound vacs [54].

These have the added benefit of removing excess intraperitoneal fluid while reducing the retraction of the fascial edges laterally and preventing adhesions to the anterior abdominal wall. All of these techniques allow for some additional expansion of the abdominal cavity as compared to primary closure of the fascia, but they are not limitless. Patients with severe inflammatory processes can redevelop ACS in the setting of an "open abdomen." In that case, the temporary closure must be removed to allow even further expansion of the intra-abdominal contents [55], i.e., letting the belt out even further.

Conclusion

The prompt diagnosis and management of IAH is critical to the management of patients at risk for ACS. Routine and frequent IAP measuring is the cornerstone of this approach. These measurements allow for prompt medical therapy and may reduce the duration of an "open abdomen" if not avoid the need for surgery altogether. Routine IAP measurements may also prove a valuable tool for monitoring the medical treatment of cardiorenal syndrome. The early recognition of IAH avoids under-resuscitation by recognizing artificially elevated filling pressures. The pathophysiological consequences of unrecognized IAH are significant and delays in diagnosis often progress to MOF and death.

Key Messages

- IAH is defined as sustained IAP ≥12 mmHg; ACS is defined as IAP ≥20 mmHg associated with new multiorgan dysfunction/failure.
- Renal dysfunction associated with IAH/ACS may be due to renal venous hypertension secondary to the collapse of the renal veins. Renal artery duplex ultrasound may be useful as a screening tool to identify early renal manifestations of IAH.
- Routine IAP monitoring using bladder pressures may help identify IAH before it progresses to ACS and its associated end organ damage.
- Medical management includes fluid management, sedation and neuromuscular blockage, and drainage of intraluminal fluids. Surgical decompression remains the gold standard for management of ACS and should not be delayed in the setting of end organ damage.
- IAH/ACS is a systemic disease. Cellular/biochemical manifestations, including the release of pro-inflammatory cytokines, can persist following surgical decompression and may lead to refractory organ dysfunction.

Acknowledgements The authors would like to thank Lynn Abell for her assistance in writing this chapter.

References

1. Coombs HC. The mechanism of the regulation of intra-abdominal pressure. Am J Physiol. 1920;61:159–63.
2. Kron IL, Harman PK, Nolan SP. The measurement of intra-abdominal pressure as a criterion for abdominal re-exploration. Ann Surg. 1984;199(1):28–30.
3. Kron IL. A simple technique to accurately determine intra-abdominal pressure. Crit Care Med. 1989;17(7):714–5.
4. Overholt RH. Intraperitoneal pressure. Arch Surg. 1931;22:691–700.
5. Li H, Qian Z, Liu Z, Liu X, Han X, Kang H. Risk factors and outcome of acute renal failure in patients with severe acute pancreatitis. J Crit Care. 2010;25(2):225–9.
6. Fritsch DE, Steinmann RA. Managing trauma patients with abdominal compartment syndrome. Crit Care Nurse. 2000;20(6):48–58.
7. Kirkpatrick AW, Roberts DJ, De Waele J, et al. Intra-abdominal hypertension and the abdominal compartment syndrome: updated consensus definitions and clinical practice guidelines from the World Society of the Abdominal Compartment Syndrome. Intensive Care Med. 2013; 39(7):1190–206.
8. Sugrue M, Jones F, Deane SA, Bishop G, Bauman A, Hillman K. Intra-abdominal hypertension is an independent cause of postoperative renal impairment. Arch Surg. 1999;134(10):1082–5.
9. Cheatham ML, Malbrain ML, Kirkpatrick A, et al. Results from the international conference of experts on intra-abdominal hypertension and abdominal compartment syndrome. II. Recommendations. Intensive Care Med. 2007;33(6):951–62.
10. Balogh Z, McKinley BA, Holcomb JB, et al. Both primary and secondary abdominal compartment syndrome can be predicted early and are harbingers of multiple organ failure. J Trauma. 2003;54(5):848–59; discussion 859–61.
11. Sugrue M, Bauman A, Jones F, et al. Clinical examination is an inaccurate predictor of intraabdominal pressure. World J Surg. 2002;26(12):1428–31.
12. Malbrain ML. Different techniques to measure intra-abdominal pressure (IAP): time for a critical re-appraisal. Intensive Care Med. 2004;30(3):357–71.
13. Malbrain M. Abdominal perfusion pressure as a prognostic marker in intraabdominal hypertension. In: Vincent J, editor. Yearbook of intensive care and emergency medicine. Berlin: Springer; 2002. p. 792–814.
14. Balogh Z, Jones F, D'Amours S, Parr M, Sugrue M. Continuous intra-abdominal pressure measurement technique. Am J Surg. 2004;188(6):679–84.
15. Al-Mufarrej F, Abell LM, Chawla LS. Understanding intra-abdominal hypertension: from the bench to the bedside. J Intensive Care Med. 2012;27(3):145–60.
16. Shah SK, Jimenez F, Letourneau PA, et al. Strategies for modulating the inflammatory response after decompression from abdominal compartment syndrome. Scand J Trauma Resusc Emerg Med. 2012;20:25.
17. Friedlander MH, Simon RJ, Ivatury R, DiRaimo R, Machiedo GW. Effect of hemorrhage on superior mesenteric artery flow during increased intra-abdominal pressures. J Trauma. 1998;45(3):433–89.
18. Koike K, Moore EE, Moore FA, Kim FJ, Carl VS, Banerjee A. Gut phospholipase A2 mediates neutrophil priming and lung injury after mesenteric ischemia-reperfusion. Am J Physiol. 1995; 268(3 Pt 1):G397–403.
19. Grotz MR, Deitch EA, Ding J, Xu D, Huang Q, Regel G. Intestinal cytokine response after gut ischemia: role of gut barrier failure. Ann Surg. 1999;229(4):478–86.
20. Rezende-Neto JB, Moore EE, Melo de Andrade MV, et al. Systemic inflammatory response secondary to abdominal compartment syndrome: stage for multiple organ failure. J Trauma. 2002;53(6):1121–8.
21. Bloomfield GL, Ridings PC, Blocher CR, Marmarou A, Sugerman HJ. A proposed relationship between increased intra-abdominal, intrathoracic, and intracranial pressure. Crit Care Med. 1997;25(3):496–503.

22. Joseph DK, Dutton RP, Aarabi B, Scalea TM. Decompressive laparotomy to treat intractable intracranial hypertension after traumatic brain injury. J Trauma. 2004;57(4):687–93; discussion 693–5.
23. Scalea TM, Bochicchio GV, Habashi N, et al. Increased intra-abdominal, intrathoracic, and intracranial pressure after severe brain injury: multiple compartment syndrome. J Trauma. 2007;62(3):647–56; discussion 656.
24. Takata M, Wise RA, Robotham JL. Effects of abdominal pressure on venous return: abdominal vascular zone conditions. J Appl Physiol. 1990;69(6):1961–72.
25. Kashtan J, Green JF, Parsons EQ, Holcroft JW. Hemodynamic effect of increased abdominal pressure. J Surg Res. 1981;30(3):249–55.
26. Luecke T, Pelosi P. Clinical review: positive end-expiratory pressure and cardiac output. Crit Care. 2005;9(6):607–21.
27. Ridings PC, Bloomfield GL, Blocher CR, Sugerman HJ. Cardiopulmonary effects of raised intra-abdominal pressure before and after intravascular volume expansion. J Trauma. 1995;39(6):1071–5.
28. Quintel M, Pelosi P, Caironi P, et al. An increase of abdominal pressure increases pulmonary edema in oleic acid-induced lung injury. Am J Respir Crit Care Med. 2004;169(4):534–41.
29. Mutoh T, Lamm WJ, Embree LJ, Hildebrandt J, Albert RK. Abdominal distension alters regional pleural pressures and chest wall mechanics in pigs in vivo. J Appl Physiol. 1991;70(6):2611–8.
30. Ivatury RR, Porter JM, Simon RJ, Islam S, John R, Stahl WM. Intra-abdominal hypertension after life-threatening penetrating abdominal trauma: prophylaxis, incidence, and clinical relevance to gastric mucosal pH and abdominal compartment syndrome. J Trauma. 1998;44(6): 1016–21; discussion 1021–3.
31. Malbrain ML, Pelosi P, De laet I, Lattuada M, Hedenstierna G. Lymphatic drainage between thorax and abdomen: please take good care of this well-performing machinery. Acta Clin Belg Suppl. 2007;1:152–61.
32. Diebel LN, Dulchavsky SA, Wilson RF. Effect of increased intra-abdominal pressure on mesenteric arterial and intestinal mucosal blood flow. J Trauma. 1992;33(1):45–8; discussion 48–9.
33. Leduc LJ, Mitchell A. Intestinal ischemia after laparoscopic cholecystectomy. JSLS. 2006; 10(2):236–8.
34. Diebel LN, Dulchavsky SA, Brown WJ. Splanchnic ischemia and bacterial translocation in the abdominal compartment syndrome. J Trauma. 1997;43(5):852–5.
35. Thorington JM, Schmidt CF. A study of urinary output and blood pressure changes resulting in experimental ascites. Am J Med Sci. 1923;165(6):880–6.
36. Harman PK, Kron IL, McLachlan HD, Freedlender AE, Nolan SP. Elevated intra-abdominal pressure and renal function. Ann Surg. 1982;196(5):594–7.
37. Kirsch AJ, Hensle TW, Chang DT, Kayton ML, Olsson CA, Sawczuk IS. Renal effects of CO2 insufflation: oliguria and acute renal dysfunction in a rat pneumoperitoneum model. Urology. 1994;43(4):453–9.
38. Doty JM, Saggi BH, Sugerman HJ, et al. Effect of increased renal venous pressure on renal function. J Trauma. 1999;47(6):1000–3.
39. Le Roith D, Bark H, Nyska M, Glick SM. The effect of abdominal pressure on plasma antidiuretic hormone levels in the dog. J Surg Res. 1982;32(1):65–9.
40. De Waele JJ, De Laet I, Kirkpatrick AW, Hoste E. Intra-abdominal hypertension and abdominal compartment syndrome. Am J Kidney Dis. 2011;57(1):159–69.
41. Mullens W, Abrahams Z, Skouri HN, et al. Elevated intra-abdominal pressure in acute decompensated heart failure: a potential contributor to worsening renal function? J Am Coll Cardiol. 2008;51(3):300–6.
42. Ross EA. Congestive renal failure: the pathophysiology and treatment of renal venous hypertension. J Card Fail. 2012;18(12):930–8.
43. Revell M, Greaves I, Porter K. Endpoints for fluid resuscitation in hemorrhagic shock. J Trauma. 2003;54(5 Suppl):S63–7.

44. Schachtrupp A, Graf J, Tons C, Hoer J, Fackeldey V, Schumpelick V. Intravascular volume depletion in a 24-hour porcine model of intra-abdominal hypertension. J Trauma. 2003;55(4): 734–40.
45. Schachtrupp A, Lawong G, Afify M, Graf J, Toens C, Schumpelick V. Fluid resuscitation preserves cardiac output but cannot prevent organ damage in a porcine model during 24 h of intraabdominal hypertension. Shock. 2005;24(2):153–8.
46. Cheatham ML, Safcsak K, Block EF, Nelson LD. Preload assessment in patients with an open abdomen. J Trauma. 1999;46(1):16–22.
47. De Waele JJ, Benoit D, Hoste E, Colardyn F. A role for muscle relaxation in patients with abdominal compartment syndrome? Intensive Care Med. 2003;29(2):332.
48. De Waele JJ, Hoste EA, Malbrain ML. Decompressive laparotomy for abdominal compartment syndrome–a critical analysis. Crit Care. 2006;10(2):R51.
49. Cullen DJ, Coyle JP, Teplick R, Long MC. Cardiovascular, pulmonary, and renal effects of massively increased intra-abdominal pressure in critically ill patients. Crit Care Med. 1989;17(2):118–21.
50. Diaz Jr JJ, Mejia V, Subhawong AP, et al. Protocol for bedside laparotomy in trauma and emergency general surgery: a low return to the operating room. Am Surg. 2005;71(11): 986–91.
51. Bloomfield GL, Blocher CR, Fakhry IF, Sica DA, Sugerman HJ. Elevated intra-abdominal pressure increases plasma renin activity and aldosterone levels. J Trauma. 1997;42(6):997–1004; discussion 1004–5.
52. Morris Jr JA, Eddy VA, Blinman TA, Rutherford EJ, Sharp KW. The staged celiotomy for trauma. Issues in unpacking and reconstruction. Ann Surg. 1993;217(5):576–84; discussion 584–6.
53. Offner PJ, de Souza AL, Moore EE, et al. Avoidance of abdominal compartment syndrome in damage-control laparotomy after trauma. Arch Surg. 2001;136(6):676–81.
54. Murdock AD. What is the standard approach to temporary abdominal closure? J Trauma. 2007;62(6 Suppl):S29.
55. Gracias VH, Braslow B, Johnson J, et al. Abdominal compartment syndrome in the open abdomen. Arch Surg. 2002;137(11):1298–300.

Chapter 13
Kidney Function and Injury After Nephrectomy for Kidney Cancer

Charuhas V. Thakar and Krishnanath Gaitonde

Objectives

- To describe approaches and techniques of kidney cancer surgeries
- To explain short-term renal complications during postoperative period
- To understand long-term renal and patient outcomes after surgery for kidney cancer
- To evaluate novel approaches to diagnose and predict kidney injury and related outcomes

Introduction

The management of renal cell carcinoma has undergone a transformation in the past few years. Surgical innovation has reduced hospital morbidity, and several novel techniques have attempted to focus on the preservation of residual renal function after

C.V. Thakar, MD, FASN (✉)
Division of Nephrology and Hypertension, University of Cincinnati, Cincinnati, OH, USA

Section of Nephrology, Cincinnati VA Medical Center, Cincinnati, OH, USA
e-mail: charuhas.thakar@uc.edu; charuhas.thakar@va.gov

K. Gaitonde, MD
Division of Urology, University of Cincinnati, Cincinnati, OH, USA

Section of Urology, Cincinnati VA Medical Center, Cincinnati, OH, USA
e-mail: gaitonk@ucmail.uc.edu

C.V. Thakar, C.R. Parikh (eds.), *Perioperative Kidney Injury: Principles of Risk Assessment, Diagnosis and Treatment*, DOI 10.1007/978-1-4939-1273-5_13

total or partial removal of nephron mass while reducing invasiveness and preserving oncological efficacy. Renal cell carcinoma (RCC) usually occurs in the elderly and is also associated with comorbid conditions such as hypertension, diabetes, or reduced renal function either due to aging or other kidney disorders. This has led to the increasing interest in studying the epidemiology of progressive chronic kidney disease (CKD) after surgery for RCC, and the pathobiological link between perioperative kidney injury and long-term clinical outcomes. The following sections will discuss the surgical treatment options for RCC, its impact on short-term and long-term renal outcomes, and innovations and discoveries in this field.

Surgical Treatment and Hospital Course

Nephrectomy for Kidney Tumors

The incidence of renal tumors is rising at 3 % per year; in 2006, more than 35,000 patients developed renal cortical tumors in the USA [1]. Detection of small (≤4 cm), localized, renal cortical tumors accounts for 60–70 % of all diagnosed renal masses [2]. Radical nephrectomy (RN) has been the gold standard treatment for localized renal tumors [3], the reasonable supposition being that if the preoperative kidney function is preserved, then the other kidney should compensate the glomerular filtration rate (GFR) for the loss of the function on the contralateral side, akin to donor nephrectomies in transplantation. However, epidemiological data indicates, in patients without preoperative chronic kidney disease (CKD), the probability of incident CKD during a 3-year follow-up can reach up to 65 % after radical nephrectomy [4]. A plausible explanation is that given the age and comorbidity profile of an average patient with RCC, the compensatory ability of the remaining kidney is limited. Hence, a partial nephrectomy (PN) provides a "nephron-sparing" approach, and increasingly, surgeons are now able to safely perform partial nephrectomy without compromising oncological efficacy [5–8] (Fig. 13.1).

Between 20 and 60 % of all renal cortical tumors (<4 cm) are preferentially treated with partial nephrectomy [9, 10]. PN is performed by a variety of surgical techniques [8, 11]. The two commonly used approaches are open and a laparoscopic/minimally invasive approach. The major techniques include either a temporary application of renal pedicle clamp and subjecting the kidney to warm or cold (induced by ice packs) ischemia during renal tumor excision and reconstruction or a non-clamp approach where the tumor removal is performed without subjecting the kidney to ischemia, by control of bleeding. Each surgical approach and technique has its own advantages and respective limitations, and of course, they also require different levels of technical expertise.

Other approaches to treat kidney cancer include thermal or cryoablation of the tumor. This approach is minimally invasive and can be repeated. However, long-term oncological effectiveness has not been well established, and some reports suggest

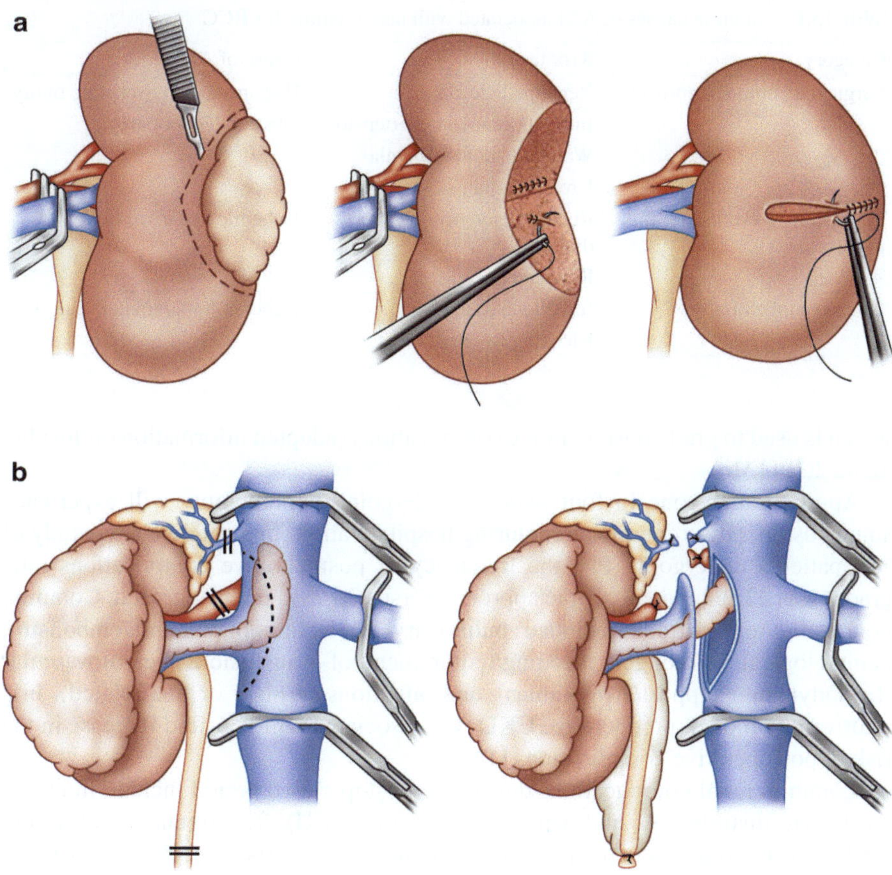

Fig. 13.1 Surgical options for kidney cancer. (**a**) Partial nephrectomy. (**b**) Radical nephrectomy

that local recurrence rates are higher than with surgical excision. Additionally, conventional surgical salvage may be required and can be complicated by fibrotic reaction, and radiographic parameters for success are also not well established. This technique is typically chosen in cases based on a careful evaluation of the risk of other surgical approaches, life expectancy, and tumor size [12].

Postoperative Complications

In patients undergoing radical or partial nephrectomy, there are several anticipated and unanticipated renal and nonrenal complications. Much of the literature that have outlined these complications or risk factors have used the Clavien approach

Table 13.1 Common causes of AKI associated with nephrectomy for RCC

Category	Risk factors	Cause of AKI
Surgical technique/approach	Renal pedicle clamp	Hypoperfusion, ischemic injury
	Intra-abdominal hypertension	Obstructive uropathy
	Warm and cold ischemia	
	Ureteral injury	
Perioperative events/ nephrotoxins	Renin-angiotensin blockers, diuretics, NSAID	Ischemic and toxic injury
	Rhabdomyolysis	
Other complications	Infection/sepsis	Ischemic/inflammatory injury
	Bleeding	

which is used to grade postoperative complications (adapted information outlined in Table 2.1) [13].

Approximately one in four patients undergoing nephrectomy will experience some postoperative complication during hospitalization. In a single-center study of 150 patients undergoing PN, the frequency of postoperative complications (any grade) was 22 % in laparoscopic approach versus 26 % in open approach. Common nonrenal complications included pulmonary (atelectasis/pneumonia/embolism), hematological (prolonged bleeding/requirement of transfusions), cardiovascular (hemodynamic support/arrhythmias), and infections (urinary or line related). In a multivariate model, preoperative CKD was associated with 4.5-fold increase in the risk of postoperative complications [14].

Common renal complications during the postoperative period include fluid and electrolyte disturbances and acute kidney injury (AKI). The frequency of severe AKI requiring dialysis is relatively low, and in most reports, it is <5 %. In patients undergoing radical or partial nephrectomy, several potential risk factors are known to be associated with AKI. These are shown in Table 13.1.

In patients undergoing PN, certain surgical approaches and techniques lead to subjecting of the kidney to warm or cold ischemia during surgery; cold ischemia is usually achieved by packing ice around the kidney. The optimal duration of ischemia that can be safely tolerated by the kidney remains unclear. Much of the current practice relies on the knowledge generated from large mammalian models of partial nephrectomy, where animals have been exposed to ischemia-reperfusion injury to assess the post-procedure renal damage [11, 15]. It is extrapolated that approximately 30–45 min of ischemia followed by reperfusion is considered to be generally safe and represents the optimal time required in achieving surgical efficacy for the treatment of these tumors. A recent study evaluating serial biopsies suggested that subjecting the human kidney to ischemia, lasting for 30 min or less, leads to mitochondrial swelling and cytological changes, which are potentially reversible [16].

Laparoscopic approaches to PN or RN, in some cases, can be associated with intra-abdominal hypertension (IAH). Typically, these procedures require induction of pneumoperitoneum to achieve pressures ranging from 20 to 25 mmHg. Experimental models that have studied the safety of this process indicate that IAH can impact the production of nitric oxide in renal microcirculation [17, 18]. Taken together, it can be hypothesized that a certain subgroup of patients may be vulnerable to sustain significant kidney injury/damage when exposed to prolonged IAH and other coexisting risk factors (e.g., preoperative CKD, intraoperative hypotension, preoperative use of drugs that may impair intrarenal hemodynamics and autoregulation). Additionally, robotic-assisted approach, which poses additional technical challenges and associated complications, can also be now used to perform minimally invasive surgery [17, 19].

Long-Term Follow-Up

In addition to oncological efficacy, surveillance, and imaging, patients undergoing radical or partial nephrectomy are at risk of incident and progressive chronic kidney disease. Several large observational cohorts have examined the renal and overall prognosis in patients undergoing radical and partial nephrectomy [4–6]. Huang and colleagues studied a single-center experience in 662 patients (1989–2005) with normal preoperative serum creatinine and two healthy kidneys undergoing elective PN or RN (~55 % underwent PN) for solitary cortical tumors of <4 cm [4]. Of note, 26 % of the 662 patients had preexisting CKD based on estimated GFR (estimated by Modification of Diet in Renal Disease [MDRD] equation) despite normal creatinine values. Over a 3-year follow-up, the probability to be free from CKD was 80 % in PN versus 35 % in those with RN. Corresponding probabilities to be free from reaching Stage IIIB CKD (eGFR <45 ml/min/1.73 m^2) were 95 % for PN and 67 % for RN. None of the patients reached end-stage renal disease (ESRD) during the follow-up in either group.

Another single-center observational cohort studied 1,004 patients who underwent PN or RN (between 1999 and 2004) [20]. Along with comparing cancer-free survival, this study also examined the impact of new-onset CKD on overall and cardiac survival. In a risk-adjusted analysis, cancer-specific survival was equivalent for PN and RN. The study confirmed the earlier findings that RN patients lost significantly more renal function than those undergoing PN. The average excess loss of renal function observed with radical nephrectomy was associated with a 25 % (95 % CI 3–73) increased risk of cardiac death and 17 % (95 % CI 12–27) increased risk of death from any cause by multivariate analysis.

Although there have been no large prospective randomized studies comparing these two treatment modalities, the observational studies make a strong case that partial nephrectomy, in selected individuals, can achieve similar oncological efficacy while preserving renal function in the long term; and preserved renal function in turn is a good prognostic indicator of overall and cardiac survival.

Assessment of Renal Function

In the preoperative period, estimated GFR and 24 h urine creatinine clearance are likely to be more reliable methods of assessing renal function in patients undergoing radical or partial nephrectomy. Use of serum creatinine alone may not be most accurate and may misclassify patients from a prognostic standpoint in the perioperative period, as suggested by large observational studies. This opinion is based on the interpretation of observational studies, as there are no studies that have compared different methods of assessing preoperative baseline renal function.

During the postoperative period, clinicians rely on the duration of ischemia or postoperative serum creatinine level as diagnostic and prognostic indicators of postoperative renal function. Given that the serum creatinine level during the postoperative period represents the compensatory changes in the contralateral kidney (along with reperfusion of the remnant kidney in PN patients), it may not be the ideal marker to assess renal function. This could be one of the surgical settings where the urine output-based definitions of AKI may be more relevant during the immediate postoperative period, as it is more likely to correspond to the changes in renal hemodynamics and intra-abdominal pressure.

Regardless of the type of surgery, patients after nephrectomy (radical or partial) are at an increased risk of incident and progressive CKD and reduced survival. The progressive loss of renal function could be due to glomerular hypertension/compensatory stress in the contralateral kidney in patients with RN. In those patients with PN, in addition to the effects on the contralateral kidney, the remnant kidney is now exposed to the consequences of ischemia-reperfusion injury. These data mirror the information derived from other experimental and clinical settings of acute kidney injury (AKI), where a single episode of ischemia-reperfusion injury (IRI) to the kidney leads to permanent changes in kidney structure and progressive loss of renal function [21–25].

Renal scintigraphy has been utilized to circumvent some of the challenges posed by biochemical measurement of pre- and postoperative renal function. In a single-center study, 54 patients undergoing laparoscopic PN underwent pre- and postoperative renal scintigraphy [26]. These patients were followed for up to 4 years, and the split renal function and effective renal plasma flow (ERPF) were evaluated by renal scintigraphy preoperatively, at 3 and 12 months postoperatively, and then yearly for up to 4 years. The split renal function (SRF) and ERPF of the affected kidneys decreased significantly at month 3 and subsequently remained stable, but below baseline, throughout the duration of follow-up. Duration of warm ischemia was the only significant risk factor that correlated with reduction in SRF and ERPF at 3 and 48 months. In this study, the serum creatinine and estimated GFR of the entire group remain statistically similar at all time points of follow-up. The data suggests that the ischemic damage sustained by the remnant kidney leads to continued deterioration of function in that kidney for up to 3 months, without any further worsening or improvement. At least in this study, the preservation of overall renal function can be attributed to compensatory increase in the GFR in the contralateral kidney, which did not experience ischemia-reperfusion injury.

Innovation and Discovery

Although animal studies of PN have described the relationship between the duration of ischemia and the subsequent renal dysfunction, direct translation of this knowledge into clinical settings is very limited [8, 11]. Assessment of kidney injury by way of measuring tissue-specific kidney injury markers in the setting of partial nephrectomy may pave the way for further improvement in our ability to improve outcomes in these patients.

Several biomarkers have been identified as tissue-specific and sensitive indicators of ischemic renal injury [27]. These have been discovered and validated in animal models of IRI, followed by validation in clinical settings of acute kidney injury (AKI) including delayed graft function after kidney transplantation [28]. Two such markers, which are easily detectable in the urine and have been validated in clinical studies, are (1) neutrophil gelatinase-associated lipocalin [NGAL] and (2) interleukin-18 [IL-18] [29–32]. These proteins are released in response to renal epithelial cell injury and can identify kidney injury within minutes to hours of inducing renal ischemia [33] (Fig. 13.2).

From the standpoint of application of biomarker research in the setting of ischemic kidney injury, the clinical model of PN offers a unique ability to validate kidney injury biomarkers. Measuring tissue-specific markers will provide direct assessment of injury sustained by the remnant kidney in "real time." As shown in

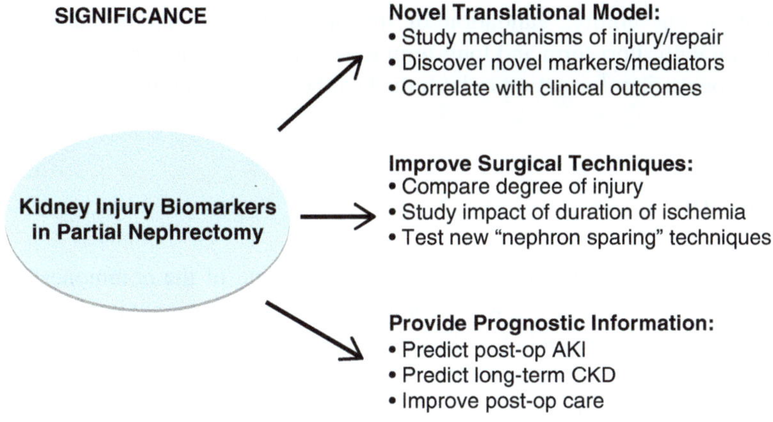

Fig. 13.2 Potential role of biomarkers

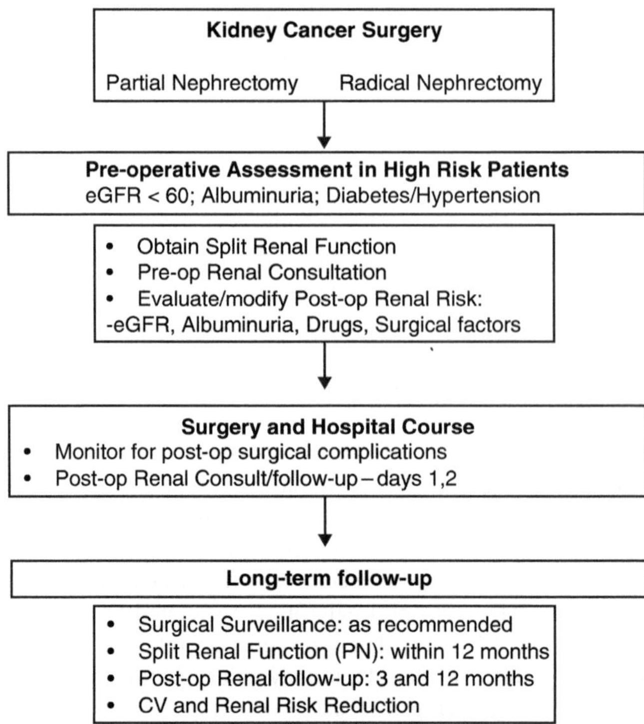

Fig. 13.3 Perioperative care schematic

Fig. 13.2, such information may allow the surgeons to improve the safety of their techniques such that the remainder of the kidney parenchyma can be preserved to the best of our ability. Validation of this and other biomarker pathways and correlation with short-term and long-term renal outcomes would result in the provision of prognostic information to both the healthcare provider and the patient.

Conclusion

Partial and radical nephrectomy for kidney cancer, one of the commonest cancers afflicting US adults, offer expected oncological efficacy. However, it is associated with perioperative impairment of kidney function, which has both short-term and long-term health consequences. Existing epidemiological studies, and prospect of application of knowledge about kidney injury biomarkers, offer hope that we may be able to deliver better care to these patients and improve health outcomes. In the following figure, the authors propose an algorithm to suggest a perioperative care paradigm. Its applicability can be customized based on local/regional resources. We believe that such care pathways will foster interdisciplinary and patient-centered perioperative care and create platforms to perform clinical and translational research (Fig. 13.3).

Key Messages

- Approximately one out of every four patients undergoing surgery for kidney cancer will experience a spectrum of immediate postoperative complications, and the risk of complications is higher in patients with preoperative CKD.
- Up to 60 % of patients will develop incident or progressive CKD after surgery for kidney cancer.
- Current methods of quantifying ischemic injury to the remnant renal tissue are suboptimal, and hence, its long-term prognostic impact remains unclear.
- Multidisciplinary approach in the perioperative period and frequent periodic monitoring in the postoperative period should be adopted to improve renal and patient outcomes.

References

1. Chow W-H, Devesa SS, Warren JL, et al. Rising incidence of renal cell cancer in the United States. JAMA. 1999;281(17):1628–31.
2. Hollingsworth JM, Miller DC, Daignault S, et al. Rising incidence of small renal masses: a need to reassess treatment effect. J Natl Cancer Inst. 2006;98(18):1331–4.
3. Robson CJ, Churchill BM, Anderson W. The results of radical nephrectomy for renal cell carcinoma. J Urol. 1969;101(3):297–301.
4. Huang WC, Levey AS, Serio AM, et al. Chronic kidney disease after nephrectomy in patients with renal cortical tumours: a retrospective cohort study. Lancet Oncol. 2006;7(9):735–40.
5. Lau WK, Blute ML, Weaver AL, et al. Matched comparison of radical nephrectomy vs nephron-sparing surgery in patients with unilateral renal cell carcinoma and a normal contralateral kidney. Mayo Clin Proc. 2000;75(12):1236–42.
6. Fergany AF, Hafez KS, Novick AC. Long-term results of nephron sparing surgery for localized renal cell carcinoma: 10-year followup. J Urol. 2000;163(2):442–5.
7. Uzzo RG, Wei JT, Hafez K, et al. Comparison of direct hospital costs and length of stay for radical nephrectomy versus nephron-sparing surgery in the management of localized renal cell carcinoma. Urology. 1999;54(6):994–8.
8. Rini BI, Campbell SC, Escudier B. Renal cell carcinoma. Lancet. 2009;373(9669):1119–32.
9. Hollenbeck BK, Taub DA, Miller DC, et al. National utilization trends of partial nephrectomy for renal cell carcinoma: a case of underutilization? Urology. 2006;67(2):254–9.
10. Miller DC, Hollingsworth JM, Hafez KS, et al. Partial nephrectomy for small renal masses: an emerging quality of care concern? J Urol. 2006;175(3 Pt 1):853–7; discussion 858.
11. Simmons MN, Schreiber MJ, Gill IS. Surgical renal ischemia: a contemporary overview. J Urol. 2008;180(1):19–30.
12. Klatte T, Shariat SF, Remzi M. Systematic review and meta-analysis of perioperative and oncological outcomes of laparoscopic cryoablation versus laparoscopic partial nephrectomy for the treatment of small renal tumors. J Urol. 2013;191(5):1209–1217.
13. Dindo D, Demartines N, Clavien PA. Classification of surgical complications: a new proposal with evaluation in a cohort of 6336 patients and results of a survey. Ann Surg. 2004;240(2): 205–13.
14. Hakimi AA, Rajpathak S, Chery L, et al. Renal insufficiency is an independent risk factor for complications after partial nephrectomy. J Urol. 2010;183(1):43–7.

15. Porpiglia F, Fiori C, Bertolo R, et al. The effects of warm ischaemia time on renal function after laparoscopic partial nephrectomy in patients with normal contralateral kidney. World J Urol. 2012;30(2):257–63.
16. Parekh DJ, Weinberg JM, Ercole B, et al. Tolerance of the human kidney to isolated controlled ischemia. J Am Soc Nephrol. 2013;24(3):506–17.
17. Wiesenthal JD, Fazio LM, Perks AE, et al. Effect of pneumoperitoneum on renal tissue oxygenation and blood flow in a rat model. Urology. 2011;77(6):1508. e9–15.
18. Dunn MD, McDougall EM. Renal physiology. Laparoscopic considerations. Urol Clin North Am. 2000;27(4):609–14.
19. Kim EH, Larson JA, Figenshau M, et al. Perioperative complications of robot-assisted partial nephrectomy. Curr Urol Rep. 2014;15(1):377.
20. Weight CJ, Larson BT, Fergany AF, et al. Nephrectomy induced chronic renal insufficiency is associated with increased risk of cardiovascular death and death from any cause in patients with localized cT1b renal masses. J Urol. 2010;183(4):1317–23.
21. Meyer TW, Rennke HG. Progressive glomerular injury after limited renal infarction in the rat. Am J Physiol. 1988;254(6 Pt 2):F856–62.
22. Basile DP, Donohoe D, Roethe K, et al. Renal ischemic injury results in permanent damage to peritubular capillaries and influences long-term function. Am J Physiol Renal Physiol. 2001;281(5):F887–99.
23. Pagtalunan ME, Olson JL, Tilney NL, et al. Late consequences of acute ischemic injury to a solitary kidney. J Am Soc Nephrol. 1999;10(2):366–73.
24. Lo LJ, Go AS, Chertow GM, et al. Dialysis-requiring acute renal failure increases the risk of progressive chronic kidney disease. Kidney Int. 2009;76(8):893–9.
25. Newsome BB, Warnock DG, McClellan WM, et al. Long-term risk of mortality and end-stage renal disease among the elderly after small increases in serum creatinine level during hospitalization for acute myocardial infarction. Arch Intern Med. 2008;168(6):609–16.
26. Porpiglia F, Fiori C, Bertolo R, et al. Long-term functional evaluation of the treated kidney in a prospective series of patients who underwent laparoscopic partial nephrectomy for small renal tumors. Eur Urol. 2012;62(1):130–5.
27. Coca SG, Yalavarthy R, Concato J, et al. Biomarkers for the diagnosis and risk stratification of acute kidney injury: a systematic review. Kidney Int. 2008;73(9):1008–16.
28. Coca SG, Parikh CR. Urinary biomarkers for acute kidney injury: perspectives on translation. Clin J Am Soc Nephrol. 2008;3(2):481–90.
29. Mishra J, Ma Q, Prada A, et al. Identification of neutrophil gelatinase-associated lipocalin as a novel early urinary biomarker for ischemic renal injury. J Am Soc Nephrol. 2003;14(10): 2534–43.
30. Parikh CR, Jani A, Mishra J, et al. Urine NGAL and IL-18 are predictive biomarkers for delayed graft function following kidney transplantation. Am J Transplant. 2006;6(7):1639–45.
31. Parikh CR, Mishra J, Thiessen-Philbrook H et al. Urinary IL-18 is an early predictive biomarker of acute kidney injury after cardiac surgery. Kidney Int. 2006;70(1):199–203
32. Mishra J, Dent C, Tarabishi R, et al. Neutrophil gelatinase-associated lipocalin (NGAL) as a biomarker for acute renal injury after cardiac surgery. Lancet. 2005;365(9466):1231–8.
33. Devarajan P. Emerging biomarkers of acute kidney injury. Contrib Nephrol. 2007;156: 203–12.

Part IV
Transplant Surgery

Chapter 14
The Kidney in Nonrenal Solid Organ Transplantation: Liver and Heart

Titte R. Srinivas and Stuart M. Flechner

Objectives

- To understand the pathophysiology of acute kidney injury in end-stage liver disease, liver transplantation, and heart transplant recipients.
- To recognize the complexities in the measurement of renal function, diagnosis of acute kidney injury, and associated complications.
- To discuss renal replacement and kidney transplant options in nonrenal solid organ transplantation settings.

Introduction

The spectrum of kidney pathology accompanying nonrenal solid organ transplantation spans the gamut from acute kidney injury (AKI) to chronic kidney disease (CKD) and end-stage renal disease (ESRD). In this chapter, based on the annual number of transplants and burden of AKI, we will primarily discuss issues relevant to the diagnosis and management of kidney injury in liver transplant candidates or recipients. We also highlight key principles related to diagnosis and management of AKI in the setting of heart transplantation.

T.R. Srinivas, MD (✉)
Section of Transplant Nephrology, Division of Nephrology, Medical University of South Carolina, 96 Jonathan Lucas Street, Suite CSB 829 MSC 629, Charleston, SC 29425, USA
e-mail: srinivat@musc.edu

S.M. Flechner, MD, FACS
Department of Urology, Glickman Urologic and Kidney Institute, Cleveland Clinic Lerner College of Medicine, 9500 Euclid Ave/Q10, Cleveland, OH 44195, USA
e-mail: flechns@ccf.org

C.V. Thakar, C.R. Parikh (eds.), *Perioperative Kidney Injury: Principles of Risk Assessment, Diagnosis and Treatment*, DOI 10.1007/978-1-4939-1273-5_14

Liver Transplantation

Measurement of Kidney Function in Cirrhotic Patients Is Complex

In cirrhotic patients, serum creatinine (SCr) is an unreliable marker of kidney function as most of these patients have low muscle mass, poor protein intake, and reduced creatinine production. About a third of patients with cirrhosis will have SCr in the "normal range" despite having measured creatinine clearances (CrCl) of 50 mL/min/1.73 m^2 or less [1]. As SCr lies in the denominator of any estimating equation for glomerular filtration rate (GFR) or CrCl, creatinine-based equations will thus systematically overestimate GFR (or CrCl). Interestingly, the six-variable Modification of Diet in Renal Disease (MDRD) study equation may perform better in cirrhotics (it incorporates albumin and urea nitrogen levels) than the four-variable MDRD study equation [2–4].

Other alternatives to measure kidney function are equally problematic: the direct measurement of GFR using 125-I iothalamate or 99mTcDTPA (technetium 99m diethylenetriamine pentaacetic acid) is also limited, because the volume of distribution of the tracer may vary based on the amount of ascites and edema. Novel markers of GFR, such as cystatin C, may be more accurate in these patients; however, concerns about assay interference with calcineurin inhibitors (CNIs) and corticosteroid therapy remain [5]. Despite this uncertainty, cystatin C-based equations presently seem more promising than creatinine-based equations.

Kidney and Electrolyte Disturbances in ESLD and Hepatorenal Syndrome (HRS)

Several hemodynamic features predispose patients with liver disease to renal dysfunction. The predominant physiological precedent to renal dysfunction is decreased renal plasma flow. Through the subsequent activation of the sympathetic nervous system and the renin-angiotensin-aldosterone system, GFR is initially preserved in the earliest stages of cirrhosis. However, as liver disease worsens, these compensatory mechanisms fail, and GFR falls with ensuing AKI [5].

A working group of the International Ascites Club and the Acute Dialysis Quality Initiative has attempted to define the spectrum of renal function decline in patients with cirrhosis as follows: AKI was defined as an acute increase in SCr ≥50 % from baseline or an increase in SCr >0.3 mg/dL in <48 h. CKD was defined as an estimated glomerular filtration rate (eGFR) <60 mL/min for >3 months using a combination of the six-variable MDRD study equation. Acute-on-chronic renal insufficiency was defined as a combination of the above [2].

A specific functional form of AKI that reflects severe renal vasoconstriction without structural kidney damage is known as HRS. This condition culminates from progressive renal vasoconstriction with advancing portal hypertension, subsequently

Table 14.1 Hepatorenal syndrome [1, 2]

Type 1
Doubling of serum creatinine to >2.5 mg/dL within 2 weeks
Type 2 HRS (progression >2 weeks)
Cirrhosis with ascites
Serum creatinine >1.5 mg/dL
No improvement in serum creatinine (decrease <1.5 mg/dL) after 2 days of diuretics and volume expansion with albumin (1 g/kg body weight up to a maximum of 100 g/d)
Absence of shock
No current or recent treatment with nephrotoxic drugs
Absence of signs of parenchymal renal disease as suggested by proteinuria (urine protein excretion >500 mg/day) or hematuria (>50 red cells/high-power field) and/or abnormal renal ultrasound

followed by rising creatinine and stages of diuretic responsive ascites, followed by diuretic resistant ascites. Though sodium avidity is regarded as an important component of HRS physiology, recent definitions summarized in Table 14.1 rely more on the tempo of serum creatinine rise and the absence of parenchymal disease. Type 1 HRS is of rapid onset with an oftentimes identifiable precipitating event such as hypovolemia, and type 2 HRS likely reflects chronic renal vasoconstriction of cirrhosis and progresses commensurately with liver disease [2].

Hyponatremia is another complication commonly encountered in ESLD patients and is of prognostic significance. While safe preoperative cutoffs for serum sodium are not known, a sodium level of <120 mEq/L may require treatment [1]. Whether preoperative correction of hyponatremia improves, liver transplant outcomes are not clear. The current mainstays of therapy are free water restriction and diuretics. Vasopressin-2 antagonists such as conivaptan and tolvaptan may confer utility in hypervolemic hyponatremic patients but offer only modest effects on serum sodium and do not impact mortality or renal function. Correction of serum sodium must be gradual in asymptomatic individuals and not exceed 8–10 mEq/L/day in order to avoid central pontine myelinolysis [1]. Along similar lines, hyponatremic patients receiving dialysis should have dialysate sodium maintained within 10 mEq/L of their serum sodium concentration to avoid rapid correction of hyponatremia.

Incidence and Risk Factors of AKI Post-Liver Transplant

The incidence of AKI during the postoperative period after liver transplant is variable and ranges between 48 and 94 % and requires renal replacement therapy (RRT) between 8 and 17 % of the time [4–7]. Some of the wide variation in the incidence is likely due to varying definitions of AKI. Recently, novel urinary biomarkers reflecting renal tubular injury have been studied for earlier and more sensitive diagnosis of AKI. For example, Wagener et al. found that urinary neutrophil gelatinase-associated lipocalin (NGAL) is able to predict postoperative AKI within 3 h after liver transplant, far before the rise in serum creatinine [8]. Whether biomarker-based early diagnosis will lead to improved outcomes remains to be examined.

Table 14.2 Temporal profile of clinical risk factors for postoperative ARF after liver transplantation

Early (<1 week postoperative)	Late (>2 <4 weeks postoperative)
Preoperative factors	
Preoperative ARF[a] *(Cr >1.5 mg/dL)*	Elective re-transplant
Lower preoperative serum albumin[a] *(<3.2 mg/dL)*	Preoperative ARF
Urgent re-transplant	
Child-Pugh score	
Hematuria and/or proteinuria	
Advanced age	
Diabetes mellitus	
Need for high doses of diuretics	
High body mass index (BMI)	
Intraoperative factors	
Increasing use of fresh frozen plasma and cryoprecipitate (surrogate for coagulopathy)[a]	Platelet units
Higher number of platelet transfusions	
Intraoperative complications	
Increased use of pressors	
Postoperative factors	
Longer duration of pressors postoperatively[a]	Mechanical ventilation
Longer duration of ventilator support[a]	*Bacterial infection*[a]
Liver allograft dysfunction[a]	*Surgical reoperation*[a]
Lower blood pressures through all aspects of the operation and postoperatively	CNI toxicity
Higher pulmonary capillary wedge pressure pre-anhepatic and lower cardiac indices post-anhepatic	
CNI toxicity	

Adapted from Cabezuelo et al. [9]

[a]Likely reflects convergence of several individual variables that confer a dominant clinical effect

Risk factors associated with AKI are listed in Table 14.2. Factors associated with AKI in the liver transplant setting are best understood in the context of the time frame after transplantation when they may be operative. Cabezuelo et al. studied factors associated with early (<1 week post transplant [TX]) and late (2–4 weeks post TX) AKI [9]. Independent risk factors for early AKI included preoperative AKI, duration of dopamine treatment, and liver allograft dysfunction [9]. A higher serum albumin was associated with a lower odds for postoperative AKI. Late AKI was associated with reoperation and bacterial infection/sepsis [9]. Approaching postoperative AKI by such risk stratification based on timing can clarify the differential diagnosis and potentially facilitate preventative and treatment measures.

Considerations for Renal Replacement Therapy (RRT) in ESLD

The milieu of hepatic failure is marked by decreased urea generation rates, which, combined with the sarcopenia of ESLD, can lead to an underestimation of the true renal dysfunction simply based on the degree of azotemia. Moreover, the choice of modality of RRT among patients awaiting liver transplantation is determined by considerations of hemodynamic stability. Intermittent RRT may take the form of either hemodialysis (HD) or peritoneal dialysis (PD) [6], which is possible even in the presence of ascites. Measures to maintain blood pressure (BP) during HD include midodrine, sodium modeling, and lowered dialysate temperatures. PD may provide better hemodynamic stability but can be complicated by protein depletion and infection. In general, PD is avoided in liver transplant candidates as peritonitis can impede transplant candidacy. A retrospective comparison between intermittent and continuous renal replacement therapy (CRRT) demonstrated that those on CRRT had inferior survival. However, such data must be interpreted with extreme caution due to the inherent bias in selecting CRRT for those patients with the greatest degree of hemodynamic instability [6]. CRRT is usually the treatment of choice in patients with renal failure and hepatic encephalopathy, as it is less likely to exacerbate the proclivity of these patients for raised intracranial pressure and brainstem herniation [6]. Regional citrate anticoagulation is applied in most centers for CRRT, and this method minimizes the added bleeding risk engendered by heparin. It is important to consider, however, that in the face of advanced liver failure, citrate may not be metabolized and lead to citrate toxicity and worsening of acidosis [10].

Intraoperative and Peri-transplant CRRT

The intraoperative use of CRRT during liver transplantation may improve hemodynamic stability and control of volume status, as enormous quantities of blood products are utilized. Large-scale randomized investigations of the utility and efficacy of intraoperative CRRT in liver transplantation have not been conducted. In a single-center study, CRRT was used intraoperatively in 41 of 636 (6.4 %) liver transplants (median model for ESLD score, 38) [11]. Patients were selected for intraoperative CRRT either for indications relating to renal failure (e.g., hyperkalemia or acidosis) or those related to liver transplantation and ESLD (e.g., transfusion volume, lactic acidosis, hyponatremia, and hypernatremia) [11]. CRRT was used over half of the total operative time with a 40 % filter clot rate; the filter clot rate did not correlate with CRRT duration. Equal or negative fluid balance was achieved in 92.7 % of cases. CRRT was discontinued in a week in 80 % of the cases, and transition to HD was successful in the majority of CRRT cases. Overall survival was 97.6 % at 1 month and 75.6 % at 1 year with a mean eGFR of 54.7 mL/min/1.73 m^2 [11].

Heart Transplant

AKI occurs in approximately 5–30 % of recipients of thoracic organ transplantations. Early postoperative AKI in cardiac transplant recipients is associated with crude hospital mortality rates ranging between 30 and 50 % [12].

Many risk factors for AKI in cardiac transplant settings are similar to other cardiac surgery patients and include atherosclerosis, valvular disease, cigarette smoking, diabetes, and abnormal baseline renal function [13]. Certain factors such as low baseline albumin and prolonged cold ischemia time are relatively unique to transplant settings only. Attention to modifiable risk factors should focus on glycemic control and lipid management. Patients with systemic atherosclerosis are particularly sensitive to hemodynamic changes as a result of decreased cardiac output or hypotension. Additionally, vascular manipulation in this population can be associated with cholesterol emboli and downstream athero-embolic disease in the kidney.

The intraoperative use of cardiopulmonary bypass also contributes to the development of AKI. These include factors specifically related to the bypass procedure itself, such as cross-clamp time and duration of bypass. Cardiopulmonary bypass is also associated with the generation of free hemoglobin and iron through hemolysis that typically occurs during the procedure [14]. Hemolysis may also be caused by cardiotomy suction, occlusive roller pumps, turbulent flow in the oxygenator, and blood return through cell saver devices. This may contribute to increased oxidative stress and renal tubular injury [15]. The relationship between the use of left ventricular assist device and renal insufficiency is beyond the scope of this discussion but is addressed elsewhere. Table 14.3 outlines organ-specific risk factors in heart transplant recipients [16].

Table 14.3 Risk factors for AKI and management in cardiac transplants

Heart transplant recipients	Risk factor management
Baseline	Baseline
Low cardiac output	Minimize IV contrast exposure
Medication toxicity	Preoperative volume optimization
Diabetes	Low oxalate diet in those at risk
Prior cardiac surgery	Consideration of candidacy for simultaneous kidney transplantation
Serum albumin	
Hepatitis C	
Intraoperative	Intraoperative
Cardiopulmonary bypass time (CB)	Minimize aortic cross-clamp/CB time as feasible
Organ ischemia time	Vasopressor support as needed
Transfusion requirement	Methylene blue, questionable benefit
Hypotension/hypoperfusion	Minimize IV contrast
Nephrotoxic agent exposure (antibiotics, radiographic contrast)	
Atheroembolism	
Hemolysis/pigment nephropathy	
Postoperative	Postoperative
CNI exposure	Avoidance of nephrotoxic antibiotics when alternatives available
Aggressive diuresis	CNI monitoring
Sepsis	Judicious volume management
Graft dysfunction	CRRT may be of benefit to optimize volume balance

Abbreviations: *CB*, *CNI* calcineurin inhibitor, *CRRT* continuous renal replacement therapy, *IV* intravenous, *CB* cardiopulmonary bypass

The risk of postoperative dialysis is slightly higher in cardiac transplant recipients than in those undergoing non-transplant surgery. However, length of stay and crude hospital mortality are similar regardless of the setting of cardiac surgery [16]. This observation emphasizes the need for additional efforts to prevent kidney injury in heart transplant recipients given its impact on both the patient and the valuable organ.

Chronic Kidney Disease Post-Solid Organ Transplant

Epidemiology

Ojo et al. studied a nationwide sample to demonstrate that the 5-year cumulative incidence of chronic renal failure—defined as an estimated glomerular filtration rate (eGFR) <30 mL/min/1.73 m^2—was 15 % among liver transplant recipients and 10 % in heart transplant recipients [17]. Factors associated with chronic renal failure were lower pre-transplant eGFR, increasing age, female sex, hypertension, diabetes mellitus, and postoperative AKI. The occurrence of chronic renal failure increased the overall mortality risk by fourfold. CNI nephrotoxicity with progressive vasculopathy and interstitial fibrosis and tubular atrophy has been implicated in the pathogenesis of chronic renal failure [18]. Other histologic entities include glomerulonephritis, diabetic nephropathy, and atherosclerotic disease, but it has been difficult to assess their attributable risk to transplantation [19].

Calcineurin Inhibitors and Posttransplant Renal Function

In addition to minimizing hemodynamic risk factors and providing prophylaxis for infection, deft management of immunosuppression is critical to preserve posttransplant renal function. Given the preeminent role of CNI toxicity both in acute and chronic kidney disease after transplantation, attempts should be made towards minimizing CNI dosing. The spectrum of CNI toxicity to the kidneys includes hemodynamic effects on renal microcirculation, their impact on the renin-angiotensin-aldosterone system, and electrolyte abnormalities such as impairments in renal handling of magnesium and potassium. At a systemic level, these agents are also associated with global endothelial injury, leading to thrombotic microangiopathy like picture, which could be apparent at any time point during their exposure.

In the immediate postoperative period, induction immunosuppression by using newer agents such as with interleukin-2 (IL-2) receptor blockade or antithymocyte globulin has been used to delay the introduction of CNI. However, this approach is fraught with some risk of propagation of opportunistic infections and progression of native disease such as viral replication among organ recipients with hepatitis C [20]. The use of inhibitors of mammalian target of rapamycin (m-TOR inhibitors) (e.g., sirolimus and everolimus) may be a promising alternative. However, their de novo use is tempered by their association with impaired wound healing and a Food and Drug Administration (FDA) advisory on the increased incidence of arterial thrombotic events. The m-TOR inhibitors also may lead to proteinuria and are best avoided in subjects that have proteinuria at baseline [21].

The application of mTOR inhibition after the immediate postoperative period to both salvage and preserve renal function among liver transplant recipients has undergone investigation. Late conversion (>1 year post transplant) to sirolimus has been reported to not confer any benefit [22]. In a more recent trial, renal function after liver transplantation was compared across three arms of immunosuppression: reduced-dose tacrolimus and everolimus versus standard tacrolimus versus tacrolimus elimination [23]. The tacrolimus elimination arm was prematurely stopped due to increased risk of liver allograft rejection. In the other two arms, although everolimus with reduced-dose tacrolimus arm led to better preservation of renal function, the long-term efficacy remains to be determined, and the long-term impact of proteinuria observed in everolimus-low-dose tacrolimus regimen remains a concern.

Kidney Transplantation After Other Solid Organ Transplant

Kidney transplantation may be a consideration among liver transplant candidates and recipients either concurrent with the liver transplant (combined liver-kidney transplant) or as a treatment for ESRD ensuing after liver transplantation (kidney after liver transplantation). Waitlist mortality for liver transplant candidates who develop ESRD is twice that expected among kidney waitlist candidates in general [24]. Successful renal transplantation among liver transplants developing ESRD halves the mortality risk when compared to those ESLD patients with ESRD remaining on dialysis over a 5-year period (relative risk, 0.56; $p=0.02$) [24].

There is a legitimate concern that some patients who are regarded as candidates for combined liver and kidney may in fact have reversible forms of renal injury, which may recover with successful liver transplant alone. Given the limitations with regard to measuring renal function, determination of the candidacy for a kidney transplant along with liver depends on establishing *plausible irreversibility* of kidney disease at the time of liver transplantation. Criteria from three different consensus groups are summarized in Table 14.4 [25, 26]. In general, the criteria aim to establish chronicity of renal dysfunction and evidence of irreversible features such as fibrosis, small kidney size, and proteinuria or substantial renal dysfunction that would be expected to worsen in the perioperative period or as a result of ongoing CNI therapy. Renal biopsy, while fraught with risk in the liver transplant population, may help make decisions based on the amount of interstitial fibrosis or glomerulosclerosis; however, histologic cutoffs used to interpret biopsy findings are derived from kidney disease other than that in liver transplant candidates [27].

Table 14.4 Guidelines on combined liver-kidney transplantation [1, 25, 26]

OPTN Kidney Transplantation Committee and the Liver and Intestinal Organ Transplantation Committee Policy 3.5.10 (2009)
Combined liver-kidney transplantation recommended for:
(a) Patients with CKD requiring dialysis as documented in CMS form 2728 indicating start of dialysis with no chance of renal recovery
(b) Patients with CKD (GFR ≤30 mL/min/1.73 sq m by MDRD study six-variable equation or direct measurement by iothalamate clearance and proteinuria >3 g/day)
(c) Patients with sustained AKI requiring dialysis for ≥6 weeks (defined as dialysis at least twice per week for 6 consecutive weeks)
(d) Patients with sustained AKI (GFR ≤25 mL/min/1.73 m^2 for ≥6 weeks by MDRD study six-variable equation or direct measurement) not requiring dialysis
(e) Patients with sustained AKI: patients may also qualify for combined liver-kidney transplantation listing for a combination of time in categories (c) and (d) for a total of 6 weeks (e.g., patients with GFR <25 mL/min/1.73 m^2 for 3 weeks followed by dialysis for 3 weeks)
(f) Patients with metabolic disease (e.g., hyperoxalosis type 1)

Abbreviations: *AKI* acute kidney injury, *CKD* chronic kidney disease, *CMS* Centers for Medicare and Medicaid Services, *eGFR* estimated glomerular filtration rate, *HRS* hepatorenal syndrome, *MDRD* Modification of Diet in Renal Disease, *OPTN* Organ Procurement and Transplantation Network, *CMS Form 2728* A form required by Medicare stating that a dialysis patient has end-stage renal disease with no chance of renal recovery

As far as heart transplantation is concerned, the approaches for dual organ transplantation are similar to those described above. Kidney transplantation is certainly a viable option for those reaching ESRD after heart transplant. Death-censored kidney allograft survival in kidney after heart transplantation is similar to solitary kidney transplantation from an expanded criteria donor [28]. This suggests that the overall decrease in kidney after heart transplant survival is due to recipient's death rather than poor graft function. Kidney graft survival is similar between kidney after heart and kidney after lung recipients who survive long term.

Conclusion

Renal insufficiency in ESLD, liver transplant, and cardiac transplant population offers multiple diagnostic and therapeutic challenges. The literature that guides us in this setting is limited, due to multiple confounders and lack of randomized trials. However, present observational studies provide some insights into preoperative risk assessment, intraoperative management, and postoperative complications of kidney and electrolyte disorders. Optimization of outcomes in this complex population demands the involvement of a transplant nephrologist as a part of a multidisciplinary team throughout the duration of patient care.

Key Messages

- Challenges in accurate estimation of renal function in patients with advanced liver disease pose serious impediments in diagnosis and management of AKI in this group of patients.
- Renal dysfunction in end-stage liver disease is typically of functional origin and may reverse with restoration of organ function.
- AKI in posttransplant period is associated with different set of risk factors in liver and cardiac transplantation.
- There is commonality in terms of risk factors of CKD after liver and cardiac transplantation.
- Candidacy for dual organ transplantation is challenging but should be considered after reasonably satisfying evidence of irreversible loss of renal function.

References

1. Gonwa TA, Wadei HM. Kidney disease in the setting of liver failure: core curriculum 2013. Am J Kidney Dis. 2013;62:1198–212.
2. Wong F, Nadim MK, Kellum JA, et al. Working party proposal for a revised classification system of renal dysfunction in patients with cirrhosis. Gut. 2011;60:702–9.
3. Gerhardt T, Poge U, Stoffel-Wagner B, Palmedo H, Sauerbruch T, Woitas RP. Creatinine-based glomerular filtration rate estimation in patients with liver disease: the new chronic kidney disease epidemiology collaboration equation is not better. Eur J Gastroenterol Hepatol. 2011;23:969–73.
4. Francoz C, Nadim MK, Baron A, et al. Glomerular filtration rate equations for liver-kidney transplantation in cirrhotic patients: validation of current recommendations. Hepatology. 2014;59(4):1514–21.
5. Mindikoglu AL, Weir MR. Current concepts in the diagnosis and classification of renal dysfunction in cirrhosis. Am J Nephrol. 2013;38:345–54.
6. Gonwa TA, Wadei HM. The challenges of providing renal replacement therapy in decompensated liver cirrhosis. Blood Purif. 2012;33:144–8.
7. Gonwa TA, McBride MA, Mai ML, Wadei HM. Kidney transplantation after previous liver transplantation: analysis of the organ procurement transplant network database. Transplantation. 2011;92:31–5.
8. Wagener G, Minhaz M, Mattis FA, Kim M, Emond JC, Lee HT. Urinary neutrophil gelatinase-associated lipocalin as a marker of acute kidney injury after orthotopic liver transplantation. Nephrol Dial Transplant. 2011;26:1717–23.
9. Cabezuelo JB, Ramirez P, Rios A, et al. Risk factors of acute renal failure after liver transplantation. Kidney Int. 2006;69:1073–80.
10. Tolwani A, Wille KM. Advances in continuous renal replacement therapy: citrate anticoagulation update. Blood Purif. 2012;34:88–93.
11. Townsend DR, Bagshaw SM, Jacka MJ, Bigam D, Cave D, Gibney RT. Intraoperative renal support during liver transplantation. Liver Transplant. 2009;15:73–8.
12. Pham PT, Slavov C, Pham PT. Acute kidney injury after liver, heart, and lung transplants: dialysis modality, predictors of renal function recovery, and impact on survival. Adv Chronic Kidney Dis. 2009;16(4):256–67.

13. Kobashigawa JA, Starling RC, Mehra MR, Kormos RL, Bhat G, Barr ML, et al. Multicenter retrospective analysis of cardiovascular risk factors affecting long-term outcome of de novo cardiac transplant recipients. J Heart Lung Transplant. 2006;25(9):1063–9.
14. Wright G. Haemolysis during cardiopulmonary bypass: update. Perfusion. 2001;16(5):345–51.
15. Baliga R, Ueda N, Walker PD, Shah SV. Oxidant mechanisms in toxic acute renal failure. Am J Kidney Dis. 1997;29(3):465–77.
16. Boyle JM, Moualla S, Arrigain S, Worley S, Bakri MH, Starling RC, Heyka R, Thakar CV. Risks and outcomes of acute kidney injury requiring dialysis after cardiac transplantation. Am J Kidney Dis. 2006;48(5):787–96.
17. Ojo AO, Held PJ, Port FK, et al. Chronic renal failure after transplantation of a nonrenal organ. N Engl J Med. 2003;349:931–40.
18. Platz KP, Mueller AR, Blumhardt G, et al. Nephrotoxicity following orthotopic liver transplantation. A comparison between cyclosporine and FK506. Transplantation. 1994;58:170–8.
19. Kim JY, Akalin E, Dikman S, et al. The variable pathology of kidney disease after liver transplantation. Transplantation. 2010;89:215–21.
20. Cassuto JR, Levine MH, Reese PP, et al. The influence of induction therapy for kidney transplantation after a non-renal transplant. Clin J Am Soc Nephrol. 2012;7:158–66.
21. Wadei HM, Zaky ZS, Keaveny AP, et al. Proteinuria following sirolimus conversion is associated with deterioration of kidney function in liver transplant recipients. Transplantation. 2012;93:1006–12.
22. Gerhardt T, Terjung B, Knipper P, et al. Renal impairment after liver transplantation – a pilot trial of calcineurin inhibitor-free vs calcineurin inhibitor sparing immunosuppression in patients with mildly impaired renal function after liver transplantation. Eur J Med Res. 2009;14:210–5.
23. Saliba F, De Simone P, Nevens F, et al. Renal function at two years in liver transplant patients receiving everolimus: results of a randomized, multicenter study. Am J Transplant. 2013;13: 1734–45.
24. Srinivas TR, Stephany BR, Budev M, et al. An emerging population: kidney transplant candidates who are placed on the waiting list after liver, heart, and lung transplantation. Clin J Am Soc Nephrol. 2010;5:1881–6.
25. Eason JD, Gonwa TA, Davis CL, Sung RS, Gerber D, Bloom RD. Proceedings of consensus conference on Simultaneous Liver Kidney transplantation (SLK). Am J Transplant. 2008;8: 2243–51.
26. Nadim MK, Sung RS, Davis CL, et al. Simultaneous liver-kidney transplantation summit: current state and future directions. Am J Transpant. 2012;12:2901–8.
27. Wadei HM, Geiger XJ, Cortese C, et al. Kidney allocation to liver transplant candidates with renal failure of undetermined etiology: role of percutaneous renal biopsy. Am J Transplant. 2008;8:2618–26.
28. Lonze B, Warren D, Stewart Z, Dagher N, Singer A, Shah A, et al. Kidney transplantation in previous heart or lung recipients. Am J Transplant. 2009;9(3):578–85.

Chapter 15
Acute Allograft Injury After Kidney Transplantation

Bernd Schröppel and Christophe Legendre

Objectives

- To outline the major biological processes implicated in ischemia and reperfusion.
- To recognize the importance of early graft function and its related complications.
- To define current and new approaches aimed to limit organ injury at the time of transplantation.

Introduction

Delayed graft function (DGF) is a common early complication following deceased donor kidney transplantation. DGF is often defined as the need for dialysis in the first week after transplantation and is primarily a consequence of ischemia/reperfusion (IR) injury resulting in postischemic acute tubular necrosis (ATN) [1]. The degree of IR injury is dependent on a complex interplay of pre-transplant injury and subsequent innate and adaptive immune responses after reperfusion [2]. The consequences of developing DGF are significant. In addition to the acute complications

B. Schröppel, MD (✉)
Division of Nephrology, University of Ulm, Albert-Einstein-Allee 23, Ulm 89081, Germany
e-mail: bernd.schroeppel@uniklinik-ulm.de

C. Legendre, MD
Department of Nephrology and Transplantation, Necker Hospital,
149 Rue de Sèvres, Paris 75015, France
e-mail: christophe.legendre@nck.aphp.fr

C.V. Thakar, C.R. Parikh (eds.), *Perioperative Kidney Injury: Principles of Risk Assessment, Diagnosis and Treatment*, DOI 10.1007/978-1-4939-1273-5_15

Table 15.1 Selected recently published randomized and controlled trials in DGF

Intervention	Target	Population	Endpoint and outcome	Ref.
Epoetin-beta	Multiple	$N=104$	No difference in DGF, SGF, and GFR at 1–3 months	[27]
Epoetin-alpha	Multiple	$N=72$	No difference in DGF, SGF, and urine NGAL/IL-18	[26]
YSPSL (rPSGL-Ig)	Blocks P-E-L selectins	$N=59$	No difference in DGF; lower serum creatinine 5 days after transplantation in the treatment group	[11]

Excluding trials investigating preservation solutions and machine perfusion

Table 15.2 Selected registered randomized and controlled DGF trials in ClinicalTrials.gov (Accessed September 3rd 2013)

Intervention	Target	Primary endpoint(s)	Stage	ClinicalTrials.gov identifier
I5NP	siRNA inhibiting p53	Safety and incidence of delayed graft function	Phase 2B	NCT00802347
Eculizumab	Terminal complement C5a and C5b-9	Hemodialysis (7 days posttransplantation)	Phase 2	NCT01919346
OPN-305	TLR2	Hemodialysis (7 days posttransplantation)	Phase 2	NCT01794663
BB3	Hepatocyte growth factor/ scatter factor	Difference in creatinine clearance over time	Phase 2	NCT01561599
Remote ischemic preconditioning	Multiple	Number of organs recovered per donor	Phase 3	NCT01515072
Alteplase	Dissolution of microthrombi by ex vivo treatment of DCD organs with rTPA	Delayed kidney graft function and primary liver graft nonfunction		NCT01197573
Etanercept	TNF-alpha inhibitor to the perfusion fluid	Hemodialysis (7 days posttransplantation)	Phase 2	NCT01731457

Abbreviations: *TNF* tumor necrosis factor

related to renal failure and the associated costs of prolonged hospitalization, the magnitude of the association between DGF and subsequent chronic allograft dysfunction is fairly strong, but it is not clear whether DGF directly affects long-term graft survival [1]. Several new drugs show promise in animal studies in preventing or ameliorating IR injury, and clinical trials are ongoing (Tables 15.1 and 15.2). The aim of this review is to summarize the clinical risk factors and consequences and the translational science investigating the mechanism of IR injury and summarize the clinical trials regarding the prevention or management of DGF.

Important Biological Processes Implicated in Brain Death, Ischemia, and Reperfusion

It is important to differentiate in models the effects of warm versus cold ischemia and isograft versus allograft. Excellent science has been generated in animal models identifying a wide range of pathological processes contribute to hypoxic and IR-associated injury (reviewed in detail [3]). We will focus here on cell death and survival programs and innate and adaptive immune activation, as these are potentially amenable to innovative therapeutic approaches.

Cell Death, Apoptosis, and Autophagy

Ischemia and reperfusion activates various programs of cell death, which can be categorized as necrosis-, apoptosis-, or autophagy-associated cell death. Autophagy is a general term for pathways by which cytoplasmic material is delivered to lysosomes for degradation [4]. The main purposes of autophagosome formation are quality control and removal of defunct organelles, provision of an energy source during starvation, and regulation of cell survival and cell death. More recently, autophagy was identified as an important effector and regulator of innate and adaptive immunity and inflammation [4]. Several studies have reported the upregulation of autophagy in tubular cells in response to acute kidney injury caused by experimental nephrotoxic, IR, or ureteral obstruction models [4], and autophagy was identified as a protective mechanism by tubular cells during stress, suggesting it is upregulated after injury in order to selectively degrade damaged mitochondria and protein aggregates [5]. While there is huge clinical interest, the lack of validated clinical markers and the absence of selective inducers and inhibitors of autophagy are challenges for successful translational research.

Innate Immunity

Important components and well studied in animal models of IR injury are toll-like receptors (TLR) and the complement system.

Toll-Like Receptors

TLRs are expressed on immune as well as nonimmune cells, and endogenous, cell-derived ligands (so-called damage-associated molecular patterns or DAMPs) can signal through specific TLRs. Among the list of DAMPs that have been described to be induced or upregulated after IR only, HMGB1 was so far mechanistically linked to the pathogenesis of IR injury [6]. HMGB1 is a nuclear protein that binds DNA and modulates transcription and chromatin modeling and dependent on its redox state also functions as an extracellular signaling molecule during sterile inflammation, providing a chemotactic and activation signal to inflammatory cells [6]. TLR4 was found to be upregulated, and tubular HMGB1 was detectable in deceased donor kidneys when compared with living donor kidneys. In addition, kidneys carrying the loss-of-function TLR4 variants (Asp299Gly and Thr399Ile), known to diminish ligand-receptor binding, were linked with better function immediately after transplantation [7]. Chimeric mice with deficiency in renal-associated TLR2 and TLR4 had less renal damage and dysfunction when compared with wild-type mice, and when comparing single $TLR2^{-/-}$ and $TLR4^{-/-}$ with the $TLR2/4^{-/-}$, no increased protection was seen, indicating that ligands prime TLR2 and TLR4 during IR injury [6].

Complement System

Studies in small and large animals revealed that terminal complement activation is a critical mediator in IR injury [8]. IR injury is abrogated in animals that are deficient in C3 (and factor B) but not C4 [8]. Using chimeric mice C3aR/C5aR on renal cells as well as leukocytes contributes to IR injury [9]. In kidneys retrieved from brain-dead donors compared to kidneys from living donors, systemic generation of C5a mediates renal inflammation via tubular C5a-C5aR interaction [10]. Overall, the data strongly support the model that IR injury leads to local (kidney derived) as well as immune cell-derived complement release and activation, which leads to acute organ injury. With eculizumab, a C5 inhibitor, agents are available and clinical trials in DGF are ongoing (Table 15.2), and therapeutic interventions already at the time of brain death might be needed for optimal effects on graft outcome.

Adaptive Immunity

IR injury elicits a robust adaptive immune response. Studies have shown that T cells (CD4 and CD8) accumulate during IR injury and mediate injury [3, 6]. The specific mechanisms underlying T cell activation in the absence of specific exogenous antigen remain to be elucidated, but data indicate antigen-specific and antigen-independent mechanisms of action [3].

Clinical Definitions of DGF

The early graft dysfunction especially using deceased donors is often classified into immediate, slow (SGF), delayed (DGF), or in the most severe cases primary nonfunction (PNF). Due to the complexity of its pathophysiology, it is complex to find one definition of early graft dysfunction explaining why currently more 18 definitions coexist [1]. The most frequent definitions are based on posttransplant dialysis requirements (most frequently one dialysis session during the first 7 days after transplantation) [1]. While useful for data reporting, this definition suffers from many pitfalls including clinical-dependent decision, dialysis required for potassium or fluid overload, residual renal function, or preemptive transplantation, which may lead to misclassification or large variations in DGF rates that were observed in multicenter trials [11]. Other definitions may rely on urine output, creatinine reduction, and analysis of urine biomarkers such as interleukin-18 (IL-18), kidney injury molecule 1 (KIM1), neutrophil gelatinase-associated lipocalin (NGAL). In order to advance in the prevention and/or treatment of DGF, it is important to isolate the diagnosis of IR-induced AKI, to dissect and evaluate the influence of factors related to the donor (age, intensive care management), to the recipient (age, quality of arteries, surgical procedure, antihuman leukocyte antigen (anti-HLA) immunization), to the transplant allocation (leading to various cold ischemia times), and finally to other causes of renal failure such as surgical complications, drug nephrotoxicity, and rejection (Fig. 15.1).

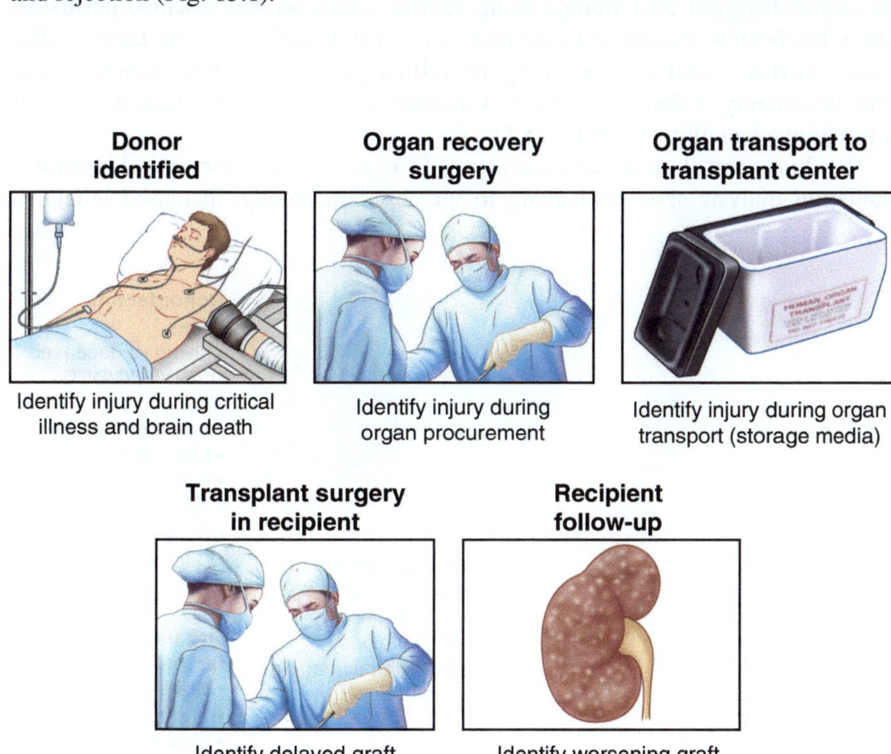

Fig. 15.1 Key time points starting with the donor identification that have the potential to induce ischemic or nonischemic injury to the kidney (Adapted from Hall and Parikh [29])

Clinical Risk Factors and Consequences

The main donor factors increasing the risk of DGF are increasing donor age, donor type, and quality of pre-kidney procurement care (Fig. 15.2). The risk of DGF (and subsequent graft failure) augments from living donor kidneys to deceased donors (standard criteria donors [SCD] < expanded criteria donors [ECD] < donation after cardiac death [DCD] < ECD/DCD) [12]. This reflects mainly the positive influence of short warm and cold ischemia time in living kidney donors and the negative influence of prolonged ischemia time after brain or cardiac death. Donor serum creatinine at time of procurement is not a sensitive marker of subsequent DGF mainly because its implication is likely to be different between SCD (ischemia reperfusion) and ECD kidneys (preexisting chronic renal damage). Related to donor age are histological markers such as arteriolar hyalinosis and atherosclerosis, which may reflect an increased sensitivity to ischemia [13]. There is a clear correlation between the length of cold ischemia time and the incidence of DGF, which is very useful since it is a highly modifiable factor. Another significant modifiable factor is the choice between cold storage using varying solutions and machine perfusion, which has been reintroduced in the past years [14]. Finally, recipient factors influencing the risk of DGF include male gender, BMI greater than 30, African-American ethnicity, history of diabetes, anti-HLA immunization, and requirement for dialysis before transplantation [15] (Fig. 15.1).

The short-term clinical consequences of DGF are the need for several posttransplantation dialysis sessions leading to increased morbidity, increased length of

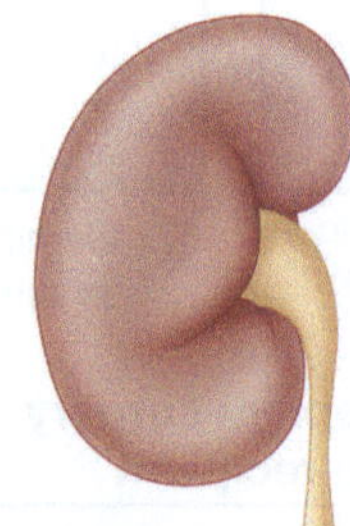

Fig. 15.2 Modifiable and non-modifiable risk factors and tools to assess initial kidney graft dysfunction

hospitalization, and hence increased cost [16]. More interesting and still a matter of debate are long-term consequences of DGF. The classical view is that postischemic ATN leads to various repair mechanisms involving both adaptive and innate immunity [3]. May be more puzzling is the most recent viewpoint suggesting that cold ischemia time may have more subtle consequences. Kayler et al. studied the impact of cold ischemia time on graft survival among ECD kidney using a paired kidney analysis (kidneys derived from the same donor but transplanted to two different recipients) [17]. Not surprisingly, the DGF incidence was higher in pairs with greater cold ischemia time difference, but the incidence of graft loss was not different even in multivariable models adjusted for recipient factors. This first analysis was followed by a second in whom the impact of cold ischemia time-induced DGF on long-term graft loss was studied in paired kidneys when one kidney experienced DGF in one recipient but not in the second [18]. The author concluded that of course the incidence of DGF increased with increasing cold time but that graft loss was similar in both groups suggesting that cold ischemia time-induced DGF may not have deleterious long-term consequences and hence that kidneys should not be discarded because of that sole reason. Another example of the complexity in the interactions between AKI and chronic kidney disease (CKD) is the fact that patients that received the kidneys from donors without a heartbeat, which was twofold more than the incidence of DGF in matched recipients that received kidneys from donors with a heartbeat (24 %), had similar long-term graft survival [19].

Prediction and Detecting DGF

In recent years, there has been a lot of interest devoted to both prediction of DGF before transplantation and early detection at time or just after kidney transplantation. Early, noninvasive, and rapid assessment of deceased donor kidney injury could drive better allocation decisions and potentially reduce the rates of posttransplant complications. It must be stressed that the rewards of prediction and early detection require that therapeutic intervention modifies the course of DGF, which is until now far from obvious. Indeed, the few useful interventions, such as reducing drastically cold ischemia time and use of machine perfusion, are able to unselectively decrease the incidence of DGF. For example, it is a strong belief that avoiding calcineurin inhibitors (CNIs) in patients at high risk of DGF would be beneficial which has never been proven when correctly tested [20]. Even more, in the Benefit [21] and Benefit Ext studies [22], patients treated with CNIs from the time of transplantation had similar incidences of DGF as patients never exposed to CNI.

It may nevertheless be useful to predict DGF for clinical trials. Irish et al. developed a risk prediction model using a multivariable logistic regression analysis [23]. These Web-based calculators are easily accessible and helpful to assess DGF risk in a population but will not be able to assess individual DGF risk.

Interventional Trials in DGF

Prevention of Organ Injury Is Superior to Treatment

Improved donor management, namely, the use of dopamine, has been shown in a randomized trial to significantly decrease dialysis requirements and hence the length of DGF but without a difference in graft failure at 3 years [24]. Moers et al. demonstrated that the use of hypothermic machine perfusion instead of cold storage was able to reduce the incidence and duration of DGF as well as improve 1-year graft survival [25]. At 3 years, the benefit was still present especially in ECD kidneys [25]. It is interesting to note that despite the lower DGF incidence in kidneys recovered after cardiac death, there was no improvement in graft survival. A recent meta-analysis concluded that hypothermic machine perfusion reduces DGF rate but does not modify primary nonfunction, acute rejection, and patient and graft survival [14]. Data on the effect of the preservation solutions (two most commonly used are histidine-tryptophan-ketoglutarate [HTK] and University of Wisconsin [UW] solution) have been inconsistent and were summarized in detail elsewhere; however, prospective adequately powered trials in high-risk kidneys are needed [12].

Published and Ongoing Interventional Trials

Most interventional strategies are recipient directed and target cell death and inflammation. These trials differ in terms of endpoint definition and donor/recipient selection (Tables 15.1 and 15.2). Recombinant P-selectin glycoprotein ligand IgG fusion protein, rPSGL-Ig, efficiently binds P- and E- selectin and prevents polymorphonuclear neutrophil (PMN) adhesion and sequestration to the site of injury. A multicenter phase 2 study found that while there were no differences in the DGF rate, fewer patients receiving the drug had serum creatinine >6.0 mg/dl on the postoperative day 5 (26 % vs 55 %, $p=0.04$) [11]. No effect on the DGF incidence (hemodialysis [HD] requirement within 1 week) of high doses of erythropoietin, with its potential antiapoptotic and regenerative effects, was seen in two trials when compared to placebo. One relatively small study applied 40,000 U of epoetin [EPO]-alpha (Procrit) as a single dose at the time of reperfusion into the ipsilateral artery proximal to the graft anastomosis [26]. Martinez and colleagues used 30,000 U EPO-beta before and three subcutaneous injections after transplantation (12 h, 7 and 14 days) of ECD kidneys [27]. It is not known whether earlier EPO administration (e.g., during cold storage) would achieve the desired effects. Based on strong preclinical data on the role of complement in IR injury, eculizumab is now being tested in a clinical pilot trial in 24 patients at high risk for DGF (NCT01919346). Another interesting target is TLR2. OPN-305 is a monoclonal antibody that blocks TLR2 and is currently tested in a multicenter trial in the USA and Europe including DCD, ECD, and SCD kidneys with a cold ischemia time greater than 18 h (NCT01794663).

Conclusion

DGF is a clinic description of a series of complex events that start during donor management and progress during organ procurement, transport, implantation, and reperfusion (Fig. 15.1). While there is ample of excellent science using animal models of IR injury, many challenges in translation from bench to bedside remain. Animal models are important to test basic pathophysiological mechanisms, but there is no reliable animal model available that mimics human AKI with or without transplantation. Indeed, the poor correlation of murine models with human inflammatory diseases supports for priority for translational medical research addressing complex human conditions [28].

Interventions that limit the short-term and long-term effects of peri-transplant injury in humans are urgently needed. Reduction of the discard rate of procured organs is also an important area for the development of new therapeutics. In the past the main focus was to dampen the injury, and more recently strategies that enhance tissue regeneration are increasing, including highly effective tools to manipulate microRNAs. Once our understanding of how microRNAs affect gene expression in hypoxic and injured tissues involves these tools are likely being integrated into clinical practice.

For clinical trial design clear defined endpoints are critical. In addition, the logistics and ethics in deceased donor intervention need to be addressed with the help of academia, transplant societies, and government. There are promising novel therapeutics in the pipeline, but any DGF intervention will be measured whether it provides improved long-term outcomes.

Key Messages

- DGF is often defined as the need for dialysis in the first week after transplantation and is primarily a consequence of ischemia/reperfusion injury resulting in postischemic ATN.
- The main donor factors increasing the risk of DGF are increasing donor age, donor type, quality of pre-kidney procurement care, and length of cold ischemia time.
- Early, noninvasive, and rapid assessment of deceased donor kidney injury could drive better allocation decisions and potentially reduce the rates of posttransplant complications.
- Most interventional strategies are recipient directed and target cell death and inflammation.

References

1. Yarlagadda SG, Coca SG, Formica Jr RN, Poggio ED, Parikh CR. Association between delayed graft function and allograft and patient survival: a systematic review and meta-analysis. Nephrol Dial Transplant. 2009;24:1039–47.
2. Cheung KP, Kasimsetty SG, McKay DB. Innate immunity in donor procurement. Curr Opin Organ Transplant. 2013;18:154–60.
3. Eltzschig HK, Eckle T. Ischemia and reperfusion – from mechanism to translation. Nat Med. 2011;17:1391–401.
4. Huber TB, Edelstein CL, Hartleben B, Inoki K, Dong Z, Koya D, Kume S, Lieberthal W, Pallet N, Quiroga A, Ravichandran K, Susztak K, Yoshida S, Dong Z. Emerging role of autophagy in kidney function, diseases and aging. Autophagy. 2012;8:1009–31.
5. Liu S, Hartleben B, Kretz O, Wiech T, Igarashi P, Mizushima N, Walz G, Huber TB. Autophagy plays a critical role in kidney tubule maintenance, aging and ischemia-reperfusion injury. Autophagy. 2012;8:826–37.
6. Leventhal JS, Schroppel B. Toll-like receptors in transplantation: sensing and reacting to injury. Kidney Int. 2012;81:826–32.
7. Kruger B, Krick S, Dhillon N, Lerner SM, Ames S, Bromberg JS, Lin M, Walsh L, Vella J, Fischereder M, Kramer BK, Colvin RB, Heeger PS, Murphy BT, Schroppel B. Donor Toll-like receptor 4 contributes to ischemia and reperfusion injury following human kidney transplantation. Proc Natl Acad Sci U S A. 2009;106:3390–5.
8. Damman J, Daha MR, van Son WJ, Leuvenink HG, Ploeg RJ, Seelen MA. Crosstalk between complement and Toll-like receptor activation in relation to donor brain death and renal ischemia-reperfusion injury. Am J Transplant. 2011;11:660–9.
9. Peng Q, Li K, Smyth LA, Xing G, Wang N, Meader L, Lu B, Sacks SH, Zhou W. C3a and C5a promote renal ischemia-reperfusion injury. J Am Soc Nephrol. 2012;23:1474–85.
10. van Werkhoven MB, Damman J, van Dijk MC, Daha MR, de Jong IJ, Leliveld A, Krikke C, Leuvenink HG, van Goor H, van Son WJ, Olinga P, Hillebrands JL, Seelen MA. Complement mediated renal inflammation induced by donor brain death: role of renal C5a-C5aR interaction. Am J Transplant. 2013;13:875–82.
11. Gaber AO, Mulgaonkar S, Kahan BD, Woodle ES, Alloway R, Bajjoka I, Jensik S, Klintmalm GB, Patton PR, Wiseman A, Lipshutz G, Kupiec-Weglinski J, Gaber LW, Katz E, Irish W, Squiers EC, Hemmerich S. YSPSL (rPSGL-Ig) for improvement of early renal allograft function: a double-blind, placebo-controlled, multi-center Phase IIa study. Clin Transplant. 2011;25: 523–33.
12. Cavaille-Coll M, Bala S, Velidedeoglu E, Hernandez A, Archdeacon P, Gonzalez G, Neuland C, Meyer J, Albrecht R. Summary of FDA workshop on ischemia reperfusion injury in kidney transplantation. Am J Transplant. 2013;13:1134–48.
13. Matignon M, Desvaux D, Noel LH, Roudot-Thoraval F, Thervet E, Audard V, Dahan K, Lang P, Grimbert P. Arteriolar hyalinization predicts delayed graft function in deceased donor renal transplantation. Transplantation. 2008;86:1002–5.
14. O'Callaghan JM, Knight SR, Morgan RD, Morris PJ. Preservation solutions for static cold storage of kidney allografts: a systematic review and meta-analysis. Am J Transplant. 2012; 12:896–906.
15. Doshi MD, Garg N, Reese PP, Parikh CR. Recipient risk factors associated with delayed graft function: a paired kidney analysis. Transplantation. 2011;91:666–71.
16. Schnitzler MA, Gheorghian A, Axelrod D, L'Italien G, Lentine KL. The cost implications of first anniversary renal function after living, standard criteria deceased and expanded criteria deceased donor kidney transplantation. J Med Econ. 2013;16:75–84.
17. Kayler LK, Magliocca J, Zendejas I, Srinivas TR, Schold JD. Impact of cold ischemia time on graft survival among ECD transplant recipients: a paired kidney analysis. Am J Transplant. 2011;11:2647–56.

18. Kayler LK, Srinivas TR, Schold JD. Influence of CIT-induced DGF on kidney transplant outcomes. Am J Transplant. 2011;11:2657–64.
19. Weber M, Dindo D, Demartines N, Ambuhl PM, Clavien PA. Kidney transplantation from donors without a heartbeat. N Engl J Med. 2002;347:248–55.
20. Kamar N, Garrigue V, Karras A, Mourad G, Lefrancois N, Charpentier B, Legendre C, Rostaing L. Impact of early or delayed cyclosporine on delayed graft function in renal transplant recipients: a randomized, multicenter study. Am J Transplant. 2006;6:1042–8.
21. Vincenti F, Charpentier B, Vanrenterghem Y, Rostaing L, Bresnahan B, Darji P, Massari P, Mondragon-Ramirez GA, Agarwal M, Di Russo G, Lin CS, Garg P, Larsen CP. A phase III study of belatacept-based immunosuppression regimens versus cyclosporine in renal transplant recipients (BENEFIT study). Am J Transplant. 2010;10:535–46.
22. Durrbach A, Pestana JM, Pearson T, Vincenti F, Garcia VD, Campistol J, Rial Mdel C, Florman S, Block A, Di Russo G, Xing J, Garg P, Grinyo J. A phase III study of belatacept versus cyclosporine in kidney transplants from extended criteria donors (BENEFIT-EXT study). Am J Transplant. 2010;10:547–57.
23. Irish WD, Ilsley JN, Schnitzler MA, Feng S, Brennan DC. A risk prediction model for delayed graft function in the current era of deceased donor renal transplantation. Am J Transplant. 2010;10:2279–86.
24. Schnuelle P, Gottmann U, Hoeger S, Boesebeck D, Lauchart W, Weiss C, Fischereder M, Jauch KW, Heemann U, Zeier M, Hugo C, Pisarski P, Kramer BK, Lopau K, Rahmel A, Benck U, Birck R, Yard BA. Effects of donor pretreatment with dopamine on graft function after kidney transplantation: a randomized controlled trial. JAMA. 2009;302:1067–75.
25. Moers C, Smits JM, Maathuis MH, Treckmann J, van Gelder F, Napieralski BP, van Kasterop-Kutz M, van der Heide JJ, Squifflet JP, van Heurn E, Kirste GR, Rahmel A, Leuvenink HG, Paul A, Pirenne J, Ploeg RJ. Machine perfusion or cold storage in deceased-donor kidney transplantation. N Engl J Med. 2009;360:7–19.
26. Sureshkumar KK, Hussain SM, Ko TY, Thai NL, Marcus RJ. Effect of high-dose erythropoietin on graft function after kidney transplantation: a randomized, double-blind clinical trial. Clin J Am Soc Nephrol. 2012;7:1498–506.
27. Martinez F, Kamar N, Pallet N, Lang P, Durrbach A, Lebranchu Y, Adem A, Barbier S, Cassuto-Viguier E, Glowaki F, Le Meur Y, Rostaing L, Legendre C, Hermine O, Choukroun G. High dose epoetin beta in the first weeks following renal transplantation and delayed graft function: results of the Neo-PDGF Study. Am J Transplant. 2010;10:1695–700.
28. Seok J, Warren HS, Cuenca AG, Mindrinos MN, Baker HV, Xu W, Richards DR, McDonald-Smith GP, Gao H, Hennessy L, Finnerty CC, Lopez CM, Honari S, Moore EE, Minei JP, Cuschieri J, Bankey PE, Johnson JL, Sperry J, Nathens AB, Billiar TR, West MA, Jeschke MG, Klein MB, Gamelli RL, Gibran NS, Brownstein BH, Miller-Graziano C, Calvano SE, Mason PH, Cobb JP, Rahme LG, Lowry SF, Maier RV, Moldawer LL, Herndon DN, Davis RW, Xiao W, Tompkins RG. Genomic responses in mouse models poorly mimic human inflammatory diseases. Proc Natl Acad Sci U S A. 2013;110:3507–12.
29. Hall IE, Parikh CR. Human models to evaluate urinary biomarkers of kidney injury. Clin J Am Soc Nephrol. 2010;5(12):2141–3.

Part V
Special Topics in Perioperative Acute Kidney Injury

Chapter 16
Trauma and Acute Kidney Injury

Krishna P. Athota and Betty J. Tsuei

Objectives

- To discuss how traumatic injuries can predispose patients to the development of acute kidney injury.
- To understand how new resuscitation protocols for patients with massive hemorrhage (trauma) or fluid losses (burns) can prevent acute kidney injury (AKI).
- To recognize risk factors for, diagnosis of, and treatment of rhabdomyolysis in the trauma patient.

Introduction

Traumatic injuries can range from improvised explosive devices and high-powered military firearms to the seemingly benign fall from standing height. While the latter sounds innocuous, a fall for an anticoagulated elderly individual who is not immediately found can result in serious morbidity and even death. The severity of injuries seen at most civilian trauma centers ranges between these extremes, but as advances in critical care have been made, more trauma patients are surviving the initial insult and increasingly at risk for organ dysfunction and failure later in their hospital course.

Renal failure is not uncommon in the trauma population, and the mortality for patients who develop renal failure is clearly higher than for those who do not [1]. While technologies exist to treat renal failure, prevention of acute kidney injury (AKI) in the trauma patient, as with most complications, is preferable and likely the area in which the biggest impact on patient outcome can be achieved.

K.P. Athota, MD • B.J. Tsuei, MD (✉)
Department of Surgery, University of Cincinnati, 231 Albert Sabin Way, Cincinnati, OH 45267, USA
e-mail: krishna.athota@uc.edu; betty.tsuei@uc.edu

C.V. Thakar, C.R. Parikh (eds.), *Perioperative Kidney Injury: Principles of Risk Assessment, Diagnosis and Treatment*, DOI 10.1007/978-1-4939-1273-5_16

Resuscitation of the Patient with Hemorrhagic Shock

AKI in injured patients is frequently multifactorial, though one of the most important causes is hypoperfusion secondary to hemorrhagic shock. Injuries with significant blood loss, which are not identified and treated promptly, can result in hypovolemia and prerenal renal failure. While hypotension indicates a blood volume loss of 30–40 % (class III shock), early clinical indicators of hypovolemia, such as tachycardia and altered mental status, may be affected by pain, brain injury, or medications, making immediate identification of hemorrhagic shock difficult.

Rapid diagnosis of hemorrhage in the injured patient, even before delineation of specific injuries, is critical for the timely initiation of resuscitation. In addition to visible external losses, significant hemorrhage can occur in the thorax, peritoneum, pelvis, retroperitoneum, and long bones of the lower extremities. Thorough clinical examination coupled with radiographic imaging can identify these potential sources of bleeding. Retroperitoneal hemorrhage, rare in patients without penetrating mechanisms of injury, however, is particularly difficult to detect and can be a pitfall in the evaluation of the trauma patient.

The most important intervention for the prevention of renal dysfunction in the trauma patient is restoration of adequate perfusion. The initial treatment consists of immediate volume expansion with crystalloids; however, the use of large volumes of normal saline for resuscitation can result in iatrogenic acidosis and has been associated with increased mortality [2]. Furthermore, patients with class III or class IV hemorrhagic shock will likely need blood product transfusions, and in these patients, efforts should be made to minimize crystalloid administration and transition to blood product resuscitation as quickly as possible. This approach, which has been termed "damage control resuscitation," has resulted in decreased length of stay and improved survival [3]. In accordance with these studies, the American College of Surgeons Advanced Trauma Life Support program has limited the recommended initial crystalloid resuscitation to one liter of fluid, with subsequent transfusion of blood if hypotension persists [4].

Recent military conflicts have provided a unique opportunity to study resuscitation in trauma patients who require massive transfusion, defined as greater than ten units of blood products in the first 24 h after injury. In these patients, red cell transfusion coupled with a more liberal use of fresh frozen plasma (FFP) improved outcomes to such a degree that administration of packed red blood cells (PRBC) and FFP in a 1:1 ratio in patients with massive transfusion requirements was adopted into military protocols [5, 6]. While this practice originated in the military setting, it has been adopted by most large civilian trauma centers and has become the standard of care. The most beneficial ratio of PRBC:FFP:PLT (platelet) transfusions has yet to be determined, but ongoing studies in the civilian trauma population, such as Pragmatic Randomized Optimal Platelet and Plasma Ratios (PROPPR), may answer that question in the near future [7].

Each institution caring for significantly injured patients should have a massive transfusion protocol in place, with criteria for inclusion, limitation of crystalloid infusion, and rapid availability of blood products. A pressing challenge of such protocols is identifying which patients require massive transfusion. Delayed recognition of these patients can result in underresuscitation, while overtriage can result in unnecessary blood product transfusion and depletion of valuable blood bank resources. Clinical triggers, such as hypotension and tachycardia, coupled with laboratory values, such as initial hemoglobin and base deficit, have been used to identify patients who may need massive transfusion, and these criteria continue to be refined [8].

Resuscitation goals vary depending on whether or not control of hemorrhage has been obtained. Animal studies have shown increased bleeding and mortality when aggressive resuscitation is initiated before hemorrhage control has been achieved [9]. Additional studies have shown that resuscitation with a mean arterial pressure (MAP) of 60 mmHg resulted in optimal survival and a minimal increase in inflammatory markers [10]. Resuscitation prior to control of bleeding should be consistent with what has been termed "permissive" or "controlled" hypotension. This technique aims to maintain adequate perfusion at the lowest level, preventing high or even "normal" blood pressure from exacerbating uncontrolled hemorrhage. The resulting short-term hypotension has not been associated with an increase in renal failure, although every effort should be made to limit this technique to as brief a period as possible [11]. Particular care should be taken in utilizing this technique in patients with traumatic brain injury, in which hypotension can worsen neurologic outcomes. Current recommendations from the Brain Trauma Foundation suggest maintaining systolic blood pressure [SBP] >90 mmHg, but a recent multicenter study has questioned whether even this level is sufficient [12, 13]. While hypotensive resuscitation may decrease blood loss and the need for transfusion, maintaining a higher blood pressure to minimize neurologic deficits may be of greater importance in patients with traumatic brain injury.

Once control of active hemorrhage has been achieved, resuscitation goals should focus on repletion of intravascular volume, reversal of coagulopathy, treatment of electrolyte abnormalities (hypocalcemia), and restoration of physiologic parameters. Thromboelastography (TEG) is a diagnostic adjunct which evaluates the entire coagulation cascade with a single study and, unlike measurements of partial thromboplastin time and prothrombin times, can determine the presence of clot lysis. A recent study has shown that a 30-min fibrinolysis of greater than 3 % is associated with the need for massive transfusion and increased mortality [14]. Thrombolysis should be treated with tranexamic acid (TXA), which completely inhibits the activation of plasminogen. Serial hemoglobin and TEG measurements can alert clinicians to recurrent bleeding, and monitoring base deficit and serum lactate can provide additional information about the restoration of tissue perfusion. Laboratory abnormalities that persist beyond 12 h have been associated with increased length of stay, infections, and mortality; and persistence of lactic acidosis at greater than 24 h has correlated with increased respiratory complications, multisystem organ failure, and death [15, 16].

Finally, as patients survive the initial traumatic injury, they become at risk for infectious complications, which are the major cause of mortality in the intensive care unit. Trauma patients who develop fever, leukocytosis, and other signs of systemic inflammation should be followed up with a systematic evaluation for possible infection and early initiation of appropriate antibiotic therapy in order to prevent sepsis and multisystem organ failure.

In summary, rapid diagnosis of hemorrhage in the injured patient allows initiation of resuscitation, even before specific injuries are identified. Crystalloid resuscitation of injured patients should be limited, and blood product administration should be initiated promptly in patients in class III or class IV hemorrhagic shock or those patients who are at risk for requiring massive transfusion. Patients requiring massive transfusion benefit from a high ratio of FFP:RBC (1:1). Trauma patients who present with hemorrhagic shock should have blood pressure maintained at a MAP of 60 or a SBP of 90 until hemorrhage control can be obtained. This MAP may need to be increased to 90 mmHg in patients with traumatic brain injury to maintain adequate cerebral perfusion. Intraoperative laboratory studies, including thromboelastography, should be used for the ongoing evaluation of resuscitation efforts and the presence of fibrinolysis, and postoperative resuscitation should target the elimination of occult hypoperfusion within 12 h of injury. Resuscitation in this manner will minimize the risk of hypovolemia-induced acute renal injury and overall organ failure.

Rhabdomyolysis

After the assaults on London during World War II, Bywaters and Beall reported a series of six patients who had been rescued from fallen buildings after sustaining crush injury [17]. Even those who appeared well with only apparent local trauma succumbed to otherwise unexplained renal failure, and autopsy results revealed brown pigmented casts, later found to be myoglobin, in the renal tubules. Although there have been numerous descriptions of rhabdomyolysis throughout history, the report by Bywaters was the first to describe the pathophysiology and major clinical sequelae of this disease [18].

Muscle injury leading to rhabdomyolysis causes the release of a number of substances, including calcium, potassium, myoglobin, and uric acid [19]. Several mechanisms of injury have been proposed, including renal tubule obstruction from myoglobin precipitation, oxidative injury from the release of iron and free radicals, and vasoconstriction-related hypoperfusion [20].

Rhabdomyolysis has been described in a number of traumatic settings. Along with direct crush injury, compartment syndrome from fractures and ischemia/reperfusion injuries are frequently associated with muscle necrosis and rhabdomyolysis. Lower extremity fractures, especially of the leg, are at increased risk for compartment syndrome, as the fasciae of the calf are well developed, and there is little room for swelling. Vascular injuries, which result in limb ischemia and reperfusion after revascularization, are particularly notable for rhabdomyolysis. The degree of muscle ischemia increases with longer arterial occlusion time, and venous injuries with impaired limb drainage can exacerbate elevated compartment pressures. Burns and high-voltage electrical injuries can also cause significant muscle damage and rhabdomyolysis, and pressure necrosis of the muscle in patients who are immobilized secondary to other injuries, such as falling while intoxicated, or even in surgical cases in which insufficient attention has been paid to patient positioning have been documented.

Monitoring for extremity compartment syndrome is based largely on physical exam. The development of paresthesia, pain, and decreased motor function should increase the suspicion for compartment syndrome in high-risk patients. Unfortunately, such clinical exams may be difficult to perform, as these patients are frequently sedated or mechanically ventilated. In these cases, measurement of compartment pressure may serve as a beneficial alternative. Differential pressure (ΔP) (defined as diastolic blood pressure (BP) – compartment pressure) of less than 30 mmHg should prompt decompression [21]. Fasciotomies should be performed in patients with compartment syndrome, and prophylactic fasciotomies in patients at significant risk should be strongly considered, as the consequences of undiagnosed compartment syndrome can be devastating.

Regardless of the etiology of the injury, early recognition of rhabdomyolysis is critical. While both serum myoglobin and creatine kinase (CK) are elevated, myoglobin has a much shorter half-life (2–3 h vs. 1.5 days) and is more rapidly cleared [22]. Thus, myoglobin may not be as sensitive for the diagnosis of rhabdomyolysis, particularly in cases with delayed presentation. Although CK elevation of over 5,000 U/l has been reported to increase the risk of AKI, some studies have suggested that a CK level as low as 1,000 U/l can be associated with a threefold increase in the odds of developing AKI in the intensive care unit (ICU); however the exact level which leads to renal toxicity is still unclear [20, 23]. Quantitative urine myoglobin may not be routinely performed in some laboratories, but the presence of urine dipstick hemoglobin without the presence of red blood cells on urine analysis strongly suggests presence of myoglobin, given the right clinical setting. Serial measurements of serum CK and urine and serum myoglobin levels have been used to evaluate the progression of rhabdomyolysis with varying sensitivity [19, 20].

The most important intervention in the treatment of rhabdomyolysis, after controlling the source of muscle necrosis, is the prevention of renal failure with early, aggressive volume resuscitation. The administration of intravenous fluid in the first 24 h to target urine output goals of 200–300 ml/h, while avoiding complications of volume overload, is the mainstay of this therapy. The use of hyperosmotic colloid for resuscitation has been associated with renal dysfunction as well as other undesirable side effects and, as such, is not recommended [24]. While alkalinization of urine to prevent the precipitation of myoglobin and the use of mannitol to promote volume expansion and vasodilation have theoretical benefits, clinical studies have not shown any advantage of adding these therapies to crystalloid administration alone [24, 25]. Bicarbonate administration may be warranted, however, if resuscitation with normal saline or renal dysfunction produces metabolic acidosis. Further, if renal injury fails to improve, renal replacement therapy may be necessary. Hyperkalemia is the most common indication for this situation, as large amounts of potassium are released from muscle breakdown. Several small studies have reported the use of renal replacement therapy in an effort to remove myoglobin from the systemic circulation, but the kinetics of myoglobin removal are complex, and the clinical utility of this therapy in preventing renal injury is unclear [26–28].

In summary, rhabdomyolysis can occur in a variety of traumatic settings and should be suspected whenever significant skeletal muscle injury or ischemia is seen. Serum CK measurements, along with monitoring of renal function and electrolyte abnormalities, are used to follow the course of this disease. Early aggressive crystalloid resuscitation with goals of maintaining urine output over 200 ml/h is the mainstay of therapy. The addition of bicarbonate should be utilized only for correction of acidosis.

Thermal and Electrical Injuries

Severe thermal injuries can frequently cause multisystem organ failure which is associated with high mortality. Fortunately, the overall incidence of patients with these devastating injuries is decreasing: the American Burn Association estimated that 1,000,000 patients required medical treatment in 2002, while only 450,000 burn injuries required medical treatment in 2012 [29].

Several prognostic scoring systems exist to predict mortality in burns. The most important criteria are age, presence of inhalational injury, and total body surface area (TBSA) of second- and third-degree burns [30]. The severity of a burn is based on two criteria – the depth of the burn and the surface area involved. First-degree burns have little systemic effects and are not included in calculations of TBSA burn. Estimation of TBSA includes the percent of second- and third-degree burns at the time of initial evaluation, as second-degree injuries may evolve and progress to third-degree burns. In adults, the percent body surface area burn can be roughly calculated by the "rule of nines": 9 % TBSA for head, each upper extremity, anterior lower extremity, and posterior lower extremity; 18 % for anterior trunk; 18 % for posterior trunk; and 1 % for genitalia (Fig. 16.1a). Burn diagrams, such as the one developed by Lund and Browder, are frequently used to document the location of burns and can be modified for children, who have different body proportion than adults (Fig. 16.1b).

The resuscitation of burn patients differs fundamentally from that of other injuries associated with hemorrhage because, although in both instances, patients may demonstrate hypovolemic shock, it is critical not to underestimate the degree of insensible losses in patients with significant burns. Classically, TBSA has been used to guide resuscitation efforts, and calculations such as the Parkland formula have been devised in an effort to ensure adequate fluid administration. The use of these formulas invariably resulted in large volume crystalloid administration which may contribute to organ failure and increased mortality. Several papers have identified that fluid administration in excess of what should be prescribed can occur in burn resuscitation – a phenomenon described as "fluid creep" [31, 32]. Paradoxically, both underresucitation leading to renal hypoperfusion and overresucitation causing abdominal compartment syndrome can both result in AKI and renal dysfunction. While there is no perfect resuscitation formula, current recommendations are for

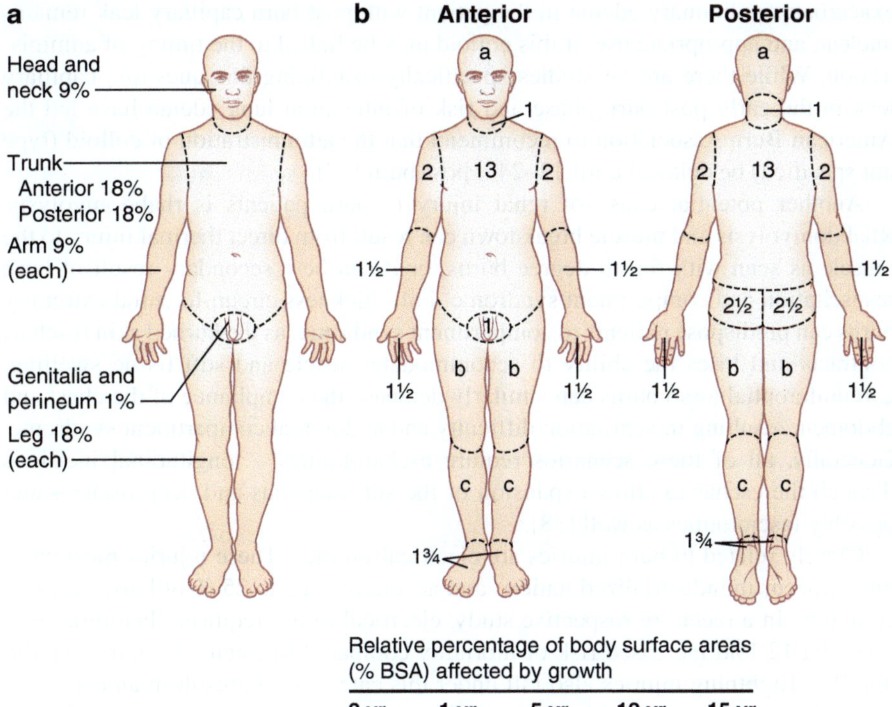

Relative percentage of body surface areas (% BSA) affected by growth

	0 yr	1 yr	5 yr	10 yr	15 yr
a – ½ of head	9½	8½	6½	5½	4½
b – ½ of 1 thigh	2¾	3¼	4	4¼	4½
c – ½ of 1 lower leg	2½	2½	2¾	3	3¼

Fig. 16.1 (**a**) Burn diagram demonstrating the "rule of nines." (**b**) Lund-Browder burn chart. This can be modified to account for different body proportions in children and infants

aggressive fluid resuscitation using these formulas as guidelines, with titration based on end organ perfusion as manifested by hourly urine output.

Studies examining the use of colloid fluids, such as hydroxyethyl starch, albumin, and plasma, in burn resuscitation have reported mixed results, with the most recent Cochrane review in 2013 showing no benefit associated with their use [33]. On the other hand, Atyieh et al. strongly recommends increased colloid use after the first 12 h of resuscitation; however, there has been no demonstrated survival advantage with this algorithm [34]. A recent prospective randomized study compared the use of hydroxyethyl starch as a colloid supplement with lactated ringers alone and found no benefit to the addition of the colloid. Although there was no decrease in fluid requirement, there was also no increase in acute respiratory distress syndrome (ARDS), length of stay (LOS), or mortality, in contrast to previous reports [35]. With regard to the use of albumin as a resuscitative colloid in burn patients, a 2012 review concluded that administration in the acute setting can decrease the amount of fluid required to achieve adequate resuscitation [36]. However, whether albumin exacerbates pulmonary edema in the patient with post-burn capillary leak remains unclear, and appropriate use of this colloid may be linked to the timing of administration. While there are no studies specifically examining this question, capillary leak in the early post-burn phase and risk of interstitial lung edema have led the American Burn Association to recommend that the administration of colloid (type not specified) be delayed until 12–24 h post-burn [37].

Another potential cause of renal injury in burn patients is rhabdomyolysis. Rhabdomyolysis and muscle breakdown can result from direct thermal injury to the muscle as seen with fourth degree burns, or it can be a secondary result of burn resuscitation and compartment syndrome. Full-thickness circumferential extremity burns can predispose patients to compartment syndrome, as the burned skin (eschar) contracts and loses the ability to accommodate muscle and soft tissue swelling. Circumferential torso burns can similarly decrease the compliance of the chest and abdomen, resulting in ventilation difficulty and abdominal compartment syndrome. Generally, all of these scenarios require escharotomies – longitudinal incisions through the eschar to allow expansion of the subcutaneous and deep tissue – and possibly fasciotomies as well [38].

Closely related to burn injuries are electrical injuries. These injuries most commonly occur in industrialized nations and account for up to 25 % of burns in those countries. In a recent retrospective study, electrical injury requiring hemofiltration carried a 12-fold increased risk of mortality compared to electrical injury that did not [39]. Lightning injuries also fall under this category and result in an estimated 1,000 deaths per year worldwide, and although an association between lightning strikes and renal failure has been described, the actual incidence is unknown due to the relatively infrequent occurrence [40]. The tissue damage from these injuries is often underappreciated and thus underresuscitated. Creatinine kinase measurements should be obtained and followed, and the rhabdomyolysis should be aggressively treated to prevent the development of renal failure as described earlier.

In summary, thermal injuries result in significant volume losses, and resuscitation efforts should be guided by percent TBSA of second- and third-degree burns and modified to support clinical parameters of resuscitation, such as hourly urine output. Circumferential eschar on the trunk and extremities should be treated with escharotomies to decrease the potential for compartment syndrome. While underresuscitation can result in poor perfusion and end organ damage, excessive fluid resuscitation in the burn patient can cause abdominal and extremity compartment syndrome. Close monitoring of end organ perfusion and resuscitation parameters should be used to adjust fluid administration in the acutely burned patient.

Urogenital Trauma

Patients with urogenital trauma account for 10 % of all trauma admissions. Because of the relatively protected location in the retroperitoneum, isolated urologic injuries, both from blunt and penetrating mechanisms, are rare. When these injuries do occur, however, they are often associated with trauma to adjacent structures (Table 16.1) [41].

Table 16.1 Common traumatic injuries to the genitourinary system

	Incidence	Comments
Kidney	1.2–3.3 % of patients with blunt trauma	Up to 7 % nephrectomy rate
Ureter	1–2.5 % of urologic trauma	High incidence of concomitant injuries, particularly vascular in blunt and penetrating trauma
Bladder	1.6 % of patients with blunt trauma	High-force injury. Pelvic fracture present in 70 % of blunt bladder injuries with an associated 10–20 % mortality rate
Urethra	4 % of urogenital trauma	65 % of these have complete disruption. Often associated with pelvic fractures

Table 16.2 Grading of renal parenchymal injuries (Adapted from Tinkoff et al. [42])

AAST renal injury grades			
Grade	Description		Mortality[a]
I	Contusion	Microscopic or gross hematuria	1.5 %
	Hematoma	Subcapsular, nonexpanding, no parenchymal laceration	
II	Hematoma	Nonexpanding, perirenal, confined to retroperitoneum	
	Laceration	<1 cm parenchymal depth of cortex only, no urinary extravasation	
III	Laceration	>1 cm parenchymal depth of cortex without collecting system injury or urinary extravasation	1.8 %
IV	Laceration	Parenchymal laceration involving the cortex, medulla, and collecting system	4.7 %
	Vascular	Main renal artery or vein injury with contained hemorrhage	
V	Laceration	Shattered kidney	10.7 %
	Vascular	Avulsion of the renal hilum that devascularizes the kidney	

Abbreviations: *AAST* American Association for the Surgery of Trauma
[a]Mortality is for isolated injury and excludes patients with severe traumatic brain injury and deaths within 24 h of emergency department arrival

Renal parenchymal lacerations are generally managed in a nonoperative fashion. Although this approach is more successful with lower-grade injuries, and higher-grade injuries have a higher associated mortality rate, as shown in Table 16.2, a recent multicenter study demonstrated that 75 % of grade IV and grade V injuries can be managed nonoperatively in hemodynamically stable patients with a low (7 %) failure rate [42, 43]. Parenchymal injuries rarely lead directly to renal failure.

Renal vascular injuries, however, are a different matter. Blunt mechanisms of injury, particularly deceleration-type injuries, can cause arterial intimal flap formation with subsequent devascularization of all or part of the kidney, even without outward signs of trauma. Long-term sequelae of these injuries can include renovascular hypertension and renal dysfunction [44]. Active hemorrhage from renal vascular injury requires operative intervention and frequently results in nephrectomy. Although operative revascularization has been attempted historically, these have resulted in mediocre long- term outcomes. Recent advances in endovascular techniques have provided a less invasive route for repair, but long- term outcomes are still not known [45].

Ureteral, bladder, and urethral injuries from a blunt mechanism are associated with significant force. Ureteral injuries frequently occur in conjunction with iliac vessel injuries, and bladder injuries are frequently found with pelvic fractures and pelvic venous plexus bleeding. While injury to the ureter and bladder does not directly affect the kidney function, hemorrhage from associated injuries can lead to hypotensive renal injury. In addition, bleeding within the urinary system and outflow obstruction can result in secondary renal insult. This possibility, while real, is rarely seen but should be considered whenever gross hematuria is present and there is evidence of oliguria and worsening renal function.

In patients with injuries to the genitourinary system, urinary extravasation can result in significant intra-abdominal fluid collections. Resorption of creatinine from the urinoma can result in an elevated serum creatinine without associated AKI. Radiographic imaging and creatinine measurements can easily identify these fluid collections as urinoma, which can be treated with appropriate drainage and stenting [46, 47].

Table 16.3 Trauma-related causes of acute kidney injury and summary of treatment options

Disease process	Key points
Hemorrhagic shock and resuscitation	Rapid diagnosis of hemorrhage in the injured patient allows initiation of resuscitation, even before specific injuries are identified
	Crystalloid resuscitation should be limited, and blood product administration should be promptly initiated in patients in class III or class IV hemorrhagic shock or patients who may require massive transfusion
	Findings of two of the following are predictive of the need for massive transfusion: INR >1.5, HR >120, SBP <90, BD >6, HGB <11, FAST (+)
	Patients requiring massive transfusion benefit from a high ratio of FFP:RBC (1:1)
	Trauma patients who present with hemorrhagic shock should have blood pressure maintained at an MAP of 60 or an SBP of 90 until hemorrhage control can be obtained. However, permissive hypotension should be used with caution in patients with suspected head injuries, and MAP >90 mmHg may improve cerebral perfusion in patients with traumatic brain injury
	Intraoperative laboratory studies, including thromboelastography, should be used to detect fibrinolysis and assess ongoing resuscitation efforts, and postoperative resuscitation should target the elimination of occult hypoperfusion within 12 h of injury
Rhabdomyolysis	Crush injury, ischemia/reperfusion, burn injuries, and electrical injuries all place patients at risk for rhabdomyolysis, which should be suspected whenever significant skeletal muscle injury or limb ischemia is present
	Fasciotomies should be performed when compartment perfusion pressures are less than 30 mmHg
	Serum CK measurements, along with monitoring of renal function and electrolyte abnormalities, are used to follow the course of this disease
	Early aggressive crystalloid resuscitation with goals of maintaining urine output over 200 ml/h is the mainstay of therapy
	The addition of bicarbonate to fluid should be utilized only for correction of acidosis, and renal replacement therapy should be initiated if clinically indicated
	Further studies need to be performed to determine if prophylactic dialysis is warranted in the treatment of rhabdomyolysis

(continued)

Table 16.3 (continued)

Disease process	Key points
Thermal and electrical injuries	Burn injuries expose patients to significant volume losses, and resuscitation efforts should be guided by percent TBSA of second- and third-degree burns and clinical parameters such as hourly urine output
	Caution should be taken in resuscitating the burn patient to prevent excess fluid administration which can cause abdominal and extremity compartment syndrome
	Circumferential eschar should be treated with escharotomies to decrease the potential for extremity or torso compartment syndrome
	Rhabdomyolysis in patients with thermal injury can result from direct muscle damage as well as overresuscitation or constricting eschar
	Close monitoring of end organ perfusion and resuscitation parameters allows for continuous adjustment in fluid administration
Urogenital trauma	AKI caused by direct urologic injury is uncommon
	Blunt and penetrating injuries to the genitourinary system are often associated with significant pelvic and vascular injuries
	Operative intervention for direct renal parenchymal injury or renal vascular injury is associated with a high incidence of nephrectomy

Abbreviations: *BD* base deficit, *CK* creatinine kinase, *FAST* focused abdominal sonography for trauma, *FFP-RBC* fresh frozen plasma-red blood cell, *HGB* hemoglobin, *INR* international normalized ratio, *HR* heart rate, *MAP* mean arterial pressure, *SBP* systolic blood pressure, *TBSA* total body surface area

Conclusion

AKI in trauma patients is rarely caused by direct urogenital injury but is common after trauma and usually multifactorial in etiology. Resuscitation with appropriate crystalloid and blood products is the mainstay of preventing AKI in patients with hemorrhagic shock. Understanding of specific traumatic entities, such as rhabdomyolysis, burn and electrical injuries, and direct trauma (Table 16.3), allows for the proactive management of trauma patients in the immediate post-injury and perioperative time period and can minimize the risk of developing acute renal failure.

Key Messages

- AKI in the setting of trauma is predominantly the result of intravascular volume loss and hypotension requiring aggressive resuscitation.
- AKI caused by direct urologic injury is uncommon. Operative intervention for direct renal parenchymal injury or renal vascular injury is associated with a high incidence of nephrectomy.
- Specific injury patterns such as crush, electrical, burn, and limb ischemia/reperfusion increase the propensity for renal failure due to endogenous toxins from rhabdomyolysis.
- Early recognition of these entities and timely treatment can minimize the risk of acute kidney injury in the trauma patient.

References

1. Ala-Kokko T, Ohtonen P, Laurila J, Martikainen M, Kaukoranta P. Development of renal failure during the initial 24 h of intensive care unit stay correlates with hospital mortality in trauma patients. Acta Anaesthesiol Scand. 2006;50(7):828–32.
2. Duchesne JC, Heaney J, Guidry C, McSwain Jr N, Meade P, Cohen M, Schreiber M, Inaba K, Skiada D, Demetriades D, Holcomb J, Wade C, Cotton B. Diluting the benefits of hemostatic resuscitation: a multi-institutional analysis. J Trauma Acute Care Surg. 2013;75(1):76–82.
3. Duchesne JC, Barbeau JM, Islam TM, Wahl G, Greiffenstein P, McSwain Jr NE. Damage control resuscitation: from emergency department to the operating room. Am Surg. 2011;77(2): 201–6.
4. Committee on Trauma, American College of Surgeons. ATLS: Advanced Trauma Life Support program for doctors. 8th ed. Chicago: American College of Surgeons; 2008.
5. Holcomb JB, Jenkins D, Rhee P, Johannigman J, Mahoney P, Mehta S, Cox ED, Gehrke MJ, Beilman GJ, Schreiber M, Flaherty SF, Grathwohl KW, Spinella PC, Perkins JG, Beekley AC, McMullin NR, Park MS, Gonzalez EA, Wade CE, Dubick MA, Schwab CW, Moore FA, Champion HR, Hoyt DB, Hess JR. Damage control resuscitation: directly addressing the early coagulopathy of trauma. J Trauma. 2007;62(2):307–10.
6. Holcomb JB, Zarzabal LA, Michalek JE, Kozar RA, Spinella PC, Perkins JG, Matijevic N, Dong JF, Pati S, Wade CE, Trauma Outcomes Group, Holcomb JB, Wade CE, Cotton BA, Kozar RA, Brasel KJ, Vercruysse GA, MacLeod JB, Dutton RP, Hess JR, Duchesne JC, McSwain NE, Muskat PC, Johannigamn JA, Cryer HM, Tillou A, Cohen MJ, Pittet JF, Knudson P, DeMoya MA, Schreiber MA, Tieu BH, Brundage SI, Napolitano LM, Brunsvold ME, Sihler KC, Beilman GJ, Peitzman AB, Zenati MS, Sperry JL, Alarcon LH, Croce MA, Minei JP, Steward RM, Cohn SM, Michalek JE, Bulger EM, Nunez TC, Ivatury RR, Meredith JW, Miller PR, Pomper GJ, Marin B. Increased platelet: RBC ratios are associated with improved survival after massive transfusion. J Trauma. 2011;71(2 Suppl 3):S318–28.
7. Holcomb JB, Pati S. Optimal trauma resuscitation with plasma as the primary resuscitative fluid: the surgeon's perspective. Hematol Am Soc Hematol Educ Program. 2013;2013:656–9.
8. Callcut RA, Cotton BA, Muskat P, Fox EE, Wade CE, Holcomb JB, Schreiber MA, Rahbar MH, Cohen MJ, Knudson MM, Brasel KJ, Bulger EM, Del Junco DJ, Myers JG, Alarcon LH, Robinson BR, PROMMTT Study Group. Defining when to initiate massive transfusion: a validation study of individual massive transfusion triggers in PROMMTT patients. J Trauma Acute Care Surg. 2013;74(1):59–65, 67–8; discussion 66–7.
9. Burris D, Rhee P, Kaufmann C, Pikoulis E, Austin B, Eror A, DeBraux S, Guzzi L, Leppäniemi A. Controlled resuscitation for uncontrolled hemorrhagic shock. J Trauma. 1999;46(2):216–23.
10. Lin GS, Chou TH, Wu CY, Wu MC, Fang CC, Yen ZS, Lee CC, Chen SC. Target blood pressure for hypotensive resuscitation. Injury. 2013;44(12):1811–5.
11. Plurad D, Brown C, Chan L, Demetriades D, Rhee P. Emergency department hypotension is not an independent risk factor for post-traumatic acute renal dysfunction. J Trauma. 2006;61(5):1120–7; discussion 1127–8.
12. Brain Trauma Foundation, American Association of Neurological Surgeons, Congress of Neurological Surgeons, Joint Section on Neurotrauma and Critical Care, AANS/CNS, Bratton SL, Chestnut RM, Ghajar J, McConnell Hammond FF, Harris OA, Hartl R, Manley GT, Nemecek A, Newell DW, Rosenthal G, Schouten J, Shutter L, Timmons SD, Ullman JS, Videtta W, Wilberger JE, Wright DW. Guidelines for the management of severe traumatic brain injury. I. Blood pressure and oxygenation. J Neurotrauma. 2007;24 Suppl 1:S7–13.
13. Fuller G, Hasler RM, Mealing N, Lawrence T, Woodford M, Juni P, Lecky F. The association between admission systolic blood pressure and mortality in significant traumatic brain injury: a multi-centre cohort study. Injury. 2013. pii: S0020-1383(13)00396-3.
14. Chapman MP, Moore EE, Ramos CR, Ghasabyan A, Harr JN, Chin TL, Stringham JR, Sauaia A, Silliman CC, Banerjee A. Fibrinolysis greater than 3% is the critical value for initiation of antifibrinolytic therapy. J Trauma Acute Care Surg. 2013;75(6):961–7; discussion 967.

15. Claridge JA, Crabtree TD, Pelletier SJ, Butler K, Sawyer RG, Young JS. Persistent occult hypoperfusion is associated with a significant increase in infection rate and mortality in major trauma patients. J Trauma. 2000;48(1):8–14; discussion 14–5.
16. Blow O, Magliore L, Claridge JA, Butler K, Young JS. The golden hour and the silver day: detection and correction of occult hypoperfusion within 24 h improves outcome from major trauma. J Trauma. 1999;47(5):964–9.
17. Bywater EGL, Beall D. Crushing injury. Br Med J. 1942;ii:643–6.
18. Shapiro M, Baldea A, Luchette FA. Rhabdomyolysis in the intensive care unit. J Intensive Care Med. 2010;27(6):335–42.
19. Zimmerman JL, Shen MC. Rhabdomyolysis. Chest. 2013;144(3):1058–65.
20. El-Abdellati E, Eyselbergs N, Sirimsi H, Van Hoof V, Wouters K, Verbrugghe W, Jorens PG. An observational study on rhabdomyolysis in the intensive care unit. Exploring its risk factors and main complication: acute kidney injury. Ann Int Care. 2013;3(8):2–8.
21. McQueen MM, Court-Brown CM. Compartment monitoring in tibial fractures: the pressure threshold for decompression. J Bone Joint Surg Br. 1996;78–B:99–104.
22. Huerta-Alardin AL, Varon J, Marik PE. Bench-to-bedside review: rhabdomyolysis – an overview for clinicians. Crit Care. 2005;9(2):158–69.
23. De Meijer AR, Fikkers BG, de Keijzer MH, van Engelen BGM, Drenth JPH. Serum creatine kinase as a predictor of clinical course in rhabdomyolysis: a 5-year intensive care survey. Intensive Care Med. 2003;29(7):1121–5.
24. Brochard L, Abroug F, Brenner M, et al. An official ATS/ERS/ESICM/SCCM/SRLF statement: prevention and management of acute renal failure in the ICU patient: an International Consensus Conference in Intensive Care Medicine. Am J Respir Crit Care Med. 2010;181(10):1128–55.
25. Brown CV, Rhee P, Chan L, Evans K, Demetriades D, Velmahos GC. Preventing renal failure in patients with rhabdomyolysis: do bicarbonate and mannitol make a difference? J Trauma. 2004;56(6):1191–6.
26. Fang S, Xu H, Zhu Y, Jiang H. Continuous veno-venous hemofiltration for massive rhabdomyolysis after malignant hyperthermia: report of 2 cases. Anesth Prog. 2013;60(1):21–4.
27. Zhang L, Kang Y, Fu P, Cao Y, Shi Y, Liu F, Hu Z, Su B, Tang W, Qin W. Myoglobin clearance by continuous venous-venous haemofiltration in rhabdomyolysis with acute kidney injury: a case series. Injury. 2012;43(5):619–23.
28. Heyne N, Guthoff M, Krieger J, Haap M, Häring HU. High cut-off renal replacement therapy for removal of myoglobin in severe rhabdomyolysis and acute kidney injury: a case series. Nephron Clin Pract. 2012;121(3–4):c159–64.
29. American Burn Association. Burn incidence and treatment in the United States: 2012 fact sheet. http://www.ameriburn.org/resources_factsheet.php. Accessed 21 Jan 2014.
30. Sheppard NN, Hemington-Gorse S, Ghanem A, Philp B, Dziewulski P, Shelley OP. The Belgian severity prediction model compared to other scoring systems in a burn intensive care population. Burns. 2010;36(8):1320–1; author reply 1318–20.
31. Pruitt Jr BA. Protection from excessive resuscitation: "pushing the pendulum back". J Trauma. 2000;49:567–8.
32. Friedrich JB, Sullivan SR, Engrav LH, Round KA, Blayney CB, Carrougher GJ, Heimbach DM, Honari S, Klein MB, Gibran NS. Is supra-Baxter resuscitation in burn patients a new phenomenon? Burns. 2004;30(5):464–6.
33. Perel P, Roberts I, Ker K. Colloids versus crystalloids for fluid resuscitation in critically ill patients. Cochrane Database Syst Rev. 2013;2:CD000567.
34. Atiyeh BS, Dibo SA, Ibrahim AE, Zgheib ER. Acute burn resuscitation and fluid creep: it is time for colloid rehabilitation. Ann Burns Fire Disasters. 2012;25(2):59–65.
35. Béchir M, Puhan MA, Fasshauer M, Schuepbach RA, Stocker R, Neff TA. Early fluid resuscitation with hydroxyethyl starch 130/0.4 (6%) in severe burn injury: a randomized, controlled, double-blind clinical trial. Crit Care. 2013;17(6):R299.
36. Cartotto R, Callum J. A review of the use of human albumin in burn patients. J Burn Care Res. 2012;33(6):702–17.

37. Pham TN, Cancio LC, Gibran NS, American Burn Association. American Burn Association practice guidelines burn shock resuscitation. J Burn Care Res. 2008;29(1):257–66.
38. Orgill DP, Piccolo N. Escharotomy and decompressive therapies in burns. J Burn Care Res. 2009;30(5):759–68.
39. Saracoglu A, Kuzucuoglu T, Yakupoglu S, Kilavuz O, Tuncay E, Ersoy B, Demirhan R. Prognostic factors in electrical burns: a review of 101 patients. Burns. 2013. pii: S0305-4179(13)00262-3.
40. Okafor UV. Lightning injuries and acute renal failure: a review. Ren Fail. 2005;27(2):129–34.
41. McGeady JB, Breyer BN. Current epidemiology of genitourinary trauma. Urol Clin North Am. 2013;40(3):323–34.
42. Tinkoff G, Esposito TJ, Reed J, Kilgo P, Fildes J, Pasquale M, Meredith JW. American Association for the Surgery of Trauma Organ Injury Scale I: spleen, liver, and kidney, validation based on the National Trauma Data Bank. J Am Coll Surg. 2008;207(5):646–55.
43. van der Wilden GM, Velmahos GC, Joseph DK, Jacobs L, Debusk MG, Adams CA, Gross R, Burkott B, Agarwal S, Maung AA, Johnson DC, Gates J, Kelly E, Michaud Y, Charash WE, Winchell RJ, Desjardins SE, Rosenblatt MS, Gupta S, Gaeta M, Chang Y, de Moya MA. Successful nonoperative management of the most severe blunt renal injuries: a multicenter study of the research consortium of New England Centers for Trauma. JAMA Surg. 2013;148(10):924–31.
44. Yashiro N, Ohtomo K, Kokubo T, Itai Y, Iio M. Traumatic occlusion of renal artery: CT and angiography. Radiat Med. 1985;3(4):204–8.
45. Abu-Gazala M, Shussman N, Abu-Gazala S, Elazary R, Bala M, Rozenberg S, Klimov A, Rivkind AI, Arbell D, Almogy G, Bloom AI. Endovascular management of blunt renal artery trauma. Isr Med Assoc J. 2013;15(5):210–5. Review.
46. Ridinger HA, Kavitt RT, Green JK. Urinary ascites and renal failure from unrecognized bladder rupture. Am J Med. 2012;125(9):e1–2.
47. Kuroki Y, Mizumasa T, Nagara T, Tsuchimoto A, Yotsueda H, Ikeda K, Takesue T, Hirakata H. Pseudorenal failure due to intraperitoneal bladder rupture after blunt trauma: usefulness of examining ascitic fluid sediment. Am J Emerg Med. 2012;30(7):1326. e1–3.

Chapter 17
Fluid-Electrolyte Imbalances and Extracorporeal Therapy in the Neurosurgical Setting

Kelly Liang and Lori Shutter

Objectives

- To explain the pathophysiology, treatment, and prognosis of common metabolic and electrolyte disorders in the neurocritical care setting, with emphasis on disorders of sodium balance
- To describe the epidemiology, outcomes, common etiologies, and treatment of acute kidney injury in the neurocritical care setting
- To discuss blood pressure and autonomic issues as well as potential useful therapies in managing neurocritical care patients

Overall Epidemiology and Outcomes of Kidney Injury in Neurocritical Care

Acute kidney injury (AKI) is defined as a rapid decline in glomerular filtration rate and increase in blood urea nitrogen (BUN) and creatinine. Urine output may or may not be affected. Most hospital-acquired acute renal failure is due to inadequate

K. Liang, MD
Renal-Electrolyte Division, Department of Medicine, University of Pittsburgh, C1102 UPMC Presbyterian Hospital, 200 Lothrop Street, Pittsburgh, PA 15213, USA
e-mail: liangk@upmc.edu

L. Shutter, MD, FCCM, FNCS (✉)
Department of Critical Care Medicine, University of Pittsburgh Medical Center, 3550 Terrace Street, Scaife Hall, Rm 646C, Pittsburgh, PA 15261, USA
e-mail: shutterla@upmc.edu

C.V. Thakar, C.R. Parikh (eds.), *Perioperative Kidney Injury: Principles of Risk Assessment, Diagnosis and Treatment*, DOI 10.1007/978-1-4939-1273-5_17

renal perfusion or acute tubular necrosis. Risk factors for developing AKI include: preexisting renal failure, volume depletion, diabetes mellitus, advanced age, postoperative patients, congestive heart failure, and urinary tract infection. Many patients in neurocritical care settings experience these risk factors due to medical comorbidities, diagnostic procedures, treatment interventions to address brain edema, and impaired mobility. Information on the incidence of renal problems in neurocritical care is difficult to find, although a few studies are available.

Li et al. reported the incidence of AKI in 136 patients after severe traumatic brain injury (TBI) using AKI network (AKIN) renal function criteria [1]. They found 31 patients (23 %) that met AKI criteria, with 21 (68 %) stratified as stage 1. Risk factors for AKI were age, lower admission Glasgow coma scale (GCS), and higher admission level creatinine and blood urea nitrogen. Patients with AKI had significantly higher mortality and worse outcomes compared to those with normal renal function [2]. Zhang et al. reported renal dysfunction in 7 % and renal failure in 0.5 % of 209 patients after severe TBI [3]. In a group of 242 patients with subarachnoid hemorrhage (SAH), Gruber et al. reported renal dysfunction in 19 % [4]. This is in contrast to a recent report of a 9 % incidence of renal dysfunction based on AKIN criteria in 736 patients with SAH [5]. Renal complications are the second most common medical complication after surgeries for intracranial neoplasms [6]. While there is no specific data on the incidence of renal complications after endovascular neurosurgery, there is no reason to suspect that the incidence of contrast-induced nephropathy (CIN) would not be similar to general data, which reports a rate of 20–30 % in high-risk patients [7].

Common Metabolic and Renal Problems in Neurocritical Care

Sodium disturbance is common in neurocritical care, and normal sodium balance depends on many factors, including neuroendocrine functions, the renin-angiotensin system, osmoregulatory systems, and iatrogenic actions.

Hyponatremia

Hyponatremia is the most important and frequently encountered electrolyte disturbance seen in the neurocritical care setting, affecting 50 % of neurosurgical patients [8] and contributing to both morbidity and mortality. There are two main causes of hyponatremia in this setting: (1) cerebral salt wasting (CSW) and (2) syndrome of inappropriate antidiuretic hormone secretion (SIADH). However, these clinical entities may form part of a spectrum prevailing at different times during the course of illness, and they are often difficult to differentiate.

Cerebral Salt Wasting (CSW)

The phenomenon of cerebral salt wasting in brain injury was first reported in 1950 with three cases of hyponatremia that corrected with salt therapy [9]. It was postulated that losing salt was a protective mechanism for brain edema. The term "cerebral salt wasting (CSW)" was coined in 1954 to describe hyponatremia associated with brain injury that has urinary sodium loss with excess water loss that is responsive to sodium chloride administration [8]. CSW is most commonly seen in patients with SAH [10].

The proposed pathophysiology of CSW is disruption of connections between the hypothalamus and proximal tubule of the kidney, with resultant direct effects that impair reabsorption of sodium. Many theories exist as to how brain injury may lead to CSW, but there are two primary thoughts. The first theory suggests that impaired sympathetic neural input to the kidneys leads to decreased proximal sodium and urate reabsorption with impaired release of renin and aldosterone. The second theory involves release of natriuretic peptides, such as brain natriuretic peptide (BNP), that decreases renal tubular sodium reabsorption and inhibits renin release [10].

The diagnosis of CSW is based on laboratory values and clinical features (Table 17.1). Treatment focuses on volume repletion with isotonic saline, but hypertonic solutions may be used in cases with hyponatremia-related neurological deterioration. Occasionally salt tablets and administration of a mineralocorticoid, such as fludrocortisone, may also be used. Long-term therapy for CSW is usually not necessary since it usually lasts only 3–4 weeks after the brain injury [10].

Table 17.1 Key features of the syndrome of inappropriate antidiuretic hormone secretion (SIADH) and cerebral salt wasting (CSW)

Feature	SIADH	CSW
Serum sodium (mmol/L)	<135	<135
Serum osmolality (mOsm/kg)	<285	<285
Urine osmolality (mOsm/kg)	>200	>200
Urinary sodium (mmol/L)	>25	>25
Extracellular fluid volume	Increased or no change	Reduced
Fluid balance	Positive	Negative
Weight	Increased	Reduced
Jugular venous distension	Yes or no	No
Blood urea nitrogen	Reduced	Increased
Serum albumin concentration	Normal	Increased
Serum potassium concentration	Decreased or no change	Increased or no change
Hematocrit	Normal or reduced	Increased
Uric acid	Reduced	Reduced
Bicarbonate	Reduced	Increased
Creatinine	Reduced	Increased or no change
Response to intravenous fluids	No (may worsen)	Yes
Response to fluid restriction	Yes	No (may worsen)

Adapted from Kirkman et al. [8]

Syndrome of Inappropriate Antidiuretic Hormone Secretion (SIADH)

SIADH was first described in two patients with brain lesions by Carter et al. in 1961 [11]. These patients had hyponatremia, clinically normal or increased extracellular volume, and low blood urea nitrogen (BUN) levels. Their hyponatremia responded to mineralocorticoid administration and fluid restriction, but not sodium chloride administration. Salt restriction and liberal (2.5 L/day) water intake worsened the hyponatremia and were associated with increased ADH secretion. Thus, it was felt that inappropriate secretion of ADH was the underlying cause of hyponatremia.

SIADH may occur in the setting of many brain lesions but is most commonly seen following SAH or TBI [12–14]. The prevalence of SIADH post-TBI ranges from 2.3 to 36.6 % [15]. SIADH is also seen after transsphenoidal pituitary surgery due to injury to the posterior pituitary, with an incidence rate of 21–35 %. It is typically most severe on postoperative day 6 or 7 and is part of a "triphasic" response where initial polyuria from central diabetes insipidus (DI) converts to transient SIADH due to the release of preformed vasopression from the intracellular granules which is finally followed by either recovery or a third phase of central DI that may be permanent [12].

SIADH secondary to brain injury likely results from stimulation of the hypothalamic supraoptic and paraventricular nuclei, which leads to abnormal release of oxytocin and vasopressin (antidiuretic hormone, or ADH). The release of ADH leads to increase in the free water reabsorption, extracellular volume expansion, and hyponatremia [8].

The diagnosis of SIADH is based on laboratory values and clinical features (Table 17.1), and treatment usually centers on addressing the underlying disease, fluid restriction, salt administration, and vasopressin receptor antagonists. However, in patients with SAH and TBI, fluid restriction contributes to cerebral vasospasm and secondary infarction. Therefore, in neurologic patients with hyponatremia due to SIADH, hypertonic saline as a continuous infusion or as intermittent boluses is used to maintain volume status and preserve cerebral perfusion. Oral sodium supplementation may also be given through dietary intake or salt tablets. Among patients with urine osmolality more than double the plasma osmolality (i.e., urine osmolality >500 mosmol/kg), a loop diuretic such as furosemide may be used to reduce urinary concentration and facilitate water excretion. Another option is vasopression receptor antagonists, which produce a selective water diuresis without affecting sodium or potassium excretion. These agents are approved for treatment of euvolemic hyponatremia due to SIADH and hypervolemic hyponatremia due to heart failure [13].

Differentiating CSW from SIADH

CSW may be difficult to distinguish from SIADH based on serum studies and urinary sodium and osmolality alone, as they share the following features:

1. Elevated urine osmolality
2. High urine sodium
3. Low serum uric acid

The key difference between CSW and SIADH lies in the patient's volume status, with CSW characterized by hypovolemia and a negative fluid balance, compared to SIADH with euvolemia or hypervolemia and a positive fluid balance. CSW patients may manifest signs of volume depletion through weight loss, hypotension, tachycardia, decreased skin turgor, increased hematocrit, or increased BUN/Cr ratio in the setting of increased urine sodium concentration. Table 17.1 summarizes some of the key features of SIADH versus CSW [8]. Differentiating these two entities is clinically very important, as treatment for CSW (sodium chloride administration) could actually worsen SIADH. Likewise, treatment for SIADH (fluid restriction) could worsen hyponatremia associated with CSW, exacerbate vasospasm, and increase the risk for delayed neurological ischemia [10, 16]. Thus, volume status must be determined prior to any corrective therapy for hyponatremia.

Hypernatremia

Hypernatremia is also commonly encountered after brain injury, with the first report in the 1950s [17]. Central DI may occur due to neurohypophysial dysfunction from either direct trauma or cerebral edema in the area of the hypothalamic paraventricular and supraoptic nucleus, pituitary stalk, or axon terminals in the posterior pituitary resulting in decreased production of ADH [14, 15]. Central DI is characterized by excessive water excretion, polyuria, dilute urine, and hypernatremia with the following parameters: (1) plasma sodium >145 mM, (2) plasma osmolality >300 mosmol/kg, (3) inappropriately dilute urine (urine/plasma osmolality ratio <2), and (4) polyuria with urine output >3.5 L/day. Agha et al. reported that 13 of 50 (26 %) moderate-to-severe TBI patients developed DI in the acute phase of injury, with a plasma sodium range of 146–159 mM [15].

Prognosis is based on the underlying etiology. If the injury producing central DI is minor or the edema transient, symptoms may improve over time. If the edema progresses to cerebral herniation, central DI may be a sign of death by brain death. Direct trauma or a lesion involving the hypothalamic-pituitary region may result in a permanent deficit. The development of central DI is associated with worse outcomes after TBI. Agha et al. reported that 5 of 13 patients (38.5 %) with acute central DI had poor outcome at 1 year, compared with 5 of 37 patients (13.5 %) without acute central DI ($p = 0.053$) [15].

Role of Hypertonic Saline Solutions in Neurocritical Care

The use of hypertonic saline (HS) is becoming common in critically ill neurologic patients. It is used in the treatment of hyponatremia due to CSW or SIADH as discussed previously. It is also frequently used in the management of cerebral edema. Theoretical advantages of HS for cerebral edema include its decreased permeability across the blood brain barrier when compared to mannitol, sustained volume expansion without subsequent diuresis, and favorable immunomodulatory properties that decrease inflammation [18]. Hypertonic saline has been used in a variety of concentrations as both bolus therapy and continuous infusions. An online survey of neurointensivists reported that 90 % use osmotic agents in the treatment of intracranial hypertension, with a fairly even split in preference for HS (55 %) versus mannitol (45 %) [19]. The use of HS to shrink brain tissue and lower intracranial pressure (ICP) was first described in 1919 [20]. Subsequent studies on the use of HS to treat elevated ICP and edema in TBI had promising results [21]. While HS may be an effective therapy, studies comparing HS to mannitol are limited due to fallacies in design or small sample size. Two meta-analyses have concluded HS may be more effective than mannitol for management of ICP [22, 23]. In contrast, a more recent prospective study found very similar effects of equi-osmolar doses of HS and mannitol in 199 episodes of ICP elevation [24].

Qureshi et al. reported that maintaining a serum sodium concentration of 145–155 mmol/L using a continuous infusion of 3 % HS was effective in reducing ICP, edema, and mass effect in patients with brain tumors and TBI [25]. In 50 patients with TBI, Roquilly et al. treated refractory ICP elevations with a continuous infusion of 20 % sodium chloride (NaCl) to maintain sodium concentrations of 145–155 mmol/L. They reported favorable effects on ICP and cerebral perfusion pressure (CPP), no rebound upon discontinuation, and no episodes of AKI or pontine myelinolysis [26]. Schwarz et al. found HS to be more effective than mannitol in treating elevated ICP after acute ischemic stroke [27]. Others have compared early use of a continuous infusion of 3 % HS to maintain sodium levels of 145–155 mmol/l in patients with cerebral edema to historical controls. Those treated with HS had fewer episodes of critically elevated ICP and lower inhospital mortality. Adverse events, including arrhythmia, heart, liver or renal dysfunction, and pulmonary edema, were similar between groups [28, 29].

Overall, the use of HS in neurocritical care patients appears safe. Froelich et al. looked for complications of HS therapy in adult patients admitted to a neurosurgical ICU and found no increase in the rate of infection, deep vein thrombosis, or renal failure [30]. To date, no specific concentration of HS has shown superiority for the treatment of cerebral edema, mass effect, or elevated ICP. Thus, the commonly accepted goal of HS therapy is to target a serum sodium concentration of 145–155 mmol/L (corresponding to a serum osmolality of 300–320 mOsm/L) [18].

Management of Blood Pressure and Autonomic Issues

Management of blood pressure in neurocritical care is crucial and varies based on the underlying neurological disease state, goals for cerebral perfusion, hemorrhagic risks, and medical comorbidities. In general, the focus of blood pressure management in this patient population is to maintain cerebral perfusion pressure while

Table 17.2 Systolic blood pressure targets in neurological conditions

Neurological condition	Target SBP (mmHg)	Reasoning	Reference
AIS, no thrombolytic therapy	<220, allow autoregulation	Maintain cerebral perfusion	[31]
AIS, thrombolytic therapy	<185	Minimize risk for hemorrhage while maintaining perfusion	[31]
ICH	<160	Minimize risk for hemorrhage	[32]
SAH, unsecured source	<160	Minimize risk for re-bleed	[33]
SAH, secured source	Autoregulation, augment up to >200 to treat vasospasm	Maintain cerebral perfusion Treat vasospasm	[33]
TBI	Avoid SBP <90; augment BP as needed to maintain CPP >60	Maintain cerebral perfusion	[34]

SBP systolic blood pressure, *AIS* acute ischemic stroke, *ICH* intracerebral hemorrhage, *SAH* subarachnoid hemorrhage, *TBI* traumatic brain injury, *BP* blood pressure, *CPP* cerebral perfusion pressure

minimizing the risk of intracranial hemorrhage. Current management guidelines discuss blood pressure targets and supporting evidence for the most common neurological conditions [31–34]. A summary of this information is presented in Table 17.2.

Extracorporeal Therapies in Neurocritical Care

Regulation of volume status is important in the neurocritical care setting to prevent hypoperfusion-related brain ischemia and severe hypertension, which increases the risk for intracranial bleeding. For this reason, when renal replacement therapy (RRT) is needed, the continuous form of RRT (CRRT) is generally preferred. CRRT is usually better tolerated hemodynamically since fluid and solute removal is slower and hypotension is less common compared to intermittent hemodialysis (IHD). CRRT includes slow continuous ultrafiltration (SCUF), continuous arteriovenous hemofiltration or hemodialysis (CAVH or CAVHD), and continuous venovenous hemofiltration or hemodialysis (CVVH or CVVHD) [35]. CVVH or CVVHD is typically chosen when patients are hemodynamically unstable and careful volume control is desired. When patients are hemodynamically stable or hypertensive, IHD may be used. Parameters for acceptable blood pressure ranges must be specified based on the clinical situation. In addition, due to the risk for intracranial bleeding in postsurgical settings or after brain injury, anticoagulation (i.e., heparin) should be avoided in the dialysis circuit. A more detailed discussion regarding dialysis modalities is covered elsewhere.

Nephrotoxic Effects of Selected Common Therapies and Special Renal Issues

Mannitol

Mannitol is used in the neurocritical care setting as an osmotic diuretic to inhibit water and sodium reabsorption in the kidney. The resultant osmotic gradient serves to decrease cerebral blood volume and edema and thus lowers ICP [36]. It is typically administered as bolus doses of 0.25–1 g/kg over 20 min in patients with signs of elevated ICP. Mannitol has been associated with development of acute tubular necrosis and renal failure, particularly if serum osmolality exceeds 320 mOsm/L or there are other predisposing risk factors for AKI. Therefore, serum osmolality should be kept <320 mOsm/L during mannitol therapy in adults and <365 mOsm/L in pediatric patients [36].

Intravenous Immune Globulin (IVIG)

Intravenous immune globulin (IVIG) is used in the neurocritical care setting to treat autoimmune conditions and may have adverse reactions in up to 20 % of infusions [37]. Although the majority of adverse reactions are minor and transient, potentially serious systemic reactions may occur in 2–6 % of patients [38]. These reactions include renal, hematologic, thrombotic, and anaphylactic reactions [39]. Renal complications of IVIG include: (1) AKI, (2) hyponatremia, and (3) pseudohyponatremia.

AKI due to IVIG occurs in <1 % of infusions and usually occurs with sucrose-containing IVIG [39, 40]. Resolution usually occurs within 4–10 days after IVIG is discontinued [40], but permanent renal failure has also been reported [39]. IVIG may also produce an acute hemolysis with resultant hemoglobinuria and AKI. Risk factors for renal complications of IVIG include preexisting renal insufficiency, diabetes mellitus, dehydration, age >65, sepsis, paraproteinemia (hyperviscosity), and concomitant use of nephrotoxic agents [39]. Levy et al. reported a 6.7 % incidence of renal impairment in 119 patients receiving IVIG for various indications, including neuropathy and Guillain-Barre syndrome. There were no significant differences in patient characteristics, dose, sucrose content, and preparation of IVIG given between those who did and did not experience AKI [41]. Patients should be well hydrated before IVIG infusions, and solutions with concentration >5 % should be avoided to minimize the risk for AKI. Fractionating large doses into smaller doses on separate days and slowing the infusion rate to <3 mg/kg/min should also be considered in patients at risk for renal compromise.

Hyponatremia may develop with IVIG therapy due to accumulation of solutes in extracellular fluid, which raises plasma osmolality and lowers plasma sodium concentration by dilution as water moves out of cells down the favorable osmotic gradient.

Pseudohyponatremia may also be seen with IVIG use due to the protein load, which increases the nonaqueous phase of plasma [39]. Since sodium concentration is physiologically regulated in the aqueous phase, but laboratory determination of sodium concentration uses total plasma volume of the sample, an artifactual dilution of sodium results. It is important to distinguish pseudohyponatremia from true hyponatremia, as incorrectly prescribing fluid restriction for hyponatremia could increase the risk for other complications of IVIG, such as AKI [39].

High-Dose Glucocorticoids

High-dose glucocorticoids (greater than 10 mg/d of prednisone or equivalent) may be used in the neurocritical care setting to treat edema related to neoplasms or surgical manipulation. High-dose steroids may have adverse effects on the renal system, including induction of fluid retention, exacerbation of hypertension, and kaliuresis. Rapid administration of high doses may result in hypokalemia and metabolic alkalosis, but clinically significant hypokalemia is uncommon with routine exogenous glucocorticoid use [42]. The benefits of high-dose glucocorticoids should be carefully weighed against its risks, and consideration should be given to using lower doses or more rapid tapering of steroids. Renal consultation for potential need for RRT or supplemental diuretics may be indicated.

Antiseizure Medications

Antiseizure medications are commonly used in the neurocritical care setting. Selected agents, such as carbamazepine, oxcarbazepine (a derivative of carbamazepine), and phenytoin, may rarely cause AKI and azotemia. In addition, carbamazepine and oxcarbazepine can cause SIADH and produce hyponatremia [12]. As noted previously, SIADH may also occur as a result of the brain injury itself, so differentiating the etiology of SIADH may be difficult. Therefore, if renal failure or SIADH develops shortly after the initiation of medications such as carbamazepine or phenytoin, consideration should be given to discontinuation of the agent and/or switching to a different agent which is less likely to cause adverse effects. Adjustments in dosing of most antiseizure medications are necessary in patients with impaired renal function.

Rhabdomyolysis

Patients admitted to the neurocritical care setting may have sustained traumatic crush injuries or experienced prolonged periods of immobility, thus placing them at risk for rhabdomyolysis. This syndrome results from skeletal muscle breakdown, which causes myoglobin, other intracellular proteins, and electrolytes to leak into the circulation, and may result in acute renal failure or AKI [43, 44]. Options to manage rhabdomyolysis include aggressive fluid therapy with isotonic fluids, sodium bicarbonate, and mannitol. Sodium bicarbonate use is thought to alkalinize the urine, although the mechanism by which urine alkalinization is protective is still uncertain. Mannitol use to prevent AKI following rhabdomyolysis is based on several proposed mechanisms, including induction of osmotic diuresis, reduction of skeletal muscle cell edema, dilation of glomerular capillaries, stimulation of prostaglandin release, reduction of tubular cell swelling, and hydroxyl radical scavenging effects [44]. Administration of intravenous fluids is protective for several reasons, primarily since fluid therapy causes volume expansion, which has been shown to restore renal blood flow and glomerular filtration rate and decrease cast formation [44]. There is no data to support a preferred fluid type or to suggest that sodium bicarbonate or mannitol is superior to fluid therapy alone. Therefore, current recommendations for management of rhabdomyolysis-induced AKI focus on rapid initiation of aggressive fluid therapy to achieve urine output in adults of 300 mL/h or more for at least 24 h. Sodium bicarbonate should be used only for the correction of profound systemic acidosis. Mannitol may be considered if additional diuresis is needed to achieve urine output of 300 mL/h or more despite aggressive fluid resuscitation [44].

Contrast-Induced Nephropathy

Patients in the neurocritical care setting often require angiography using intravenous iodinated contrast CT or MRI imaging with contrast, all of which may put them at risk for CIN. Patients with a serum Cr ≥1.5 mg/dL, with an estimated glomerular filtration rate <60 mL/min/1.73 m^2, or who have a history of diabetes mellitus are at increased risk of CIN. Volume depletion or concomitant use of nonsteroidal anti-inflammatory drugs also increases the risk. In addition, studies suggest that patients on an angiotensin-converting enzyme (ACE) inhibitor or angiotensin receptor blocker (ARB) are at higher risk for CIN, but withholding ACE inhibitor and/or ARB has not been shown to prevent CIN [45].

Several strategies are recommended to prevent CIN [46]. Avoidance of high-osmolal agents (1,400–1,800 mosmol/kg), and use of iodixanol or nonionic low-osmolal agents such as iopamidol or ioversol rather than iohexol, has been shown to reduce the incidence of CIN. In addition, use of the lowest dose of contrast and avoidance of repetitive, closely spaced studies (e.g., <48 h apart) are recommended. Volume expansion with intravenous fluids (IVF) is recommended as long as there are no contraindications, as IVF has been shown to be more efficacious than oral hydration [46]. The optimal type and timing of fluid administration are not well established. Two potential options include: (1) isotonic bicarbonate administered as a bolus of 3 mL/kg 1 h prior to the procedure and continued at a rate of 1 mL/kg/h for 6 h after the procedure and (2) isotonic saline at a rate of 1 mL/kg/h begun at least 2 and preferably 6–12 h prior to the procedure and continued for 6–12 h after the procedure. N-acetylcysteine (NAC) at a dose of 1,200 mg orally twice daily may also be administered the day before and the day of the procedure. Though data conflict on the efficacy of NAC for prevention of CIN, its low toxicity and cost and potential for benefit make it a reasonable recommendation in this setting. Prophylactic use of mannitol and other diuretics is not recommended. In addition, prophylactic hemofiltration or hemodialysis after contrast exposure is not recommended for any stage of chronic kidney disease (CKD) [46]. Several agents that prevent renal vasoconstriction have been studied, including theophylline, aminophylline, nifedipine, captopril, prostaglandin E or I2, low-dose dopamine, and fenoldopam, but evidence regarding efficacy of these agents is not strong enough to routinely recommend them for prevention of CIN [46].

Conclusion

Disturbances in sodium and water balance are a common problem in the neurocritical care setting. Management requires awareness of the unique fluid, blood pressure, and cerebral blood flow issues present in this patient population. Treatment must often be modified to optimize the overall goals of care. While the incidence of acute renal impairment is rare in these patients, if it develops, the impact on long-term neurological and patient outcomes can be significant.

Key Messages

- Fluid-electrolyte imbalances are important causes of morbidity and mortality in the neurocritical care setting.
- Hyponatremia is the most frequent sodium disorder in the neurocritical care setting, occurring due to either cerebral salt wasting or SIADH. Hypernatremia can occur from central diabetes insipidus due to hypothalamic-pituitary injury.
- The use of hypertonic saline to maintain a serum sodium concentration of 145–155 mmol/L has been shown to improve cerebral perfusion.
- Management of blood pressure (BP) and autonomic issues differs based on the underlying neurological condition.
- Acute kidney injury (AKI) occurs at variable rates after neurological injury, and many medications used in the care of these patients have nephrotoxic effects. If renal replacement therapy (RRT) is needed, continuous RRT is usually the preferred modality of choice.

References

1. Mehta RL, Kellum JA, Shah SV, Molitoris BA, Ronco C, Warnock DG, et al. Acute kidney injury network: report of an initiative to improve outcome in acute kidney injury. Crit Care. 2007;11:R31.
2. Li N, Zhao W, Zhang W. Acute kidney injury in patients with severe traumatic brain injury: implementation of the Acute Kidney Injury Network stage system. Neurocrit Care. 2011;14: 377–81.
3. Zygun DA, Kortbeek JB, Fick GH, Laupland KB, Doig CJ. Non-neurologic organ dysfunction in severe traumatic brain injury. Crit Care Med. 2005;33:654–60.
4. Gruber A, Reinprecht A, Illievich UM, Fitzgerald R, Dietrich W, Czech T, et al. Extracerebral organ dysfunction and neurologic outcome after aneurysmal subarachnoid hemorrhage. Crit Care Med. 1999;27:505–14.
5. Kumar A, et al. Acute kidney injury following subarachnoid hemorrhage – incidence, risk factors and outcomes. Oral Presentation. 43rd Critical Care Congress, San Francisco, 2014.
6. Wong JM, Panchmatia JR, Ziewacz JE, Bader AM, Dunn IF, Laws ER, et al. Patterns in neurosurgical adverse events: intracranial neoplasm surgery. Neurosurg Focus. 2012;33:E16.
7. Wong JM, Ziewacz JE, Panchmatia JR, Bader AM, Pandey AS, Thompson BG, et al. Patterns in neurosurgical adverse events: endovascular neurosurgery. Neurosurg Focus. 2012;33:E14.
8. Kirkman MA, Albert AF, Ibrahim A, Doberenz D. Hyponatremia and brain injury: historical and contemporary perspectives. Neurocrit Care. 2013;18:406–16.
9. Peters JP, Welt LG, Sims EA, Orloff J, Needham J. A salt-wasting syndrome associated with cerebral disease. Trans Assoc Am Phys. 1950;63:57–64.
10. Palmer BF. Cerebral salt-wasting. In: Sterns RH, editor. UpToDate. Waltham: UpToDate; 2013. Accessed 30 Jul 2013.
11. Carter NW, Rector Jr FC, Seldin DW. Hyponatremia in cerebral disease resulting from the inappropriate secretion of antidiuretic hormone. N Engl J Med. 1961;275:67–72.
12. Sterns RH. Pathophysiology and etiology of the syndrome of inappropriate antidiuretic hormone secretion (SIADH). In: Emmett M, editor. UpToDate. Waltham: UpToDate; 2012. Accessed 30 Jul 2013.
13. Sterns RH. Treatment of hyponatremia: syndrome of inappropriate antidiuretic hormone secretion (SIADH) and reset osmostat. In: Emmett M, editor. UpToDate. Waltham: UpToDate; 2013. Accessed 30 Jul 2013.
14. Powner DJ, Boccalandro C, Alp MS, Vollmer DG. Endocrine failure after traumatic brain injury in adults. Neurocrit Care. 2006;5:61–70.
15. Agha A, Sherlock M, Phillips J, Tormey W, Thompson CJ. The natural history of post-traumatic neurohypophysial dysfunction. Eur J Endocrinol. 2005;152:371–7.
16. Gutierrez OM, Lin HY. Refractory hyponatremia. Kidney Int. 2007;71:79–82.
17. Gordon GL, Goldner F. Hypernatremia, azotemia and acidosis after cerebral injury. Am J Med. 1957;23(4):543–53.
18. Ogden AT, Mayer SA, Connolly ES Jr. Hyperosmolar agents in neurosurgical practice: the evolving role of hypertonic saline. Neurosurgery. 2005;57:207–15.
19. Hays AN, Lazaridis C, Neyens R, Nicholas J, Gay S, Chalela JA. Osmotherapy: use among neurointensivists. Neurocrit Care. 2011;14:222–8.
20. Weed LH, McKibbens PR. Experimental alterations of brain bulk. Am J Physiol. 1919;48: 512–30.
21. Wakai A, Roberts I, Schierhout G. Mannitol for acute traumatic brain injury. Cochrane Database Syst Rev. 2007;(1):CD001049.
22. Kamel H, Navi BB, Nakagawa K, Hemphill JC 3rd, Ko NU. Hypertonic saline versus mannitol for the treatment of elevated intracranial pressure: a meta-analysis of randomized clinical trials. Crit Care Med. 2011;39:554–9.

23. Mortazavi MM, Romeo AK, Deep A, Griessenauer CJ, Shoja MM, Tubbs S, et al. Hypertonic saline for treating raised intracranial pressure: literature review with meta-analysis. J Neurosurg. 2012;116:210–21.
24. Sakellaridis N, Pavlou E, Karatzas S, Chroni D, Vlachos K, Chatzopoulos K, et al. Comparison of mannitol and hypertonic saline in the treatment of severe brain injuries. J Neurosurg. 2011;114:545–8.
25. Qureshi AI, Suarez JI, Bhardwaj A, Mirski M, Schnitzer MS, Hanley DF, et al. Use of hypertonic (3%) saline/acetate infusion in the treatment of cerebral edema: effect on intracranial pressure and lateral displacement of the brain. Crit Care Med. 1998;26:440–6.
26. Roquilly A, Mahe PJ, Latte DD, Loutrel O, Champin P, Di Falco C, et al. Continuous controlled-infusion of hypertonic saline solution in traumatic brain-injured patients: a 9-year retrospective study. Crit Care. 2011;15:R260.
27. Schwarz S, Georgiadis D, Aschoff A, Schwab S. Effects of hypertonic (10%) saline in patients with raised intracranial pressure after stroke. Stroke. 2002;33:136–40.
28. Hauer EM, Stark D, Staykov D, Steigleder T, Schwab S, Bardutzky J. Early continuous hypertonic saline infusion in patients with severe cerebrovascular disease. Crit Care Med. 2011;39:1766–72.
29. Wagner I, Hauer EM, Staykov D, Volbers B, Dörfler A, Schwab S, et al. Effects of continuous hypertonic saline infusion on perihemorrhagic edema evolution. Stroke. 2011;42:1540–5.
30. Froelich M, Ni Q, Wess C, Ougorets I, Härtl R. Continuous hypertonic saline therapy and the occurrence of complications in neurocritically ill patients. Crit Care Med. 2009;37:1433–41.
31. Jauch EC, Saver JL, Adams Jr HP, Bruno A, Connors JJ, Demaerschalk BM, et al. Guidelines for the early management of patients with acute ischemic stroke: a guideline for healthcare professionals from the American Heart Association/American Stroke Association. Stroke. 2013;44:870–947.
32. Morgenstern LB, Hemphill 3rd JC, Anderson C, Becker K, Broderick JP, Connolly Jr ES, et al. Guidelines for the management of spontaneous intracerebral hemorrhage: a guideline for healthcare professionals from the American Heart Association/American Stroke Association. Stroke. 2010;41:2108–29.
33. Connolly ES, Rabinstein AA, Carhuapoma JR, Derdeyn CP, Dion J, Higashida RT, et al. Guidelines for the management of aneurysmal subarachnoid hemorrhage: a guideline for healthcare professionals from the American Heart Association/American Stroke Association. Stroke. 2012;43:1711–37.
34. Brain Trauma Foundation, American Association of Neurological Surgeons, Congress of Neurological Surgeons, Joint Section on Neurotrauma and Critical Care, AANS/CNS, Bratton SL, et al. Guidelines for the management of severe traumatic brain injury. J Neurotrauma. 2007;24 Suppl 1:S7–S13; S59–64.
35. Golper TA. Continuous renal replacement therapy in acute kidney injury (acute renal failure). In: Schwab SJ, editor. UpToDate. Waltham: UpToDate; 2012. Accessed 5 Aug 2013.
36. Rhoney DH. Considerations in fluids and electrolytes after traumatic brain injury. Nutr Clin Pract. 2006;21:462–78.
37. Pierce LR, Jain N. Risks associated with the use of intravenous immunoglobulin. Transfus Med Rev. 2003;17:241.
38. Orange JS, Hossny EM, Weiler CR, Ballow M, Berger M, Bonilla FA, et al. Use of intravenous immunoglobulin in human disease: a review of evidence by members of the Primary Immunodeficiency Committee of the American Academy of Allergy, Asthma and Immunology. J Allergy Clin Immunol. 2006; 117:S525.
39. Silvergleid AJ, Berger M. Intravenous immune globulin: adverse effects. In: Stiehm ER, editor. UpToDate. Waltham: UpToDate; 2013. Accessed 31 Jul 2013.
40. Fakhouri F. Intravenous immunoglobulins and acute renal failure: mechanism and prevention. Rev Med Interne. 2007;28(Spec No. 1):4.
41. Levy JB, Pusey CD. Nephrotoxicity of intravenous immunoglobulin. Q J Med. 2000;93:751–5.
42. Saag KG, Furst DE. Major side effects of systemic glucocorticoids. In: Matteson EL, editor. UpToDate. Waltham: UpToDate; 2013. Accessed 6 Aug 2013.

43. Bagley WH, Yang H, Shah KH. Rhabdomyolysis. Intern Emerg Med. 2007;2:210–8.
44. Scharman EJ, Troutman WG. Prevention of kidney injury following rhabdomyolysis: a systematic review. Ann Pharmacother. 2013;47:90–105.
45. Rosenstock JL, Bruno R, Kim JK, Lubarsky L, Schaller R, Panagopoulos G, et al. The effect of withdrawal of ACE inhibitors or angiotensin receptor blockers prior to coronary angiography on the incidence of contrast-induced nephropathy. Int Urol Nephrol. 2008;40:749.
46. Rudnick MR. Prevention of contrast-induced nephropathy. In: Palevsky PM, editor. UpToDate. Waltham: UpToDate; 2013. Accessed 19 Aug 2013.

Chapter 18
Nutrition in Perioperative Patients with Kidney Failure

T. Alp Ikizler and Edward D. Siew

Objectives

- To recognize the prevalence and extent of protein energy wasting (PEW) in perioperative patients with acute kidney injury (AKI)
- To describe the causes and consequences of PEW in perioperative patients with AKI
- To understand the nutrient requirements for optimal nutritional management of perioperative patients with underlying chronic kidney disease (CKD) or AKI

Assessment of Nutritional Status in Perioperative Patients with AKI

Evaluating nutritional status can be difficult in perioperative patients with AKI (Table 18.1) [1]. Traditional anthropometric (body mass index or BMI, body weight, triceps skinfold) and biochemical measures (albumin, prealbumin, transferrin) are often confounded by volume status, which can easily obscure losses in lean body mass in these patients. While several tools have been employed to characterize nutritional abnormalities in the setting of AKI and define metabolic requirements

T.A. Ikizler, MD (✉)
Division of Nephrology, Department of Medicine, Vanderbilt University Medical Center, 1161 21st Avenue South MCN-S3306, Nashville, TN 37232-2372, USA
e-mail: alp.ikizler@vanderbilt.edu

E.D. Siew, MD, MSCI
Division of Nephrology and Hypertension, Department of Medicine, Vanderbilt University Medical Center, 1161 21st Avenue South, Nashville, TN 37232-2372, USA
e-mail: edward.siew@vanderbilt.edu

C.V. Thakar, C.R. Parikh (eds.), *Perioperative Kidney Injury: Principles of Risk Assessment, Diagnosis and Treatment*, DOI 10.1007/978-1-4939-1273-5_18

Table 18.1 Limitations in the assessment of nutritional markers in AKI

Nutritional parameters	Limitations
Albumin, prealbumin, cholesterol	May be reduced due to inflammation and/or volume overload, independently from PEW
Body weight changes	Total body water is disproportionally increased in AKI
Anthropometric measurements	Fluid overload can mask changes in body mass changes
Energy expenditure	Formulas to predict energy expenditure not reliable (often based on body weight)
Nutritional scoring systems (SGA)	Limited data in patients with AKI
Body mass and body composition assessments (total body nitrogen, bioimpedance analysis, CT/MRI)	No data on AKI; tools are cumbersome, costly, and/or invasive

Reprinted with permission from Fiaccadori et al. [1]. © 2011 Wiley Periodicals, Inc.

accordingly, none are without limitation. The Subjective Global Assessment (SGA) is a tool composed of historical elements of the patient's dietary habits, medical history, and physical exam. It has been used in AKI patients to diagnose nutritional derangements and predict poor outcomes, but is not widely employed and can be difficult to administer in an intensive care unit (ICU) setting. Bioelectrical impedance analysis (BIA) has been useful in assessing body composition in patients with kidney disease; however, it does not appear to predict acute changes in body water resulting from dialysis or fluid overload and has not been well studied in the perioperative patients with AKI.

Given its sensitivity and robust prognostic power in almost every disease state, serum albumin is likely to be the most commonly used serum biomarker in the setting of perioperative AKI. When interpreting serum albumin concentrations, clinicians should be mindful that its concentration is the net result of its synthesis, breakdown, volume of distribution, and exchange between intra- and extravascular spaces, as well as losses [2]. Dietary protein intake (DPI) has direct influence on serum albumin concentrations, and inadequate DPI is characterized by a decrease in the rate of albumin synthesis, which may have little impact on serum albumin levels in the short term. Yet in stark contrast to decreased DPI, numerous conditions and diseases applicable to perioperative patients, such as inflammatory disorders, AKI, wounds, burns, and peritonitis, can also lead to hypoalbuminemia in a very short period of time. Despite its sensitivity as a screening tool, serum albumin provides limited information about the complex nature of the underlying problem, and it is crucial that the appropriate nutritional assessment should also include a thorough physical exam and include complimentary nutritional markers including, but not limited to, serum concentrations of prealbumin, C-reactive protein, and cholesterol.

Estimating equations including the Harris-Benedict and Schofield formulas have also been used to assess energy requirements and can be useful during the perioperative period for prescribing and monitoring nutritional supplementation. Of note, these equations are also weight based and originally validated in healthy individuals. In certain circumstances, they have been found to generally underestimate measured energy expenditure and require the addition of arbitrary "stress factor" multipliers [3]. Indirect calorimetry is considered the gold standard in critically ill patients and is preferred over estimating equations though widespread use may be limited by availability of a metabolic cart, expertise, and cost [4]. Measurements made by indirect calorimetry may also be affected by variations in ventilator and oxygen settings, patient agitation/thermogenesis, hypothermia (especially during continuous renal replacement therapy or CRRT), and loss of carbon dioxide via dialysis or ventilator/cuff leak.

Epidemiology of Nutritional Abnormalities in Perioperative Patients with AKI

Observational studies of hospitalized patients with acute or chronic kidney disease have found nutritional abnormalities to be highly prevalent at the time of disease presentation and an important predictor of morbidity and mortality. In a study of 309 patients with AKI admitted to a renal intermediate care unit, severe preexisting malnutrition, as assessed by SGA, was found in 42 % of patients [5]. These patients experienced a higher likelihood of in-hospital death, complications, and healthcare resource utilization. In another study of 100 retrospectively identified AKI patients, hypoalbuminemia (3.5 g/dl) and hypocholesterolemia (<150 mg/dl) at hospital admission independently predicted in-hospital mortality [6]. A longitudinal study of 161 patients with AKI showed that low serum prealbumin (<11 mg/dl) independently predicted in-hospital mortality after adjustment for severity of illness; Risk, Injury, Failure, Loss and End-Stage Kidney Disease (RIFLE) class; and AKI treatment [7]. For every 5 mg/dl increase in prealbumin level, there was additional 29 % decrease in hospital mortality observed (HR 0.71; 95 % CI 0.52–0.96) suggesting its potential as a prognostic marker. While these studies examined a heterogeneous group of patients, a significant portion were perioperative patients with kidney injury.

Etiology of PEW in the Hospitalized AKI and CKD Patients

Kidney disease, acute or chronic, directly challenges the ability of the body's metabolism to augment recovery from illness. Following surgery, there are multiple contributors to poor nutritional state that relate to both the effects of surgery and hospitalization as well as "renal-specific" factors that relate to loss of kidney function and the response to injury. Among these include the catabolic effects of systemic inflammation, insulin resistance, metabolic acidosis, resistance to actions of anabolic hormones, hyper- or hypocortisolemia, insufficient intake or prescription of dietary protein and energy requirements, and nutrient loss during renal replacement therapy (RRT) (Fig. 18.1).

The kidneys play an important role in the metabolism of several key nutrients. One important example includes its role in glucose metabolism. As kidney function declines, diminished clearance of insulin coupled with decreased glucose utilization due to loss of target organ function likely contributes to the insulin resistance

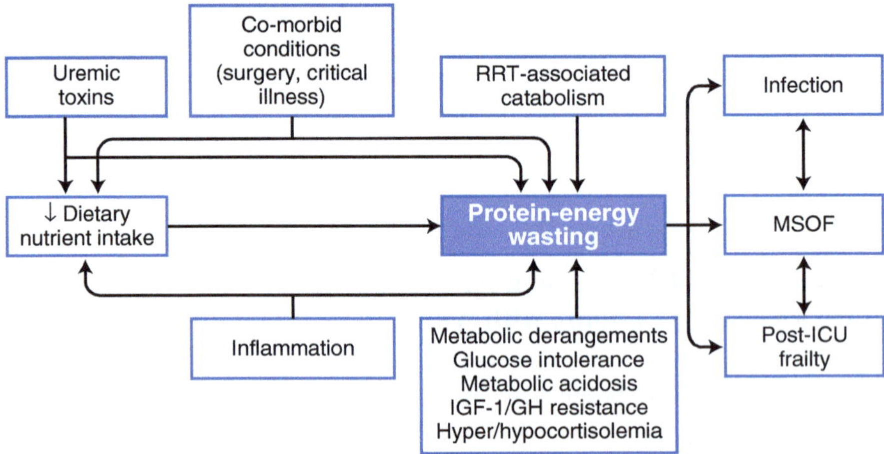

Fig. 18.1 The causes and consequences of nutritional abnormalities in perioperative patients with AKI. *RRT* renal replacement therapy, *MSOF* multisystem organ failure, *IGF-1/GH* insulin-like growth factor 1/growth hormone, *ICU* intensive care unit

observed in advanced kidney disease. Hyperglycemia, along with other aspects of insulin resistance, is a hallmark of the "diabetes of injury" observed in critically ill patients with and without AKI that is an important determinant of death and morbidity [8]. While insulin resistance and hyperglycemia are a part of an overall adaptive response to increase substrate and energy availability during physiologic stress, it has become clear that these responses are unregulated and maladaptive and may contribute to organ dysfunction, infection, polyneuropathy of critical illness, and mortality. A compelling finding from the two largest randomized controlled trials of intensive insulin therapy in the critically ill patients including perioperative patients was a significant reduction in the occurrence of AKI patients receiving treatment [9]. The mechanisms by which uncontrolled insulin resistance ultimately leads to poor outcomes in critical illness are not fully established. However, the anabolic effects of insulin are known to extend beyond simple glucose metabolism and seem to play an important role in the incorporation of other nutrients including amino acids.

Normal protein homeostasis is also altered in acute illness and AKI and is characterized by enhanced protein catabolism in the skeletal muscle resulting in hyperaminoacidemia and negative nitrogen balance. Daily protein catabolic rates in severe AKI have been reported to be 1.4–1.8 g/kg/day in several studies [10]. In addition, there is a decrement in amino acid transport into skeletal muscle for protein synthesis, partly due to hepatic extraction to support gluconeogenesis and the synthesis of acute phase proteins. The resulting imbalances in the utilization and clearance of both plasma and intracellular amino acid pools support this observed negative nitrogen balance, which is a sign of poor prognosis in patients with AKI [11]. Furthermore, recent evidence suggests that deranged protein catabolism may also directly impair endothelial function, increase oxidative stress, and weaken the immune response.

Renal replacement therapy also engenders negative nitrogen balance through the losses of amino acids into the dialysate. Losses as high as 8 g during conventional dialysis and even more during continuous therapies with between 1.2 and 15 g/day lost and with some studies observing losses as high as 20–30 g/day are reported. Consequently, adjustments to the provision of parental nutrition need to be made in this population as up to 17 % of amino acids received may be lost during treatment [12].

Inflammation appears to be a key mediator in the pathogenesis of enhanced protein catabolism in critical illness and kidney disease [13]. Acute illness often causes dramatic elevations of cytokines such as interleukin-6 (IL-6), which may be further elevated in AKI and highly predictive of mortality in this population [14]. Interleukin-6 has been demonstrated to be associated with accelerated muscle atrophy through direct upregulation of the ubiquitin-proteasome pathway and attenuated by administration of IL-6 receptor antibody. Experimental infusion studies with tumor necrosis factor-α (TNF-α) have demonstrated an enhanced proteolytic effect on muscle protein as well as a reduction in protein synthesis. Elevated IL-1 levels both induce profound anorexia and appear to enhance muscle protein breakdown in animal models, which may improve with pharmacologic blockade. Inflammation may also contribute to the production of counterregulatory hormones thereby affecting insulin signaling, which is a key modulator of the protein homeostasis. The net result of this profound catabolic state is an ongoing negative nitrogen balance and loss of lean body mass with potential consequences for immune or organ function, liberation from mechanical ventilation, wound healing, and endothelial function.

Several studies suggest that lipid metabolism is also profoundly altered in the setting of critical illness and kidney disease [15]. In particular, the triglyceride content of lipoproteins is increased, while cholesterol content is decreased. This is true for low-density lipoprotein (LDL) and high-density lipoprotein (HDL). The major cause of impairment in lipid metabolism appears to be the inhibition of lipolytic enzyme function, including peripheral lipoprotein lipase and hepatic triglyceride lipase. As a result of diminished lipolytic function, fat elimination is impaired. For example, if lipid is administered intravenously as part of parenteral nutrition, clearance of fat emulsion is reduced by as much as 50 %. This includes clearance of both long- and medium-chain triglycerides. Although not well studied, it also appears that plasma concentration of many fat-soluble vitamins (including vitamin A, vitamin D, and vitamin E) may be decreased in the setting of AKI. In contrast vitamin K stores appear to be replete in this clinical setting.

Provision of Nutritional Support in Hospitalized Patients with Kidney Disease

Several issues complicate the provision of nutritional support to perioperative patients with AKI [16]. For example, AKI patients are especially prone to fluid and solute overload from aggressive resuscitation, diminished clearance of uremic toxins, and third spacing from underlying illness. On the other hand, targeted goals of supplementation are often unmet in the perioperative period and are associated with

Table 18.2 Issues related to studies examining the efficacy of nutritional support in hospitalized patients with kidney disease

Small number of subjects
Suboptimal selection of study patients
Heterogeneity of patient population and disease state
No stratification for severity of illness or preexisting nutritional status
Design issues
Mostly retrospective data
Use of historical controls or no controls at all
Quantitative and qualitative inadequacy of kcal and/or N intake
Inadequate duration of nutritional support

Table 18.3 ESPEN Guidelines for nutritional requirements in adult patients with AKI

Nutritional requirements in patients with ARF (nonprotein calories)	
Energy	20–30 kcal/kgBW/day[a]
Carbohydrates	3–5 (max. 7) g/kgBW/day
Fat	0.8–1.2 (max. 1.5) g/kgBW/day
Protein (essential nonessential amino acids)	
Conservative therapy	0.6–0.8 (max. 1.0) g/kgBW/day
Extracorporeal therapy	1.0–1.5 g/kgBW/day
CCRT, in hypercatabolism	Up to maximum 1.7 g/kgBW/day

Abbreviation: *ARF* acute renal failure
[a]Adapted to individual needs in case of underweight or obesity

adverse clinical outcomes [17]. Currently, the provision of nutritional support in the perioperative patients with AKI remains hindered by a paucity of adequately executed trials targeting hard clinical outcomes. Table 18.2 lists some of the limitations of the available studies in this patient population. Accordingly, consensus guidelines are largely based on expert opinion such as one from the European Society for Clinical Nutrition and Metabolism (ESPEN) [15] (Table 18.3).

Macro- and Micronutrient Requirements

Observational studies using indirect calorimetry suggest that resting energy expenditure in AKI appears to be principally determined by the extent of the inciting event rather than by the loss of kidney function per se [18]. Based on the few available studies, ESPEN has recently recommended an energy intake of 20–30 kcal/kg/day (nonprotein calories) depending on estimated requirement, but no more than 1.3 times the basal energy expenditure [15]. When determining the needs, weight should be estimated by adjusted body weight, which is calculated by adding ideal body weight and 0.25 times the difference between actual body weight and ideal body weight. The nonprotein calories should be provided one-third as lipids and two-thirds as glucose and should not exceed 25 kcal/kg/day. In addition, additional calories (citrate, lactate, and glucose) from dialysis/hemofiltration fluids should be added to the energy balance of the patient to avoid overfeeding. These additional calories can be as high as 1,200 kcal/day.

Optimal protein requirement in perioperative patients with AKI is a matter of debate. Preexisting CKD, AKI, or the need for RRT markedly enhances protein catabolism with normalized protein catabolic rates (nPCR) of between 1.4 and 1.8 g per kilogram per day (g/kg/day) [19]. In the presence of diminished utilization due to altered metabolic state as well as diminished clearance due to decreased renal function, excessive protein supplementation will result in excessive accumulation of end products of protein and amino acid metabolism. In an observation of 40 patients on CRRT, increases in the dose of protein supplementation were also accompanied by an increase in protein catabolism though perhaps somewhat less so with lower energy intakes (25–35 kcal/kg/day). A nonrandomized study of AKI patients on CRRT compared a higher dose of dietary protein supplementation 2.5 g/kg/day to a group of patients receiving standard of care 1.2 g/kg/day with both receiving equal amount of calories [20]. Patients receiving the higher dose of protein were more likely to achieve a positive nitrogen balance at any time during follow-up (53.6 % vs. 36.7 %; $p<0.05$) and trended towards having less overall negative nitrogen balance but required more CRRT due to azotemia. In a detailed metabolic study, it was reported that AKI patients that received 2.0 g protein/kg had improved nitrogen balance compared to those receiving 1.5 g protein/kg. Interestingly, increasing calorie intake of 10–15 to 30 cal/kg benefited those patients with decreased protein intake (0.6–0.8 g/kg) but not ones receiving increased protein. Patients that were overfed (40–60 total calories/kg) had increased nPCR and worsened nitrogen balance. Based on the above data, ESPEN recommends protein dosing based on the expected degree of catabolism with 0.6–0.8 g/kg/day for conservative therapy, 1–1.5 g/kg/day for extracorporeal treatment, and a maximum of 1.7 g/kg/day in "hypercatabolism" [15].

Impaired lipolysis characterizes the main lipid abnormality of perioperative period and AKI resulting in hypertriglyceridemia, elevated very-low-density lipoprotein (VLDL) and LDL levels, and diminished HDL levels. Consequently, it has been recommended that supplementation remains between 0.8 and 1.2 g/kg/day [21] with general recommendations that total caloric intake from fat calories does not exceed 25–35 %, which can be achieved with 10–30 % lipid formulations of parenteral nutrition. The benefits of medium-chain triglycerides in parenteral nutrition (PN) formulations compared to long-chain triglycerides remain unclear and are not widely available. Frequent monitoring of triglyceride levels and liver function is recommended to avoid problems associated with hypertriglyceridemia.

Alterations in the metabolism of vitamins and trace elements in AKI patients have not been well studied. In patients receiving CRRT, replacement of vitamin C has been recommended not to exceed 30–50 mg/day [22]. Vitamin A is known to accumulate in renal impairment and ESPEN recommends monitoring for signs and symptoms of vitamin A toxicity during supplementation though variable levels have been observed. Thiamine (vitamin B1), vitamin B_6, selenium, zinc, and copper losses have also been reported in patients undergoing CRRT with suggestions for replacement at doses greater than the recommended dietary allowance [23]. A more recent complication of CRRT is the profound losses of phosphorus, especially when the procedure is performed over a long period of time. It is critical to check serum phosphorus levels and supplement as needed in these patients.

Route, Timing, and Type of Nutritional Supplementation

Enteral nutrition (EN) is the preferred route of supplementation in the perioperative patients with potential benefits of maintenance of intestinal mucosa to minimize bacterial translocation, less infectious risk, and lower cost [24]. While systemic reviews of the trials comparing parenteral nutrition (PN) versus EN have failed to demonstrate a clear mortality benefit with the latter, infectious complications do appear to be significantly reduced possibly due to a higher incidence of hyperglycemia and the need for central access with PN [25]. While few studies have addressed this question specifically in perioperative patients with AKI, EN appears to be safe in patients with kidney disease. For those who are unable to receive EN or meet their predicted energy requirements with EN alone, PN may serve a useful adjunctive role in meeting metabolic demand though must be balanced against the attendant infectious and hyperglycemic risks [26].

An important aspect of artificial feeding is the timing, i.e., when to initiate nutrition support. Large randomized studies in critically ill including perioperative patients have shown that late initiation of artificial support and permissive feeding is clinically and financially better compared to early initiation. In the largest randomized clinical trial performed in critically ill patients (The Early Parenteral Nutrition Completing Enteral Nutrition in Adult Critically Ill Patients, or EPaNIC), which included perioperative patients, subjects were randomized to early (48 h after ICU admission) versus late (8 days after ICU admission) parenteral nutrition. This study conclusively demonstrated that late initiation of parenteral nutrition was associated with faster recovery, fewer complications, and more cost savings, as compared with early initiation [27]. Both groups received EN as needed to reach targeted nutrition goals. In a subsequent subgroup analysis of the same trial, investigators showed that there were no differences in AKI-related outcomes between groups suggesting that late initiation is safe and more cost-effective in the setting of AKI or for the risk of development of AKI.

Standard enteral formulas used broadly in perioperative patients with AKI are generally whole-protein solutions. While many are sufficient in protein content, they are often accompanied by a larger electrolyte burden, which may represent issues in patients with kidney disease. Several enteral formulas with mixed essential and nonessential amino acids have been adapted for use in patients with AKI, largely based on lower electrolyte content (potassium/phosphorous) [15]. The use of key additives to enteral nutrition designed to modulate inflammatory or immune response including glutamine, arginine, and omega-3 fatty acids did not demonstrate differences in clinical outcome in a relatively larger randomized clinical trial of 597 critically ill adults. Meta-analyses have also failed to suggest mortality benefit though suggestion of a potential reduction in infectious complication rate exists [28]. Even less is known about their role in AKI. Significant losses of glutamine (3.5–3.6 g/day) have been demonstrated in patients on CRRT suggesting the need for supplementation though dose and safety remain undetermined. The lack of compelling evidence for immunomodulatory nutrition regimens has made them difficult to recommend for routine use in the critically ill or in AKI [15].

Conclusion

In conclusion, perioperative patients with AKI are exposed to a wide array of metabolic and nutritional derangements. These mostly result from loss of kidney function, the therapies it often engenders (i.e., RRT), and the concurrent metabolic effects of acute surgery and associated critical illness. The cumulative effects manifest as a significantly catabolic state ultimately leading to delayed cellular recovery, increased susceptibility to infections, prolonged hospitalizations, and increased risk for mortality. Adequately designed and powered studies examining the optimal approach to metabolic and nutritional support in perioperative patients with AKI are lacking. Consequently, frequent ascertainment of the nutritional and metabolic demands of these patients is warranted with an individualized therapeutic approach coupling the best available evidence and guidelines.

Key Messages

- The etiology of nutritional abnormalities in the setting of perioperative kidney disease is complex and includes a number of factors related to loss of kidney function, concurrent illnesses, surgical complications, adverse effects of ongoing therapies, and multiple metabolic derangements.
- While artificial nutrition is considered as a key component of therapy in perioperative AKI patients, there is paucity of data regarding the characteristics or efficacy of artificial nutrition in these settings.
- The recommended levels of energy and protein intake for perioperative patients with AKI are no more than 25–30 kcal/kg/day and 1.5–1.7 g/kg/day, the higher levels administered to ones on renal replacement therapies.
- Enteral nutrition should be the initial modality for artificial nutrition in perioperative patients with AKI; in certain cases it can be integrated with PN to achieve nutrition needs.

References

1. Fiaccadori E, Cremaschi E, Regolisti G. Nutritional assessment and delivery in renal replacement therapy patients. Semin Dial. 2011;24:169–75.
2. Jeejeebhoy KN. Nutritional assessment. Gastroenterol Clin North Am. 1998;27:347–69.
3. Faisy C, Guerot E, Diehl JL, Labrousse J, Fagon JY. Assessment of resting energy expenditure in mechanically ventilated patients. Am J Clin Nutr. 2003;78:241–9.
4. Wooley JA, Btaiche IF, Good KL. Metabolic and nutritional aspects of acute renal failure in critically ill patients requiring continuous renal replacement therapy. Nutr Clin Pract. 2005; 20:176–91.
5. Fiaccadori E, Lombardi M, Leonardi S, Rotelli CF, Tortorella G, Borghetti A. Prevalence and clinical outcome associated with preexisting malnutrition in acute renal failure: a prospective cohort study. J Am Soc Nephrol. 1999;10:581–93.
6. Obialo CI, Okonofua EC, Nzerue MC, Tayade AS, Riley LJ. Role of hypoalbuminemia and hypocholesterolemia as copredictors of mortality in acute renal failure. Kidney Int. 1999; 56:1058–63.
7. Perez Valdivieso JR, Bes-Rastrollo M, Monedero P, de Irala J, Lavilla FJ. Impact of prealbumin levels on mortality in patients with acute kidney injury: an observational cohort study. J Ren Nutr. 2008;18:262–8.
8. Van den Berghe G. How does blood glucose control with insulin save lives in intensive care? J Clin Invest. 2004;114:1187–95.
9. Schetz M, Vanhorebeek I, Wouters PJ, Wilmer A, Van den Berghe G. Tight blood glucose control is renoprotective in critically ill patients. J Am Soc Nephrol. 2008;19:571–8.
10. Clark WR, Mueller BA, Alaka KJ, Macias WL. A comparison of metabolic control by continuous and intermittent therapies in acute renal failure. J Am Soc Nephrol. 1994;4:1413–20.
11. Scheinkestel CD, Kar L, Marshall K, Bailey M, Davies A, Nyulasi I, Tuxen DV. Prospective randomized trial to assess caloric and protein needs of critically Ill, anuric, ventilated patients requiring continuous renal replacement therapy. Nutrition. 2003;19:909–16.
12. Scheinkestel CD, Adams F, Mahony L, Bailey M, Davies AR, Nyulasi I, Tuxen DV. Impact of increasing parenteral protein loads on amino acid levels and balance in critically ill anuric patients on continuous renal replacement therapy. Nutrition. 2003;19:733–40.
13. Himmelfarb J, Ikizler TA. Acute kidney injury: changing lexicography, definitions, and epidemiology. Kidney Int. 2007;71:971–6.
14. Simmons EM, Himmelfarb J, Sezer MT, Chertow GM, Mehta RL, Paganini EP, Soroko S, Freedman S, Becker K, Spratt D, Shyr Y, Ikizler TA. Plasma cytokine levels predict mortality in patients with acute renal failure. Kidney Int. 2004;65:1357–65.
15. Cano N, Fiaccadori E, Tesinsky P, Toigo G, Druml W, Kuhlmann M, Mann H, Horl WH. ESPEN guidelines on enteral nutrition: adult renal failure. Clin Nutr. 2006;25:295–310.
16. Fiaccadori E, Maggiore U, Cabassi A, Morabito S, Castellano G, Regolisti G. Nutritional evaluation and management of AKI patients. J Ren Nutr. 2013;23:255–8.
17. De Jonghe B, Appere-De-Vechi C, Fournier M, Tran B, Merrer J, Melchior JC, Outin H. A prospective survey of nutritional support practices in intensive care unit patients: what is prescribed? What is delivered? Crit Care Med. 2001;29:8–12.
18. Schneeweiss B, Graninger W, Stockenhuber F, Druml W, Ferenci P, Eichinger S, Grimm G, Laggner AN, Lenz K. Energy metabolism in acute and chronic renal failure. Am J Clin Nutr. 1990;52:596–601.
19. Chima CS, Meyer L, Hummell AC, Bosworth C, Heyka R, Paganini EP, Werynski A. Protein catabolic rate in patients with acute renal failure on continuous arteriovenous hemofiltration and total parenteral nutrition. J Am Soc Nephrol. 1993;3:1516–21.
20. Bellomo R, Seacombe J, Daskalakis M, Farmer M, Wright C, Parkin G, Boyce N. A prospective comparative study of moderate versus high protein intake for critically ill patients with acute renal failure. Ren Fail. 1997;19:111–20.

21. Fiaccadori E, Maggiore U, Rotelli C, Giacosa R, Picetti E, Parenti E, Meschi T, Borghi L, Tagliavini D, Cabassi A. Effects of different energy intakes on nitrogen balance in patients with acute renal failure: a pilot study. Nephrol Dial Transplant. 2005;20:1976–80.
22. Story DA, Ronco C, Bellomo R. Trace element and vitamin concentrations and losses in critically ill patients treated with continuous venovenous hemofiltration. Crit Care Med. 1999;27:220–3.
23. Klein CJ, Moser-Veillon PB, Schweitzer A, Douglass LW, Reynolds HN, Patterson KY, Veillon C. Magnesium, calcium, zinc, and nitrogen loss in trauma patients during continuous renal replacement therapy. JPEN J Parenter Enter Nutrr. 2002;26:77–92. discussion 92–73.
24. Marik PE. Death by TPN… the final chapter? Crit Care Med. 2008;36:1964–5.
25. Gramlich L, Kichian K, Pinilla J, Rodych NJ, Dhaliwal R, Heyland DK. Does enteral nutrition compared to parenteral nutrition result in better outcomes in critically ill adult patients? A systematic review of the literature. Nutrition. 2004;20:843–8.
26. Cano NJ, Aparicio M, Brunori G, Carrero JJ, Cianciaruso B, Fiaccadori E, Lindholm B, Teplan V, Fouque D, Guarnieri G. ESPEN guidelines on parenteral nutrition: adult renal failure. Clin Nutr. 2009;28:401–14.
27. Gunst J, Vanhorebeek I, Casaer MP, Hermans G, Wouters PJ, Dubois J, Claes K, Schetz M, Van den Berghe G. Impact of early parenteral nutrition on metabolism and kidney injury. J Am Soc Nephrol. 2013;24:995–1005.
28. Montejo JC, Zarazaga A, Lopez-Martinez J, Urrutia G, Roque M, Blesa AL, Celaya S, Conejero R, Galban C, Garcia de Lorenzo A, Grau T, Mesejo A, Ortiz-Leyba C, Planas M, Ordonez J, Jimenez FJ. Immunonutrition in the intensive care unit. A systematic review and consensus statement. Clin Nutr. 2003;22:221–33.

List of Common Abbreviations

AAA	Abdominal aortic aneurysm
ACE	Angiotensin-converting enzyme
ACS	Abdominal compartment syndrome
ADH	Antidiuretic hormone
AKI	Acute kidney injury
AKICS	Acute kidney injury after cardiac surgery
AKIN	Acute Kidney Injury Network
ANP	A-type natriuretic peptide
anti-HLA	Antihuman leukocyte antigen
ANZICS	Australian and New Zealand Intensive Care Society
APACHE II	Acute Physiology and Chronic Health Evaluation II
APP	Abdominal perfusion pressure
ARB	Angiotensin receptor blockers
ARDS	Acute respiratory distress syndrome
ARF	Acute renal failure
ATN	Acute tubular necrosis
BIA	Bioelectrical impedance analysis
BIVAD	Biventricular assist device
BMI	Body mass index
BNP	Brain natriuretic peptide
BP	Blood pressure
BTT	Bridge to transplant
BUN	Blood urea nitrogen
CABG	Coronary artery bypass graft
CAM	Confusion Assessment Method
CAVH	Continuous arteriovenous hemofiltration
CAVHD	Continuous arteriovenous hemodialysis
CF	Continuous flow
CI	Cardiac index
CIAKI	Contrast-induced acute kidney injury

C.V. Thakar, C.R. Parikh (eds.), *Perioperative Kidney Injury: Principles of Risk Assessment, Diagnosis and Treatment*, DOI 10.1007/978-1-4939-1273-5

CIAP	Continuous intra-abdominal pressure
CICSS	Continuous Improvement in Cardiac Surgery Study
CIN	Contrast-induced nephropathy
CK	Creatine kinase
CKD	Chronic kidney disease
CNIs	Calcineurin inhibitors
CO	Cardiac output
COPD	Chronic obstructive pulmonary disease
CORONARY	CABG Off or ON Pump Revascularization Study
COX 2i	Cyclooxygenase-2 inhibitors
CPB	Cardiopulmonary bypass
Cr	Serum creatinine
CrCl	Creatinine clearance
CRRT	Continuous renal replacement therapy
CSA-AKI	Cardiac surgery-associated acute kidney injury
CSW	Cerebral salt wasting
CT	Computed tomography
CVD	Cardiovascular disease
CVP	Central venous pressure
CVVH	Continuous venovenous hemofiltration
CVVHD	Continuous venovenous hemodialysis
CVVHDF	Continuous venovenous hemodiafiltration
CyC	Cystatin C
DA	Dopamine
DA-1	Dopamine-1
DA-2	Dopamine-2
DCD	Donation after cardiac death
DGF	Delayed graft function
DI	Diabetes insipidus
DL	Decompressive laparotomy
DO2	Oxygen delivery
DPI	Dietary protein intake
DREAM	Dutch Randomized Endovascular Aneurysm Repair
DT	Destination therapy
DVT	Deep vein thrombosis
eCCl	Estimated creatinine clearance
ECD	Expanded criteria donors
EDD	Extended daily dialysis
EF	Ejection fraction
eGFR	Estimated glomerular filtration rate
EKG	Electrocardiogram
EPaNIC	Early Parenteral Nutrition to Supplement Insufficient Enteral Nutrition in Intensive Care
EPO	Epoetin

ER	Emergency room
ERPF	Effective renal plasma flow
ESLD	End-stage liver disease
ESPEN	European Society for Clinical Nutrition and Metabolism
ESRD	End-stage renal disease
EVAR	Endovascular aneurysm repair
FDA	Food and Drug Administration
FeNa	Fractional excretion of sodium
FFP	Fresh frozen plasma
FRC	Functional residual capacity
GCS	Glasgow coma scale
GDT	Goal-directed fluid therapy
GEDVI	Global end-diastolic volume index
GFR	Glomerular filtration rate
GH	Growth hormone
GI	Gastrointestinal
HAF	Hepatic arterial flow
HD	Hemodialysis
HDL	High-density lipoprotein
HES	Hydroxyethylstarch
HF	Heart failure
HIT	Heparin-induced thrombocytopenia
HITT	Heparin-induced thrombocytopenia and thrombosis
HMF	Hepatic microcirculatory flow
HRS	Hepatorenal syndrome
HTK	Histidine-tryptophan-ketoglutarate
IABP	Intra-aortic balloon pump
IAH	Intra-abdominal hypertension
IAP	Intra-abdominal pressure
ICH	Intracranial hemorrhage
ICNARC	Intensive Care National Audit and Research Centre
ICP	Intracranial pressure
ICU	Intensive care unit
IGF-I	Insulin-like growth factor I
IHD	Intermittent hemodialysis
IIAP	Intermittent intra-abdominal pressure
IL-1	Interleukin-1
IL-1β	Interleukin-1β
IL-2	Interleukin-2
IL-6	Interleukin-6
IL-18	Interleukin-18
IMF	Intestinal mucosal flow
INTERMACS	Interagency Registry for Mechanically Assisted Circulatory Support
IR	Ischemia/reperfusion
IRF	Improvement in renal function

IRI	Ischemia reperfusion injury
ITBV	Intrathoracic blood volume
ITP	Intrathoracic pressure
IV	Intravenous
IVC	Inferior vena cava
IVF	Intravenous fluid
IVIG	Intravenous immune globulin
KDIGO	Kidney Disease: Improving Global Outcomes
KIM-1	Kidney injury molecule-1
LDL	Low-density lipoprotein
L-FABP	Liver-type fatty acid-binding protein
LOS	Length of stay
LR	Lactated Ringer's
LVADs	Left ventricular assist devices
MAF	Mesenteric arterial flow
MAP	Mean arterial pressure
McSPI	Multicenter Study of Perioperative Ischemia
MDRD	Modification of Diet in Renal Disease
MI	Myocardial infarction
MOF	Multiorgan failure
MRI	Magnetic resonance imaging
MSOF	Multisystem organ failure
NAC	N-acetylcysteine
NaCl	Sodium chloride
NAG	N-acetyl-B-(D)-glucosaminidase
NCEPOD	National Confidential Enquiry into Patient Outcome and Death
NGAL	Neutrophil gelatinase-associated lipocalin
NIH/NHLBI	National Institutes of Health/National Heart, Lung, and Blood Institute
NIS	National Inpatient Sample
NNECDSG	Northern New England Cardiovascular Disease Study Group
nPCR	Normalized protein catabolic rates
NRI	Net reclassification index
NSAIDs	Nonsteroidal antiinflammatory drugs
NYHA	New York Heart Association Functional Classification
OPCAB	Off pump coronary artery bypass graft
OPTIMISE	Optimization of perioperative cardiovascular management to improve surgical outcome
OR	Odds ratio
OR	Operating room
OVER	Open surgery vs. endovascular repair
PAD	Peripheral vascular disease
PAOP	Pulmonary artery occlusion pressure
PAP	Pulmonary artery pressure
PCI	Percutaneous coronary intervention
PCWP	Pulmonary capillary wedge pressure

PD	Peritoneal dialysis
PDSA	Plan-Do-Study-Act
PEEP	Positive end-expiratory pressure
PEW	Protein energy wasting
PGE1	Prostaglandin E1
PIRRT	Prolonged intermittent renal replacement therapy
PMN	Polymorphonuclear neutrophil
PN	Partial nephrectomy
PNF	Primary nonfunction
PO_2	Partial pressure of oxygen
pRBCs	Packed red blood cells
pRIFLE	Pediatric risk, injury, failure, loss, and end-stage renal disease
PROPPR	Pragmatic Randomized Optimal Platelet and Plasma Ratios
PVD	Peripheral vascular disease
PVF	Portal venous blood flow
RACHS	Risk Adjustment for Congenital Heart Surgery
RCA	Regional citrate anticoagulation
RCC	Renal cell carcinoma
RCTs	Randomized controlled trials
RD	Renal dysfunction
RENAL	Randomized Evaluation of Normal versus Augmented level Renal Replacement Therapy trial
RIFLE	Risk, injury, failure, loss, and end-stage kidney disease
RN	Radical nephrectomy
rPSGL-Ig	Recombinant P-selectin glycoprotein ligand IgG fusion protein
RRT	Renal replacement therapy
RV	Right ventricle
RVEDVI	Right ventricular end-diastolic volume index
SAFE	Saline vs. Albumin Fluid Evaluation trial
SAH	Subarachnoid hemorrhage
SBP	Systolic blood pressure
SCD	Standard criteria donors
Scr	Serum creatinine
SCUF	Slow continuous ultrafiltration
SGA	Subjective Global Assessment
SGF	Slow graft function
SIADH	Syndrome of inappropriate antidiuretic hormone secretion
SLED	Sustained low-efficiency dialysis
SNa	Serum concentration of sodium
SOFA	Sequential organ failure assessment
SRF	Split renal function
SRI	Simplified Renal Index
STS	Society for Thoracic Surgeons
SVR	Systemic vascular resistance
SVV	Stroke volume variation

TAA	Thoracic aortic aneurysm
TBI	Traumatic brain injury
TBSA	Total body surface area
99mTc-DTPA	Technetium diethylenetriamine pentaacetic acid
TEG	Thromboelastography
TGF-β	Transforming growth factor-β
TLR	Toll-like receptors
TNF-α	Tumor necrosis factor-α
TRIBE-AKI	Translational Research Investigating Biomarker End-Points in Acute Kidney Injury
TTKG	Transtubular potassium gradient
TX	Transplant
TXA	Tranexamic acid
UFH	Unfractionated heparin
UK	Urinary excretion of potassium
UNa	Urinary excretion of sodium
UOP	Urine output
UTI	Urinary tract infection
UW	University of Wisconsin
VADs	Ventricular assist devices
VISEP	Volume Substitution and Insulin Therapy in Severe Sepsis study
VLDL	Very-low-density lipoprotein
WBC	White blood cell count
WSACS	World Society of the Abdominal Compartment Syndrome

Index

C.V. Thakar, C.R. Parikh (eds.), *Perioperative Kidney Injury: Principles of Risk Assessment, Diagnosis and Treatment*, DOI 10.1007/978-1-4939-1273-5

R

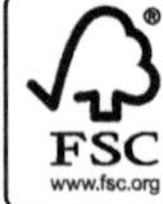

MIX
Papier aus verantwortungsvollen Quellen
Paper from responsible sources
FSC® C105338

If you have any concerns about our products, you can contact us on
ProductSafety@springernature.com

In case Publisher is established outside the EU, the EU authorized representative is:
Springer Nature Customer Service Center GmbH
Europaplatz 3, 69115 Heidelberg, Germany

Printed by Libri Plureos GmbH
in Hamburg, Germany